Pitfalls in Rheumatology

Eleftherios Pelechas • Panagiota Karagianni
Evripidis Kaltsonoudis

Pitfalls in Rheumatology

From Diagnosis to Management

Springer

Eleftherios Pelechas
Rheumatology Department
Hatzikosta General Hospital of Ioannina
Ioannina, Greece

Panagiota Karagianni
Biopathology Department
University Hospital of Ioannina
Ioannina, Greece

Evripidis Kaltsonoudis
Rheumatology Department
Hatzikosta General Hospital of Ioannina
Ioannina, Greece

ISBN 978-3-031-98670-3 ISBN 978-3-031-98671-0 (eBook)
https://doi.org/10.1007/978-3-031-98671-0

This Springer imprint is published by the registered company Springer Nature Switzerland AG
The registered company address is: Gewerbestrasse 11, 6330 Cham, Switzerland

"To my sons, Alexandros and George,
May this work inspire you to pursue knowledge,
strive for excellence,
and embrace the endless possibilities ahead.
With gratitude and love"

—Eleftherios Pelechas

"To our patients who courageously battle their ailments and teach us every day through their strength and resilience.
We are forever grateful for the wisdom and inspiration you provide"

—The authors

Preface

Rheumatology is a field of medicine that addresses the diagnosis and management of a broad spectrum of diseases affecting the musculoskeletal system and connective tissue. These conditions often exhibit chronicity, with many patients enduring a lifelong journey of managing their illness. Rheumatic diseases can present with a diverse array of symptoms, ranging from joint pain and swelling to systemic manifestations that may involve the skin, eyes, lungs, heart, kidneys, etc. This variability in presentation, even within the same disease, makes things harder and adds to the complexity of diagnosing and treating these conditions.

One of the most significant challenges in rheumatology is differentiating between diseases that share overlapping clinical and laboratory features, which in some instances may be common between them. Conditions such as rheumatoid arthritis, systemic lupus erythematosus and spondyloarthropathies can manifest with similar symptoms, leading to diagnostic dilemmas and, at times, wrong diagnoses and mismanagement. The multifaceted nature of rheumatic diseases is both a source of fascination and frustration for clinicians, as even experienced specialists can encounter diagnostic and therapeutic pitfalls. It is within this context that the need for a dedicated resource addressing these challenges becomes evident.

This book, *Pitfalls in Rheumatology: From Diagnosis to Management*, is born out of a desire to bridge this critical gap in the literature. Or journey began with the publication of the *Illustrated Handbook of Rheumatic and Musculo-Skeletal Diseases*, a comprehensive guide that was recognised and awarded by the National Academy of Athens for its clarity and utility. The positive reception of that work inspired us to delve deeper into the nuances of rheumatology and create a book specifically focused on the common pitfalls encountered in this field.

Unlike existing resources, *Pitfalls in Rheumatology* provides a systematic approach to identifying and addressing the diagnostic and management challenges in rheumatology. Each chapter is structured uniformly to ensure ease of use, guiding the reader through the clinical presentations, diagnostic considerations and therapeutic strategies of various rheumatic diseases. Special emphasis is placed on the differential diagnosis and the subtle clues that can help avoid common errors. Furthermore, we have included a list of abbreviations in each chapter to facilitate quick reference and enhance the reader's experience.

We envision this book as an invaluable tool not only for medical residents and rheumatology fellows but also for seasoned rheumatologists seeking to refine their diagnostic acumen. Additionally, practitioners from other specialties, including general medicine, internal medicine, orthopaedics and medical students, will find this resource beneficial in navigating the complexities of rheumatologic care.

Our hope is that this book serves as a trusted companion for healthcare providers, empowering them to deliver accurate diagnoses and effective management for patients with rheumatic diseases. By addressing the pitfalls inherent in this challenging yet rewarding specialty, we aim to improve outcomes and enhance the quality of care for patients living with these conditions.

Ioannina, Greece Eleftherios Pelechas
Ioannina, Greece Panagiota Karagianni
Ioannina, Greece Evripidis Kaltsonoudis

Competing Interests The authors have no competing interests to declare that are relevant to the content of this manuscript.

Acknowledgements

We would like to express our gratitude to all our expert contributors for their support and excellent advice, which were instrumental in bringing this book to life.

We also extend our sincere thanks to Stavroula Pelecha and Christina Vlachou for their invaluable assistance in language editing, ensuring the clarity and precision of the text.

List of our contributors:
Athanasios Kavvadias
Gastroenterologist
General Hospital of Corfu, Greece
Christos Tsironis
Neurologist
University Hospital of Ioannina, Greece
Dimitrios Venetis
Cardiologist
Hatzikosta General Hospital of Ioannina, Greece
Fotios Tsogkas
Ophthalmologist
Moorfields Eye Hospital, London, UK
Ilias Papadimitriou
Dermatologist
Aristotle University of Thessaloniki, Greece
Ilias Papanikolaou
Head of Respiratory Medicine
General Hospital of Corfu, Greece
Nikolaos Koletsos
Rheumatologist
Aristotle University of Thessaloniki, Greece
Tereza Memi
Rheumatologist
University Hospital of Ioannina, Greece

Contents

About the Authors

Eleftherios Pelechas MD received his MSc in Healthcare Management and PhD in Epidemiology. He has worked in various hospitals in the UK and Greece. He is a Rheumatologist and a research associate at the "Chatzikosta" General Hospital of Ioannina, Greece and the director of the Rheumatology outpatient clinics "Arthritis.gr". Certified in Musculoskeletal Ultrasonography by the Central Health Board of Greece, Dr. Pelechas has contributed extensively to medical literature, serving on the editorial boards of several journal. His contribution includes research articles, book chapters and books. He is the main author of the book *Illustrated Handbook of Rheumatic and Musculo-Skeletal Diseases* which has been awarded by the National Academy of Athens. He has also participated in several national and international congresses as well as in several research studies with several distinctions. Dr. Pelechas is a member of several prestigious Medical Associations. His research interests include: Epidemiology of the rheumatic diseases, autoimmune rheumatic diseases.

Panagiota Karagianni MD, PhD is a medical Biopathologist with extensive experience in both clinical and academic settings. She has worked in several prominent hospitals across Greece. Her expertise spans various aspects of biopathology, with a particular interest in the laboratory evaluation of rheumatic diseases. She has authored numerous research articles and book chapters and has taken part in national and international congresses. Her research interests include: Laboratory evaluation of rheumatic diseases with an interest in systemic lupus erythematosus and rheumatoid arthritis.

Evripidis Kaltsonoudis MD received his PhD in Rheumatology. Currently, he is the director of the Rheumatology Department at the "Chatzikosta" General Hospital of Ioannina, Greece. He has participated in several national and international congresses with many distinctions, as well as several research studies. He has authored many articles with an interest to newer therapeutic targets in autoimmune diseases and a particular interest in neurological adverse events after anti-TNF therapy. He has also been one of the main authors of the book *Illustrated Handbook of Rheumatic and Musculo-Skeletal diseases*. Dr. Kaltsonoudis is a member of the Medical Association of Ioannina (Greece), Hellenic Association of Rheumatologists. Research interests: Autoimmune and auto-inflammatory diseases.

Abbreviations

AAV	ANCA-associated vasculitis
ACA	Anti-centromere antibodies
ACE	Angiotensin-converting enzyme
ACL	Anterior cruciate ligament
aCL	Anticardiolipin antibodies
ACPA	Anti-citrullinated protein antibodies
ACR	American College of Rheumatology
ACTH	Adrenocorticotropic hormone
AHA	Autoimmune haemolytic anaemia
AIDs	Autoinflammatory diseases
AIH	Autoimmune hepatitis
AIP	Autoimmune pancreatitis
ALL	Anterior longitudinal ligament
ALP	Alkaline phosphatase
ALS	Amyotrophic lateral sclerosis
ANA	Antinuclear antibodies
ANCA	Anti-neutrophil cytoplasmic antibodies
anti-CCP	Anti-cyclic citrullinated peptide
anti-dsDNA	Anti-double stranded DNA
anti-Sm	Anti-Smith
anti-β2-GPI	Anti-bet-2 glycoprotein I antibodies
AOSD	Adult-onset Still's disease
aPL	Antiphospholipid antibodies
APS	Antiphospholipid syndrome
AS	Ankylosing spondylitis
ASAS	Assessment of SpondyloArthritis international Society
AZA	Azathioprine
bDMARDs	Biologic disease-modifying anti-rheumatic drugs
BLM	Belimumab
BMD	Bone mineral density
cANCA	Cytoplasmic ANCA
CAPS	Cryopyrin-associated periodic syndromes
CCP	Cyclic citrullinated peptide
CD	Colour Doppler

CHCC	Chapel Hill Consensus Conference
CK	Creatinine kinase
CKD	Chronic kidney disease
CNS	Central nervous system
CP	Cyclophosphamide
CPPD	Calcium pyrophosphate deposition
CRP	C-reactive protein
CS	Corticosteroids
CsA	Cyclosporine
csDMARDs	Conventional synthetic disease-modifying anti-rheumatic drugs
CT	Computed tomography
CTA	CT angiography
CTD	Connective tissue disease
CVD	Cardiovascular disease
CVID	Common variable immunodeficiency
dcSScl	Diffuse cutaneous systemic sclerosis
DDD	Degenerative disc disease
DEXA	Dual-energy X-ray absorptiometry
DIL	Drug-induced lupus
DISH	Diffuse idiopathic skeletal hyperostosis
DM	Dermatomyositis
DMARDs	Disease-modifying anti-rheumatic drugs
DNA	Deoxyribonucleic acid
dsSScl	Diffuse cutaneous systemic sclerosis
ECG	Electrocardiogram
ELISA	Enzyme-linked immunosorbent assays
EMA	European Medicines Agency
EMG	Electromyography
ESR	Erythrocyte sedimentation rate
ESRD	End-stage renal disease
EULAR	European League Against Rheumatism
FBC	Full blood count
Fc	Fragment crystallisable
FDA	Food and Drug Administration
FMF	Familial Mediterranean fever
FRAX	Fracture risk assessment tool
GCA	Giant cell arteritis
GI	Gastrointestinal
GN	Glomerulonephritis
GOERD	Gastroesophageal reflux disease
GPA	Granulomatosis with polyangiitis
HBV	Hepatitis B virus
HCQ	Hydroxychloroquine
HCV	Hepatitis C virus
HIV	Human immunodeficiency virus

HL	Hodgkin lymphoma
HLA	Human leucocyte antigen
HLH	Haemophagocytic lymphohistiocytosis
HPF	High-power field
HRCT	High-resolution computed tomography
HZV	Herpes zoster virus
i.v.	Intravenous
IA	Inflammatory arthritis
IBD	Inflammatory bowel disease
IBM	Inclusion body myositis
IBP	Inflammatory back pain
Ig	Immunoglobulin
IgG4-RD	Immunoglobulin G4-related disease
IL	Interleukin
IL-17i	Interleukin-17 inhibitors
IL-6i	Interleukin 6 inhibitors
ILD	Interstitial lung disease
IM	Inflammatory markers
IM	Inflammatory myopathies
IRT	Immunoglobulin replacement therapy
ITP	Immune thrombocytopaenic purpura
IVIG	Intravenous immunoglobulin
JAKi	Janus kinase inhibitors
JDM	Juvenile dermatomyositis
JIA	Juvenile idiopathic arthritis
LA	Lupus anticoagulant
LBP	Low back pain
lcSScl	Limited cutaneous systemic sclerosis
LDA	Low disease activity
LEF	Leflunomide
LFTs	Liver function tests
LN	Lupus nephritis
LVV	Large-vessel vasculitis
MALT	Mucosa-associated lymphoid tissue
MCTD	Mixed connective tissue disease
MEFV	Mediterranean fever gene
MMF	Mycophenolate mofetil
MPA	Microscopic polyangiitis
MRA	MRI angiography
MRI	Magnetic resonance imaging
MSAs	Myositis-specific autoantibodies
MSK	Musculoskeletal
MSKUS	Musculoskeletal ultrasound
MTP	Metatarsophalangeal
MTX	Methotrexate

MUC	Monosodium urate crystals
MVV	Medium-vessel vasculitis
NAM	Necrotising autoimmune myopathy
NGS	Next-generation sequencing
NHL	Non-Hodgkin lymphoma
NLRP3	Nucleotide-binding domain, leucine-rich-containing family, pyrin domain-containing-3 inflammasome
NSAIDs	Non-steroidal anti-inflammatory drugs
NVC	Nailfold videocapillaroscopy
OA	Osteoarthritis
OMERACT	Outcome Measures in Rheumatology
OP	Osteoporosis
OTC	Over-the-counter
p.o.	Per os
PAH	Pulmonary arterial hypertension
pANCA	Perinuclear ANCA
PCL	Posterior cruciate ligament
PD	Paget's disease
PDE-5	Phosphodiesterase-5
PEST	Psoriasis epidemiology screening tool
PET-CT	Positron emission tomography–computed tomography
PFTs	Pulmonary function tests
PIDs	Primary immunodeficiencies
PJP	Pneumocystis jirovecii pneumonia
PM	Polymyositis
PMR	Polymyalgia rheumatica
PROs	Patient-reported outcomes
pRP	Primary Raynaud's phenomenon
PsA	Psoriatic arthritis
pSS	Primary SS
QoL	Quality of life
RA	Rheumatoid arthritis
RBC	Red blood cell
RF	Rheumatoid factor
RMDs	Rheumatic diseases
RNA	Ribonucleic acid
ROM	Range of motion
RP	Raynaud's phenomenon
RPGN	Rapidly progressive glomerulonephritis
RTX	Rituximab
s.c.	Subcutaneous
SAA	Serum amyloid A
SI	Sacroiliac
SLE	Systemic lupus erythematosus
SLEDAI	Systemic lupus erythematosus disease activity index

SNRI	Serotonin-norepinephrine reuptake inhibitor
SOB	Shortness of breath
SpA	Spondyloarthropathies
sRP	Secondary RP
SRP	Signal recognition particle
SS	Sjögren's syndrome
SScl	Systemic sclerosis
sSS	Secondary SS
SVV	Small-vessel vasculitis
T2T	Treat-to-target
TA	Takayasu arteritis
TAB	Temporal artery biopsy
TB	Tuberculosis
TCZ	Tocilizumab
TNFi	Tumour necrosis factor α inhibitors
TNFRSF1A	Tumour necrosis factor receptor superfamily member 1A
TRAPS	Tumour necrosis factor receptor-associated periodic syndrome
tsDMARDs	Targeted synthetic DMARDs
ULT	Urate-lowering therapy
US	Ultrasound
VUS	Variants of uncertain significance
WES	Whole exome sequencing
WGS	Whole genome sequencing
XLA	X-linked agammaglobulinaemia

Introduction: Pitfalls in the Diagnosis of Rheumatic Diseases

1

Abbreviations

ANA	Antinuclear antibodies
ANCA	Anti-neutrophil cytoplasmic antibodies
aPL	Antiphospholipid antibodies
AS	Ankylosing spondylitis
bDMARDs	Biologic DMARDs
CCP	Cyclic citrullinated peptide
CRP	c-Reactive protein
CS	Corticosteroids
csDMARDs	Conventional synthetic DMARDs
CSF	Cerebrospinal fluid
DM	Dermatomyositis
DMARDs	Disease-modifying anti-rheumatic drugs
ESR	Erythrocyte sedimentation rate
IBP	Inflammatory back pain
MCTD	Mixed connective tissue disease
MRI	Magnetic resonance imaging
NSAIDs	Non-steroidal anti-inflammatory drugs
PMR	Polymyalgia rheumatica
PsA	Psoriatic arthritis
RA	Rheumatoid arthritis
RF	Rheumatoid factor
RMDs	Rheumatic diseases
SI	Sacroiliac
SLE	Systemic lupus erythematosus
SpA	Spondyloarthropathies
SScl	Systemic sclerosis
TB	Tuberculosis

E. Pelechas et al., *Pitfalls in Rheumatology*,
https://doi.org/10.1007/978-3-031-98671-0_1

1.1 Misinterpreting Early or Atypical Symptoms

RMDs often present with vague, non-specific symptoms in their early stages, such as weakness, malaise, fatigue, low-grade fever, generalised pain or stiffness [1]. These symptoms can be mistaken for common viral infections, overuse injuries (Fig. 1.1) or age-related musculoskeletal discomfort [1]. Furthermore, atypical presentations of well-known RMDs can lead to diagnostic delays or misdiagnosis.

Consequences (a) *Delayed diagnosis*: patients may experience significant delays in diagnosis, leading to progressive joint damage or organ involvement, as seen in RA or SLE [2]; (b) *misdiagnosis*: early symptoms can be attributed to other conditions, such as fibromyalgia [3], chronic fatigue syndrome, carpal tunnel syndrome or even psychiatric disorders, resulting in improper treatment and persistent disease activity, which in some instances may lead to irreversible organ damage.

How to Avoid This Pitfall (a) *High index of suspicion*: clinicians should maintain a high level of suspicion for RMDs in patients with chronic or unexplained musculoskeletal pain, stiffness or fatigue, particularly if symptoms persist for more than 6 weeks or are associated with morning stiffness or systemic symptoms [4]; (b) *detailed history and physical examination*: a thorough history and physical examination can help identify key clues, such as symmetric joint swelling in RA, photosensitive rashes in SLE or back pain that improves with activity in AS; (c) *early referral*: if symptoms are persistent or unclear, early referral to a rheumatologist is critical [5]. Rheumatologists are equipped to evaluate subtle signs of the disease and order appropriate diagnostic tests.

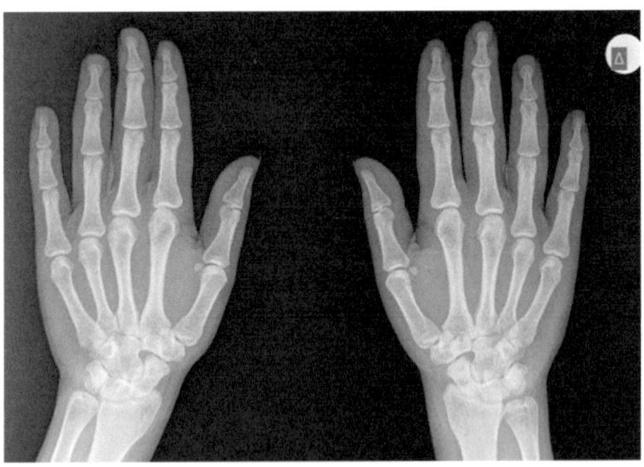

Fig. 1.1 Hand X-ray of a 34-year-old female with soft tissue oedema of the fingers and stiffens. Due to her job (manual worker), the diagnosis was overuse injury of the hands, but the laboratory exams came back positive for anti-CCP and RF

1.2 Over-Reliance of Serologic Testing

Serologic tests, such as RF, anti-CCP, ANA, aPL and ANCA, are important tools in the diagnosis of RMDs. However, over-reliance on these tests without correlating clinical findings can lead to misdiagnosis. Many serologic markers are non-specific and can be positive in healthy individuals or in those with other conditions [6].

Consequences (a) *False positives*: a positive RF or ANA can be seen in healthy individuals, particularly in older adults, or in non-RMD conditions such as chronic infections or malignancies [7, 8]. This can lead to overdiagnosis leading to unnecessary treatment or further testing; (b) *missed diagnosis*: a negative result for serologic markers, such as RF or anti-CCP, especially in early RA or negative ANA in early SLE, can lead to false reassurance and delayed diagnosis.

How to Avoid This Pitfall (a) *Clinical correlation*: serologic tests should be used as supportive tools in conjunction with a minute clinical history and thorough clinical evaluation [9]. A positive test result should only reinforce a diagnosis that is already suspected based on clinical findings; (b) *understanding sensitivity and specificity*: physicians must be familiar with the limitations of these tests, including their sensitivity and specificity [10]. For example, ANA testing is highly sensitive but not specific for SLE, and a negative result, in a small proportion of patients, does not rule out the disease; (c) *testing in the appropriate context*: avoid ordering broad panels of serologic tests without clinical indications. Serologic testing should be focused on confirming a suspected diagnosis based on history and physical examination.

1.3 Failure to Recognise Rheumatic Disease Mimickers

Many non-RMD conditions, such as infections, malignancies and metabolic or endocrine disorders, can mimic RMDs. These conditions may present with fever, joint pain or systemic inflammation, leading to misdiagnosis as a primary rheumatologic disorder.

Common Mimickers (a) *Infections*: bacterial endocarditis, TB, viral infections (e.g., parvovirus, hepatitis) and fungal infections can all present with joint pain, fever and systemic symptoms that mimic diseases like RA [11] or vasculitis; (b) *malignancies*: paraneoplastic syndromes associated with cancers can present with PMR symptoms [12], arthritis (Fig. 1.2), vasculitis-like symptoms or DM-like rashes [13]; (c) *endocrine disorders*: hypothyroidism, hyperthyroidism, diabetes mellitus and vitamin D deficiency can cause musculoskeletal symptoms, including joint pain, muscle weakness and fatigue, which can resemble RMD [14].

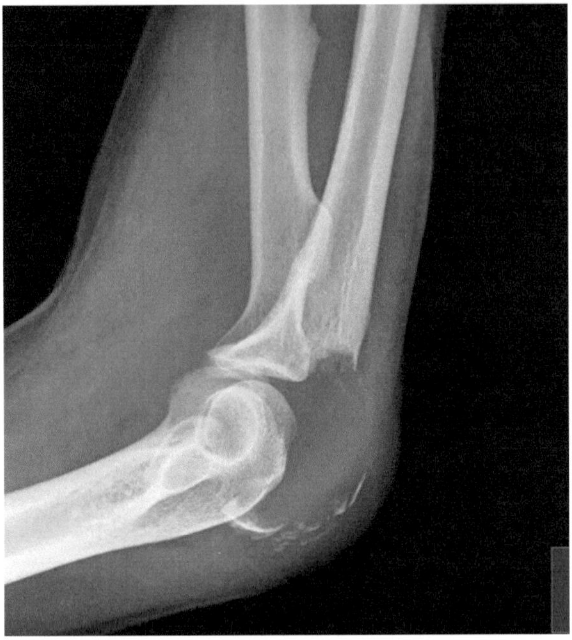

Fig. 1.2 Bone metastasis of the right elbow of a patient suffering from lung cancer

Consequences (a) *Inappropriate treatment*: treating an infection or malignancy with immunosuppressive medications can worsen the underlying condition and delay proper diagnosis and treatment; (b) *missed opportunity for early detection*: failure to recognise a mimicker can delay the diagnosis of life-threatening conditions like malignancy or infection, leading to poor outcomes.

How to Avoid This Pitfall (a) *Broad differential diagnosis*: always consider non-RMD conditions in patients presenting with rheumatic symptoms, especially if they have atypical features [15], unusual disease progression or a poor response to treatment; (b) *use of diagnostic imaging, cultures and biopsy*: in cases of uncertainty, imaging studies, cultures or tissue biopsy can be crucial for ruling out mimickers. For example, bone scans or MRIs can help identify infections or malignancies, while biopsies can confirm or rule out vasculitis or malignancy. In addition, negative cultures from blood, urine, synovial fluid and other serous fluids (pleural CSF, etc.) rule out infections that may be involved in or coexist with RMDs [16]; (c) *close collaboration*: collaborating with infectious disease specialists, oncologists or endocrinologists can be essential when evaluating patients with atypical presentations or suspected mimickers.

1.4 Neglecting Inflammatory Back Pain in Young Adults

IBP in young adults is a key feature of SpA, including AS, PsA and reactive arthritis [17]. However, IBP is often mistaken for mechanical or non-specific low back pain [18], leading to diagnostic delays. In non-specific low back pain, genetic conditions such as Bertolotti syndrome (sacralisation of the L1) (Fig. 1.3) or lumbarisation of the S1 are not uncommon reasons (Fig. 1.4).

Consequences (a) *Missed diagnosis of SpA*: mislabelling IBP as mechanical back pain can result in a delayed diagnosis of AS or other SpA, allowing for progressive spinal damage and functional impairment; (b) *inadequate treatment*: patients with SpA may receive inappropriate treatments, such as physical therapy focused on mechanical causes, simple analgesics or short-term NSAIDs, rather than the DMARDs to control disease progression [19].

How to Avoid This Pitfall (a) *Recognising features of IBP*: IBP typically improves with activity and worsens with rest and is associated with morning stiffness lasting more than 30 min [20]. It often presents before the age of 40 and may be associated with peripheral arthritis, enthesitis, IBD or uveitis; (b) *early imaging*: in patients with suspected SpA, consider ordering MRI of the SI joints, which can reveal early signs of sacroiliitis [21] before it is visible on plain radiographs; (c) *genetic testing*: for the detection of the HLA-B27 antigen, the positivity of which—particularly in AS—confers high sensitivity and specificity [22]; (d) *referring to rheumatology*: prompt referral to a rheumatologist is important for early diagnosis and initiation of appropriate therapy, including bDMARDs, in patients with suspected SpA.

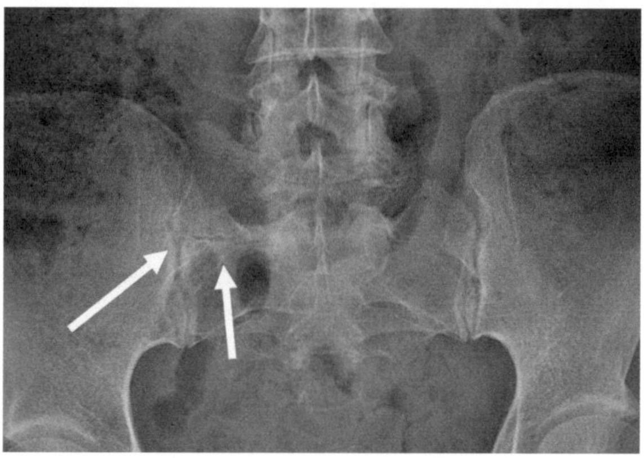

Fig. 1.3 Bertolotti syndrome or sacralization of the L5 vertebra or lumbosacral transitional vertebra. X-ray showing a right transverse mega-apophysis of L5 with pseudoarticulation with the sacral bone

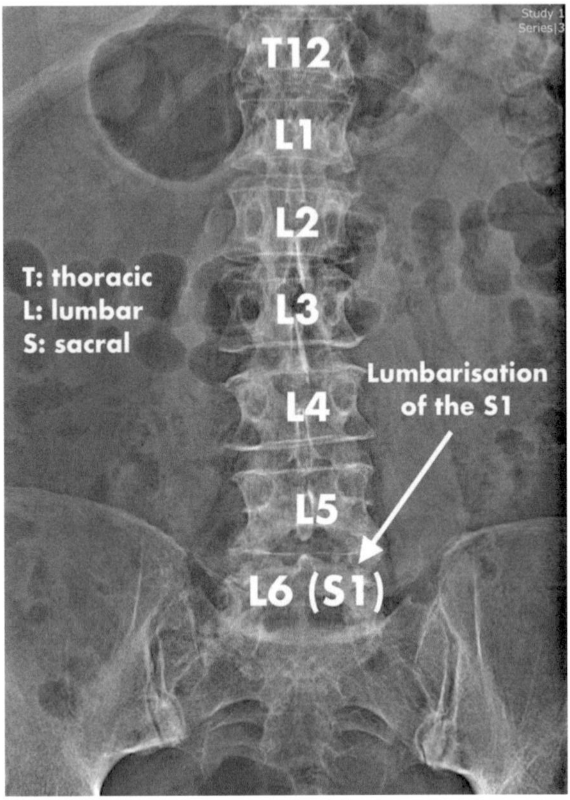

Fig. 1.4 X-ray showing lumbarization of the S1 vertebra. Lumbarization occurs when the S1 of the sacral bone is separated and the lumbar spine appears to have 6 vertebrae instead of 5. This condition is prone to lumbar spine injury and sometimes, patients referring symptoms such as inflammatory back pain

1.5 Misdiagnosing Fibromyalgia as an Inflammatory Disease

Fibromyalgia is a chronic pain syndrome characterised by widespread musculoskeletal pain, fatigue, tender points and other non-pain symptoms, including poor sleep and cognitive impairment, but without evidence of joint inflammation or systemic involvement. These symptoms are common but non-specific. They can be present in other disorders that may overlap with fibromyalgia, often without clear boundaries, while their nature makes objective assessment and quantification challenging. However, its symptoms overlap with many inflammatory RMDs, and it is often misdiagnosed as RA, SLE or another inflammatory condition, leading to unnecessary and potentially harmful treatment with immunosuppressive drugs [23].

Consequences (a) *Inappropriate and unnecessary use of immunosuppressants*: patients with fibromyalgia may be treated with csDMARDs, bDMARDs or CS intended for inflammatory diseases, which are not effective in fibromyalgia and can cause significant side effects; (b) *persistent symptoms*: treating fibromyalgia as an inflammatory disease can result in continued pain and frustration for patients, as the underlying condition is not addressed [24].

How to Avoid This Pitfall (a) *Clear diagnostic criteria*: recognise the diagnostic criteria for fibromyalgia [25], which include widespread pain for at least 3 months and the absence of underlying inflammation or joint swelling. A minute clinical history is necessary and can reveal sleep disorders or other psychological disturbances. Laboratory markers such as ESR and CRP are typically normal in fibromyalgia, but essential laboratory testing to rule out other causes that may mimic the symptomatology of fibromyalgia, such as thyroid disorders and vitamin deficiencies, should be carried out [26]; (b) *avoid overuse of testing*: avoid overtesting in patients with clinical features of fibromyalgia, as this can lead to false positives and confusion; (c) *multidisciplinary management*: fibromyalgia management focuses on non-pharmacologic treatments such as exercise, cognitive behavioural therapy and pain management strategies. Medications like antidepressants or anticonvulsants may also be helpful, but immunosuppressants are not indicated [27].

1.6 Failure to Recognise Overlap Syndromes

It is a fact that some patients present with features of more than one RMD, a situation referred to as an "overlap syndrome" [28]. Common overlap syndromes include MCTD, overlap between RA and SLE or overlap between SLE and myositis. Failure to recognise these overlap syndromes can lead to incomplete diagnosis and suboptimal treatment.

Consequences (a) *Incomplete diagnosis*: if overlap syndromes are not recognised, patients may only receive treatment for one component of their disease, leading to incomplete control of symptoms and disease activity; furthermore, some medications with proven efficacy in one disease may be contraindicated in the other; (b) *inadequate monitoring*: overlap syndromes often involve multiple organ systems, requiring more comprehensive monitoring and a multidisciplinary approach to care.

How to Avoid This Pitfall (a) *Recognising patterns of overlap*: be alert for signs of multiple RMDs [29], such as RA features in a patient with SLE, or myositis features in a patient with SScl; (b) *broad serologic testing*: in patients with suspected overlap syndromes, a broader panel of serologic tests may be needed, including anti-U1RNP antibodies, which are pathognomonic of MCTD; (c) *multidisciplinary care*: in cases of overlap syndromes, consider involving multiple specialists, such as dermatologists, pulmonologists or nephrologists, to ensure comprehensive care.

1.7 Conclusion

The diagnosis of RMDs is complex, requiring careful evaluation of a patient's medical history, clinical findings, judicious use of diagnostic tests and consideration of non-RMD mimickers. By avoiding common pitfalls such as over-reliance on serologic tests, misinterpretation of early symptoms and failure to recognise mimic conditions or overlap syndromes, clinicians can improve diagnostic accuracy and ultimately enhance patient outcomes. Early and accurate diagnosis, followed by appropriate treatment, remains the key to preventing long-term disability and preserving quality of life in patients with RMDs.

References

1. Katz JD, Walitt B. Rheumatic diseases in oder adults. Clin Geriatr Med. 2017;33:ix–x. https://doi.org/10.1016/j.cger.2016.10.001.
2. Al-Mehmadi BA, Alelaiwi MMM, Alnumayr HAS, Alghamdi BS, Alomari BA, Alzahrani HS. Knowledge of common symptoms of rheumatic diseases and causes of delayed diagnosis in Saudi Arabia. Patient Prefer Adherence. 2024;18:635–47. https://doi.org/10.2147/PPA.S448999.
3. Daoud KF, Barkhuizen A. Rheumatic mimics and selected triggers of fibromyalgia. Curr Pain Headache Rep. 2022;6:284–8. https://doi.org/10.1007/s11916-0049-y.
4. Niemantsverdriet E, Dougados M, Combe B, van der Helm-van Mil AHM. Referring early arthritis patients within 6 weeks versus 12 weeks after symptom onset: an observational cohort study. Lancet Rheumatol. 2020;2:e332–8. https://doi.org/10.1016/S2665-9913(20)30061-8.
5. Fautrel B, Benhamou M, Foltz V, Rincheval N, Rat AC, Combe B, et al. Early referral to the rheumatologist for early arthritis patients: evidence for suboptimal care. Results from the ESPOIR cohort. Rheumatology (Oxford). 2010;49:147–55. https://doi.org/10.1093/rheumatology/kep340.
6. Suresh E. Laboratory tests in rheumatology: a rational approach. Cleve Clin J Med. 2019;86:198–210. https://doi.org/10.3949/ccjm.86a.18076.
7. Ingegnoli F, Castelli R, Gualtierotti R. Rheumatoid factors: clinical applications. Dis Markers. 2013;35:727–34. https://doi.org/10.1155/2013/726598.
8. Grygiel-Górniak B, Rogacka N, Puszczewicz M. Antinuclear antibodies in healthy people and non-rheumatic diseases—diagnostic and clinical implications. Reumatologia. 2018;56:243–8. https://doi.org/10.5114/reum.2018.77976.
9. Habash-Bseiso DE, Yale SH, Glurich I, Goldberg JW. Serologic testing in connective tissue diseases. Clin Med Res. 2005;3:190–3. https://doi.org/10.3121/cmr.3.3.190.
10. Van Boekel MAM, Vossenaar ER, van den Hoogen FHJ, van Venrooij WJ. Autoantibody systems in rheumatoid arthritis: specificity, sensitivity and diagnostic value. Arthritis Res. 2001;4:87–93. https://doi.org/10.1186/ar395.
11. Sharma V, Sharma A. Infectious mimics of rheumatoid arthritis. Best Pract Res Clin Rheumatol. 2022;36:101736. https://doi.org/10.1016/j.berh.2021.101736.
12. Ide Y, Yuki T, Taooka Y, Higashi Y, Tachiyama Y. Malignant peritoneal mesothelioma presenting with polymyalgia rheumatica-like syndrome. Intern Med. 2020;59:2629–32. https://doi.org/10.2169/internalmedicine.4809-20.
13. Racanelli V, Prete M, Minoia C, Favoino E, Perosa F. Rheumatic disorders as paraneoplastic syndromes. Autoimmun Rev. 2008;7:352–8. https://doi.org/10.1016/j.autrev.2008.02.001.
14. Chakravarty SD, Markenson JA. Rheumatic manifestations of endocrine disease. Curr Opin Rheumatol. 2013;25:37–43. https://doi.org/10.1097/BOR.0b013e32835b4f3f.

15. Cappelli LC, Shah AA. The relationships between cancer and autoimmune rheumatic diseases. Best Pract Res Clin Rheumatol. 2020;34:101472. https://doi.org/10.1016/j.berh.2019.101472.
16. Fragoulis GE, Nikiphorou E, Dey M, Zhao SS, Courvoisier DS, Arnaud L, et al. 2022 EULAR recommendations for screening and prophylaxis of chronic and opportunistic infections in adults with autoimmune inflammatory rheumatic diseases. Ann Rheum Dis. 2023;82:742–53. https://doi.org/10.1136/ard-2022-223335.
17. Pelechas E, Kaltsonoudis E, Voulgari PV, Drosos AA. Spondyloarthropathies. In: Illustrated handbook of rheumatic and musculo-skeletal diseases. Cham: Springer; 2023. https://doi.org/10.1007/978-3-031-47379-1_7.
18. Pelechas E, Kosta P, Voulgari PV, Drosos AA. Bertolotti syndrome: a not-to-miss cause of chronic low back pain in young adults. Acta Reumatol Port. 2020;45:58–60.
19. Gibbs D, McGalan BG, Ropper AE, Xu DS. Back pain: differential diagnosis and management. Neurol Clin. 2023;41:61–76. https://doi.org/10.1016/j.ncl.2022.07.002.
20. Coath FL, Gaffney K. Inflammatory back pain: a concept, not a diagnosis. Curr Opin Rheumatol. 2021;33:319–25. https://doi.org/10.1097/BOR.0000000000000807.
21. Ramiro S, Nikiphorou E, Sepriano A, Ortolan A, Webers C, Baraliakos X, et al. ASAS-EULAR recommendations for the management of axial spondyloarthritis: 2022 update. Ann Rheum Dis. 2023;82:19–34. https://doi.org/10.1136/ard-2022-223296.
22. Khan MA, Yong SB, Wei JC. Ankylosing spondylitis: history, epidemiology, and HLA-B27. Int Rheum Dis. 2023;26:413–4. https://doi.org/10.1111/1756-185X.14547.
23. Atzeni F, Cazzola M, Benucci M, Di Franco M, Salaffi F, Sarzi-Puttini P. Chronic widespread pain in the spectrum of rheumatological diseases. Best Pract Res Clin Rheumatol. 2011;25:165–71. https://doi.org/10.1016/j.berh.2010.01.011.
24. Salaffi F, Farah S, Bianchi B, Lommano MG, Di Carlo M. Delay in fibromyalgia diagnosis and its impact on the severity and outcome: a large cohort study. Clin Exp Rheumatol. 2024;42:1198–204. https://doi.org/10.55563/clinexprheumatol/ta9xtc.
25. Arnold LM, Bennett RM, Crofford LJ, Dean LE, Clauw DJ, Goldenberg DL, et al. AAPT Diagnostic criteria for fibromyalgia. J Pain. 2019;20:611–28. https://doi.org/10.1016/j.jpain.2018.10.008.
26. Cure O, Kizilkaya B, Ciftel S, Klisic A, Ciftel E, Mercantepe F. Effect of fibromyalgia on demographic, biochemical, metabolic and inflammatory profiles: a single-centre retrospective study. Clin Exp Rheumatol. 2024;42:1205–14. https://doi.org/10.55563/clinexprheumatol/oo5zjo.
27. Jones EA, Asaad F, Patel N, Jain E, Abd-Elsayed A. Management of fibromyalgia: an update. Biomedicines. 2024;12:1266. https://doi.org/10.3390/biomedicines12061266.
28. Fiori G, Pignone A, Matucci-Cerinic M. Overlap syndromes. Reumatizam. 2002;49:12–5.
29. Pepmueller PH. Undifferentiated connective tissue disease, mixed connective tissue disease, and overlap syndromes in rheumatology. Mo Med. 2016;113:136–40.

Pitfalls in the Interpretation of Inflammatory Markers in Rheumatology

2

Abbreviations

anti-dsDNA	Anti-double-stranded DNA
AOSD	Adult-onset Still's disease
CRP	C-Reactive protein
CS	Corticosteroids
DISH	Diffuse idiopathic skeletal hyperostosis
DMARDs	Disease-modifying anti-rheumatic drugs
ESR	Erythrocyte sedimentation rate
FMF	Familial Mediterranean fever
GCA	Giant cell arteritis
HLH	Haemophagocytic lymphohistiocytosis
IM	Inflammatory markers
MRI	Magnetic resonance imaging
MSKUS	Musculoskeletal ultrasound
NSAIDs	Non-steroidal anti-inflammatory drugs
PFTs	Pulmonary function tests
PMR	Polymyalgia rheumatica
RA	Rheumatoid arthritis
RBC	Red blood cell
RMDs	Rheumatic diseases
SAA	Serum amyloid A
SLE	Systemic lupus erythematosus
SpA	Spondyloarthropathy
SS	Sjögren's syndrome
SScl	Systemic sclerosis

E. Pelechas et al., *Pitfalls in Rheumatology*,
https://doi.org/10.1007/978-3-031-98671-0_2

2.1 Over-Reliance on Inflammatory Markers for Diagnosis

One of the most significant pitfalls is the over-reliance on IMs for making a diagnosis. While elevated ESR and CRP are commonly associated with RMDs such as RA, GCA, PMR and SLE, they are not pathognomonic [1]. ESR and CRP can be elevated in many non-rheumatic conditions, including infections, malignancies, metabolic disorders and even normal aging [2]. Conversely, some patients with active RMD may have normal IMs, especially in early disease.

How to Avoid This Pitfall (a) *Clinical correlation*: always interpret ESR and CRP in the context of the patient's clinical presentation. RMDs should be suspected based on characteristic symptoms (polyarthritis, morning stiffness, systemic symptoms or organ-specific involvement) rather than IMs alone; (b) *consider differential diagnoses*: in cases of elevated IMs, consider non-rheumatologic causes such as infections, malignancies [3], metabolic and other systemic conditions; (c) *use as an adjunct*: ESR and CRP should be considered as supportive evidence for diagnosis rather than primary diagnostic tools [4]. A thorough clinical evaluation and additional diagnostic tests are essential to confirm the underlying diagnosis.

2.2 Misinterpreting Normal Inflammatory Markers as Disease Exclusion

Another common pitfall is assuming that normal ESR and CRP levels rule out active RMDs [5]. Certain conditions, such as early-stage RA [6], SLE with no serositis [7] or SpAs [8], may present with little or no elevations in IMs despite significant clinical disease activity. In conditions like fibromyalgia, DISH or other non-inflammatory and degenerative arthritides, patients may have severe pain and disability, but normal IMs, leading to diagnostic confusion [9].

How to Avoid This Pitfall (a) *Recognise variability/heterogeneity*: not all RMDs cause marked elevations in ESR or CRP. Clinical suspicion should remain high in the presence of characteristic symptoms even if markers are normal; (b) *disease-specific knowledge*: in some conditions like SLE, disease activity may not correlate with IMs but instead with other markers like complement levels, anti-dsDNA antibodies [10] or specific organ involvement [11]; (c) *consider alternative markers*: for conditions with normal ESR and CRP, focus on other diagnostic tools such as autoantibody profiles, imaging studies (MSKUS, MRI for synovitis), synovial fluid analysis (where possible) or direct tissue sampling such as synovial biopsy in RA [12].

2.3 Failure to Recognise False Positives

IMs can be elevated for reasons unrelated to underlying RMD, leading to false positives. Conditions like infections, trauma and malignancies [13] or coexisting conditions can increase both ESR and CRP levels. Similarly, certain physiologic states (pregnancy and obesity) [14, 15] or medications (CS and NSAIDs) can influence these markers [16]. In the elderly and patients with anaemia, particularly ESR may be elevated due to age-related changes or decreased red blood cell mass without significant inflammatory disease [17].

How to Avoid This Pitfall (a) *Consider the full clinical picture*: elevated IMs should prompt consideration of alternative causes, especially when the clinical presentation does not clearly point to an RMD; (b) *review patient history*: assess for recent infections, trauma or chronic conditions like cancer that may elevate ESR and CRP levels. Evaluate the potential impact of medications; (c) *use additional diagnostic tools*: if the clinical presentation is unclear, utilise more specific tests such as imaging, biopsy or specific serologic markers, to confirm or exclude an RMD.

2.4 Misinterpretation of ESR in Certain Conditions

ESR is influenced by several factors, including age, gender and RBC count, making it less specific than CRP in some cases [18]. Anaemia, in particular, can falsely elevate ESR, while polycythaemia or other conditions that increase plasma viscosity can lower it [19]. Moreover, kidney disease can affect the ESR levels [20]. The ESR also rises with age and is generally higher in females, making it less reliable as a sole indicator for inflammation, especially in elderly patients or those with coexisting conditions.

How to Avoid This Pitfall (a) *Understanding the limitations of ESR*: ESR is less sensitive and specific than CRP for detecting acute inflammation. It should be interpreted with caution, particularly in the context of age-related changes or haematologic conditions like anaemia; (b) *use ESR with other markers*: combine ESR with CRP and other laboratory and clinical indicators of inflammation to increase diagnostic accuracy. When both markers are elevated, the likelihood of systemic inflammation is higher; (c) *correct for anaemia*: be aware that anaemia can artificially elevate ESR, and its interpretation should be adjusted accordingly in anaemic patients [21].

2.5 Underappreciating the Rapid Response of CRP

CRP has a short half-life and responds quickly to changes in the inflammatory state [22], making it a useful marker for monitoring disease activity and treatment response in RMDs. However, clinicians may underestimate the rapid fluctuations in

CRP levels, leading to incorrect conclusions about disease activity or treatment efficacy. For instance, CRP can rise dramatically during an acute infection [23] or injury, potentially overshadowing the underlying RMD process.

How to Avoid This Pitfall (a) *Monitor trends over time*: CRP levels should be monitored serially rather than relying on a single measurement, especially when evaluating response to treatment or disease activity. Acute fluctuations may reflect temporary non-rheumatologic factors such as infections or trauma; (b) *assess clinical context*: use CRP in conjunction with clinical assessments to gauge disease activity. A sudden rise in CRP may indicate an intercurrent illness rather than worsening of the underlying RMD; (c) *use CRP as a dynamic marker*: in a disease like PMR [24] or RA [25], a rapid decrease in CRP following CS or DMARDs can confirm effective treatment, whereas persistent elevation suggests ongoing inflammation. On the other hand, drugs that interfere with the hepatic metabolism of hepcidin may rapidly and falsely lower CRP levels, without this truly reflecting disease activity, which may still persist [26].

2.6 Neglecting to Use Other Markers of Inflammation

In certain RMDs, ESR and CRP alone may not provide a full picture of the inflammatory process. Other markers, such as ferritin [27], fibrinogen [28], white blood cells [29] and SAA [30], can be helpful in specific situations. For example, elevated ferritin levels are a hallmark of AOSD and HLH, whereas SAA is used to monitor amyloidosis risk in patients with chronic inflammatory conditions like FMF.

How to Avoid This Pitfall (a) *Consider disease-specific markers*: for diseases such as AOSD [31], HLH or FMF [32], use additional IMs such as ferritin, white blood cell count or SAA, to confirm diagnosis and monitor disease activity; (b) *use a multimodal approach*: combine clinical assessments, ESR/CRP and other disease-specific markers to get a comprehensive understanding of the inflammatory process; (c) *tailor testing to the disease*: different RMDs may require different markers for monitoring. For instance, monitoring white blood cell count and complement levels is critical in SLE [33], while SAA may be more important in FMF or systemic amyloidosis risk.

2.7 Inappropriate Use of Inflammatory Markers for Monitoring in Certain Diseases

Some RMDs, such as SScl and SS, are characterised by chronic inflammation, but elevated ESR or CRP levels may not correlate well with the disease activity. Overreliance on these markers for monitoring can lead to undertreatment or inappropriate treatment. For instance, in SScl and SS, CRP may remain low despite active disease and organ involvement [34].

How to Avoid This Pitfall (a) *Disease-specific monitoring*: for diseases like SScl and SS, clinical features and specific organ-based tests (PFTs and echocardiograms) are often more informative than ESR or CRP levels; (b) *focus on clinical symptoms*: in conditions where IMs are less reliable, the focus should be on patient-reported outcomes, physical examination findings and targeted imaging or organ-specific evaluations; (c) *be cautious in treatment decisions*: in patients with diseases where IMs are less helpful, avoid basing treatment decisions solely on ESR or CRP levels. Clinical judgement and disease-specific assessments are crucial.

2.8 Conclusion

IMs, particularly ESR and CRP, play a central role in the diagnosis, management and follow-up of RMDs, but they have limitations. Misinterpretation of these markers can lead to misdiagnosis, inappropriate treatment and unnecessary delays in care. Clinicians must use IMs as part of a broader diagnostic and monitoring strategy, considering clinical context, patient history and disease-specific features. By recognising the pitfalls outlined in this chapter, clinicians can avoid common mistakes and make more informed decisions, improving outcomes for patients with RMDs. In Fig. 2.1, a schematic flow is presented in order to approach a patient with high inflammatory markers.

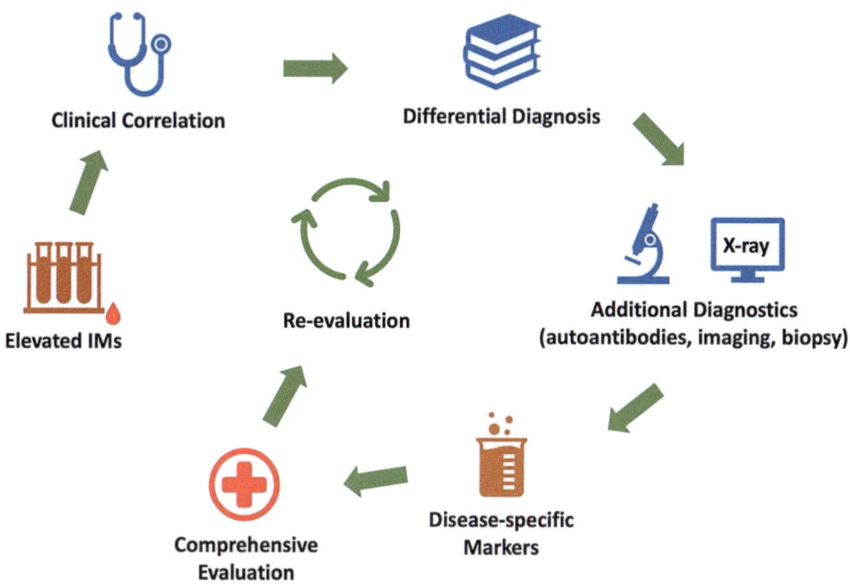

Fig. 2.1 Schematic representation of the approach for a patient with elevated inflammatory markers and a potential autoimmune disease

References

1. Pelechas E, Kaltsonoudis E, Voulgari PV, Drosos AA. Autoimmune rheumatic diseases: pathophysiology and laboratory tests. In: Illustrated handbook of rheumatic and musculo-skeletal diseases. Cham: Springer; 2023. https://doi.org/10.1007/978-3-031-47379-1_2.
2. Bitik B, Mercan R, Tufan A, Tezcan E, Küçük H, Ilhan M, et al. Differential diagnosis of elevated erythrocyte sedimentation rate and C-reactive protein levels: a rheumatology perspective. Eur J Rheumatol. 2015;2:131–4. https://doi.org/10.5152/eurjrheum.2015/0113.
3. Ozsoy Z, Bilgin E, Aksun MS, Eroglu I, Kalyoncu U. Extremely high erythrocyte sedimentation rate revisited in rheumatic diseases: a single-center experience. Turk J Med Sci. 2022;52:1889–99. https://doi.org/10.55730/1300-0144.5536.
4. Siva C, Larson EC, Barnett M. Rational use of blood tests in the evaluation of rheumatic diseases. Mo Med. 2012;109:59–63.
5. Birtane M, Yavuz S, Tastekin N. Laboratory evaluation in rheumatic diseases. World J Methodol. 2017;7:1–8. https://doi.org/10.5662/wjm.v7.i1.1.
6. Suresh E. Diagnosis of early rheumatoid arthritis: what the non-specialist needs to know. J R Soc Med. 2004;97:421–4. https://doi.org/10.1258/jrsm.97.9.421.
7. Aringer M. Inflammatory markers in systemic lupus erythematosus. J Autoimmun. 2020;110:102374. https://doi.org/10.1016/j.jaut.2019.102374.
8. Maksymowych WP. Biomarkers for diagnosis of axial spondyloarthritis, disease activity, prognosis, and prediction of response to therapy. Front Immunol. 2019;10:305. https://doi.org/10.3389/fimmu.2019.00305.
9. El-Sawy EA, Hakim MMA, El-Zohiery A, Salama SM. Significance of inflammatory markers in primary fibromyalgia syndrome and their relation in assessing the disease severity. Egypt J Immunol. 2024;31:67–74.
10. Gómez-Bañuelos E, Fava A, Andrade F. An update on autoantibodies in systemic lupus erythematosus. Curr Opin Rheumatol. 2022;35:61–7. https://doi.org/10.1097/BOR.0000000000000922.
11. Kyttaris VC. Systemic lupus erythematosus: from genes to organ damage. Methods Mol Biol. 2010;662:265–83. https://doi.org/10.1007/978-1-60761-800-3_13.
12. Orr C, Vieira-Sousa E, Boyle DL, Buch MH, Buckley CD, Cañete JD, et al. Synovial tissue research: a state-of-the-art review. Nat Rev Rheumatol. 2017;13:463–75. https://doi.org/10.1038/nrrheum.2017.115.
13. Il'yasova D, Colbert LH, Harris TB, Newman AB, Bauer DC, Stterfield S, et al. Circulating levels of inflammatory markers and cancer risk in the health aging and body composition cohort. Cancer Epidemiol Biomarkers Prev. 2005;14:2413–8. https://doi.org/10.1158/1055-9965.EPI-05-0316.
14. Ellulu MS, Patimah I, Khaza'ai H, Rahmat A, Abed Y. Obesity and inflammation: the linking mechanism and the complications. Arch Med Sci. 2016;13:851–63. https://doi.org/10.5114/aoms.2016.58928.
15. Jancsura MK, Schmella MJ, Helsabeck N, Gillespie SL, Roberts JM, Conley YP, et al. Inflammatory markers are elevated in early pregnancy, but not late pregnancy, in women with overweight and obesity that later develop preeclampsia. Am J Reprod Immunol. 2023;90:e13763. https://doi.org/10.1111/aji.13763.
16. Tarp S, Bartels EM, Bliddal H, Furst DE, Boers M, Danneskiold-Samsøe B, et al. Effect of nonsteroidal anti-inflammatory drugs on the C-reactive protein level in rheumatoid arthritis: a meta-analysis of randomized controlled trials. Arthritis Rheum. 2012;64:3511–21. https://doi.org/10.1002/art.34644.
17. Cankurtaran M, Ulger Z, Halil M, Yavuz BB, Onal IK, Unal S, et al. How to assess high erythrocyte sedimentation rate (ESR) in elderly? Arch Gerontol Geriatr. 2010;50:323–6. https://doi.org/10.1016/j.archger.2009.05.008.
18. Harrison M. Erythrocyte sedimentation rate an C-reactive protein. Aust Prescr. 2015;38:93–4. https://doi.org/10.18773/autprescr.2015.034.

19. Cuthbert D, Stain BL. Polycythemia vera-associated complications: pathogenesis, clinical manifestations, and effects on outcomes. J Blood Med. 2019;10:359–71. https://doi.org/10.2147/JBM.S189922.
20. Poole JCF, Summers GAC. Correction of ESR in anaemia. Br Med J. 1952;1:353–6. https://doi.org/10.1136/bmj.1.4753.353.
21. Buckenmayer A, Dahmen L, Hoyer J, Kamalanabhaiah S, Haas CS. Erythrocyte sedimentation rate in patients with renal insufficiency and renal replacement therapy. Lab Med. 2022;53:483–7. https://doi.org/10.1093/labmed/lmac018.
22. Pepys MB, Hirschfield GM. C-reactive protein: a critical update. J Clin Invest. 2003;111:1805–12. https://doi.org/10.1172/JCI18921.
23. Sproston NR, Ashworth JJ. Role of C-reactive protein at sites of inflammation and infection. Front Immunol. 2018;9:754. https://doi.org/10.3389/fimmu.2018.00754.
24. Mallya RK, Hind CR, Berry H, Pepys MB. Serum C-reactive protein in polymyalgia rheumatica. A prospective serial study. Arthritis Rheum. 1985;28:383–7. https://doi.org/10.1002/art.1780280405.
25. Pope JE, Choy EH. C-reactive protein and implications in rheumatoid arthritis and associated comorbidities. Semin Arthritis Rheum. 2021;51:219–29. https://doi.org/10.1016/j.semarthrit.2020.11.005.
26. Nakayama Y, Hashimoto M, Watanabe R, Murakami K, Murata K, Tanaka M, et al. Favorable clinical response and drug retention of anti-IL-6 receptor inhibitor in rheumatoid arthritis with high CRP levels: the ANSWER cohort study. Scand J Rheumatol. 2022;51:431–40. https://doi.org/10.1080/03009742.2021.1947005.
27. Cansu DU, Teke HU, Cancu G, Korkmaz C. Evaluation of hyperferritinemia causes in rheumatology practice: a retrospective, single-center experience. Rheumatol Int. 2021;41:1617–24. https://doi.org/10.1007/s00296-021-04935-y.
28. Rooney T, Scherzer R, Shigenaga JK, Graf J, Imboden JB, Grunfeld C. Levels of plasma fibrinogen are elevated in well-controlled rheumatoid arthritis. Rheumatology (Oxford). 2011;50:1458–65. https://doi.org/10.1093/rheumatology/ker011.
29. Vaitinadin NS, Stein C, Mosley JD, Kawai VK. Genetic susceptibility for autoimmune diseases and white blood cell count. Sci Rep. 2023;13:5852. https://doi.org/10.1038/s41598-023-32799-8.
30. Targońka-Stępniak B, Majdan M. Serum amyloid A as a marker of persistent inflammation and an indicator of cardiovascular and renal involvement in patients with rheumatoid arthritis. Mediat Inflamm. 2014;2014:793628. https://doi.org/10.1155/2014/793628.
31. Guerber A, Garneret E, El Jammal T, Zaepfel S, Gerfaud-Valentin M, Sève P, et al. Evaluation of glycosylated ferritin in Adult-onset Still's disease and differential diagnoses. J Clin Med. 2022;11:5012. https://doi.org/10.3390/jcm11175012.
32. Çakan M, Ayaz NA, Keskindermirci G, Karadag SG, Tanatar A, Sönmez HE. Serum amyloid A as a biomarker in differentiating attacks of familial Mediterranean fever from acute febrile infections. Clin Rheumatol. 2020;39(1):249–53.
33. Tanaka Y. Complement as a biomarker for systemic lupus erythematosus. Biomolecules. 2023;13:367. https://doi.org/10.3390/biom13020367.
34. Feldmann D, Jandova I, Heilmeier U, Kollert F, Voll RE, Finzel S. Inflammatory arthritis in systemic sclerosis is associated with elevated C-reactive protein and requires musculoskeletal ultrasound for reliable detection. Front Med (Lausanne). 2023;9:933809. https://doi.org/10.3389/fmed.2022.933809.

3 Pitfalls of Interpreting Rheumatoid Factor in Rheumatic Diseases

Abbreviations

ACPA	Anti-citrullinated protein antibodies
ACR	American College of Rheumatology
anti-CCP	Anti-cyclic citrullinated peptide
Fc	Fragment crystallisable
HCV	Hepatitis C virus
Ig	Immunoglobulin
MCTD	Mixed connective tissue disease
OA	Osteoarthritis
RA	Rheumatoid arthritis
RF	Rheumatoid factor
RMDs	Rheumatic diseases
SLE	Systemic lupus erythematosus
SS	Sjögren's syndrome
SScl	Systemic sclerosis
TB	Tuberculosis

3.1 Understanding Rheumatoid Factor

RF refers to autoantibodies, most commonly of the IgM class, that target the Fc region of IgG antibodies (Fig. 3.1) [1]. While RF is most often associated with RA, its presence is not exclusive to this condition. It can be detected in a variety of other diseases, including other autoimmune diseases, chronic infections and even in a proportion of the healthy population, particularly in the elderly. RF's initial use in medicine dates back to the 1940s when it was recognised as a marker

E. Pelechas et al., *Pitfalls in Rheumatology*,
https://doi.org/10.1007/978-3-031-98671-0_3

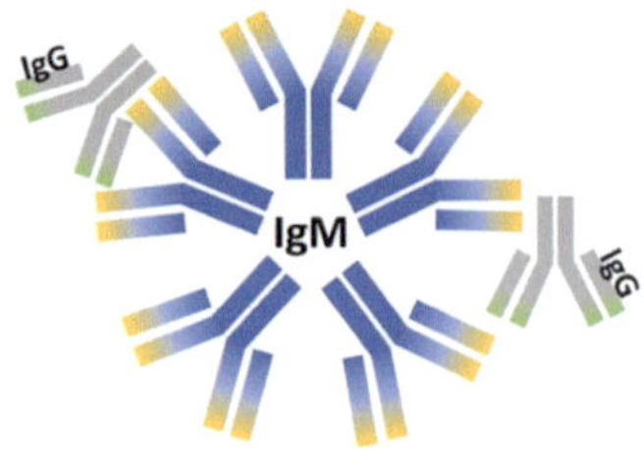

Fig. 3.1 Schematic representation of the Rheumatoid Factor

for RA. However, while the detection of RF is part of the diagnostic criteria for RA, it is not disease-specific, and its presence alone is insufficient to make a definitive diagnosis. This non-specific nature is the root of several pitfalls in interpretation.

3.2 False Positives

One of the most significant challenges with RF testing is its propensity for false positives. While elevated RF levels are present in approximately 70–80% of patients with RA, they can also be found in individuals without RA, leading to potential diagnostic errors [2, 3]. In Table 3.1 are summarised all possible reasons of a positive RF with the known mechanisms so far.

Other Autoimmune Diseases RF can be elevated in various autoimmune diseases beyond RA, including SLE [4], SS [5], MCTD [6], cryoglobulinaemia [7] and SScl [8]. In SS, RF positivity can be as high as 70%, mirroring the rates seen in RA. The overlap of RF positivity in these conditions can create confusion, particularly when patients present with non-specific symptoms.

Chronic Infections Chronic infections, such as HCV [9], TB [10] and endocarditis [11], are notorious for causing false-positive RF results. In these cases, the presence of RF is due to immune activation, rather than the underlying autoimmune disease. Clinicians may be misled by RF positivity in patients with chronic infections, especially if other rheumatic symptoms, such as joint pain or fatigue, are present.

The Elderly Population Aging itself can be associated with low-level RF positivity. Up to 10% of elderly individuals may have detectable, low RF levels without any evidence of underlying autoimmune or inflammatory disease. This finding complicates the use of RF as a diagnostic tool in older adults, where it may simply reflect an age-related phaenomenon rather than pathology [12].

Table 3.1 Conditions that the rheumatoid factor may be positive

Category	Condition	Mechanism of RF positivity
Autoimmune diseases	Rheumatoid arthritis	Autoantibody production against the Fc portion of IgG
	Sjögren's syndrome	Chronic B-cell activation and hypergammaglobulinaemia
	Systemic lupus erythematosus	Autoimmune dysregulation and B-cell hyperactivity
	Systemic sclerosis	Immune activation in connective tissue
	Mixed connective tissue disease	Overlapping features of autoimmune conditions, leading to RF production
	Polymyositis dermatomyositis	Chronic immune system activation
	Cryoglobulinaemia	Immune complex formation and chronic inflammation
Infectious diseases	Hepatitis C	Chronic immune stimulation by viral infection
	Hepatitis B	Persistent immune activation due to viral antigens
	Tuberculosis	Immune complex formation and chronic granulomatous inflammation
	Syphilis	Chronic infection leading to polyclonal B-cell activation
	Infective endocarditis	Persistent antigenic stimulation from bacterial infections
	Malaria	Chronic immune stimulation by parasitic infection
	Leprosy	Chronic inflammation and immune complex formation
	Viral infections such as Epstein–Barr virus and HIV	Immune activation and polyclonal antibody production
Other diseases	Interstitial pulmonary fibrosis	Immune dysregulation and tissue damage
	Primary biliary cirrhosis	Autoimmune attack on biliary epithelial cells
	Sarcoidosis	Granulomatous inflammation triggering immune response
	Monoclonal gammopathy	Aberrant monoclonal antibody production
	Multiple myeloma	Production of abnormal immunoglobulins
	Waldenströms macroglobulinaemia	Overproduction of monoclonal IgM antibodies
Healthy individuals	Mostly elderly	Age-related immune system changes and mild polyclonal B-cell activation

3.3 False Negatives

While much attention is given to the potential for false positives, false negatives also pose a challenge in clinical practice. Approximately 20–30% of patients with RA are seronegative, meaning that they do not have detectable RF [13]. This group can present with clinical symptoms typical of RA, including joint pain, swelling and stiffness but may be missed if RF testing is heavily relied upon.

Seronegative Rheumatoid Arthritis Seronegative RA, while less common, can be just as severe and progressive as seropositive RA [14]. Without RF positivity, clinicians must rely more heavily on clinical findings and imaging studies to make a diagnosis. Failure to recognise this variant can lead to delays in treatment, with potential harmful consequences for patients.

Early Disease In the early stages of RA, RF may not yet be detectable. It is estimated that RF levels can take months or even years to become elevated in some individuals. This delay in seroconversion means that patients with early disease may be misclassified as non-RA, particularly if RF testing is heavily emphasized in the diagnostic process.

3.4 Over-Reliance on RF in Diagnosis

The tendency to over-rely on RF as a diagnostic tool can lead to misdiagnosis, particularly in primary care settings where non-rheumatologists may have limited experience with RMDs. While RF is a helpful marker, it is only one piece of the diagnostic puzzle and should always be interpreted in the context of clinical findings and other laboratory results [15].

Clinical Context Is Key The diagnosis of RA and other RMDs requires a comprehensive evaluation that includes a thorough patient history, physical examination, imaging studies and additional laboratory tests, such as ACPA. RF positivity should never be used in isolation to make a diagnosis, as this can lead to overdiagnosis of RA in patients who may have other conditions.

Differentiating from Other Arthritides Patients with OA or crystal-induced arthropathies such as gout may present with joint pain and swelling, and if RF is detected, there is potential for misclassification as RA. These diseases, while also affecting the joints, have different pathophysiological mechanisms and require different treatment strategies. Thus, clinicians must carefully consider the entire clinical picture before making a diagnosis based on RF positivity alone [16].

3.5 Misinterpretation of RF Levels

Interpreting RF is not just about whether the test is positive or negative. The titre, or level, of RF in the bloodstream can also be misleading if not interpreted correctly.

High RF Titres Do Not Always Indicate Severe Disease Although higher RF titres are generally associated with more aggressive disease and worse prognosis in RA [17], this is not a hard-and-fast rule. Some patients with low RF titres can have severe, erosive disease, while others with very high titres may have mild or moderate disease activity. Thus, RF titre should not be used as the sole marker for disease severity. On the other hand, immunological phenomena are considered minor criteria in the modified Duke criteria for endocarditis due to positive IgM RF. Therefore, among patients with the clinical suspicion of endocarditis, the recommended systematic evaluation for immunological phenomena should include RF testing [18].

Variability in Testing Methods There is variability in the sensitivity and specificity of different RF assays, leading to differences in test results between laboratories [19]. Clinicians should be aware of the testing methods used and interpret results accordingly, as well as considering retesting in cases where the clinical suspicion remains high, but the initial RF result is negative.

3.6 Evolution of Diagnostic Criteria

RF was a cornerstone of the 1987 ACR criteria for RA [20], but newer criteria developed in 2010 [21] emphasize the combination of clinical features, joint involvement and additional markers, such as ACPA, for diagnosis. While RF remains important, the updated criteria reflect the recognition that it is not as specific or sensitive as previously thought. Clinicians must stay current with evolving diagnostic standards and avoid using outdated paradigms that overemphasize RF.

3.7 Role of Anti-CCP and Other Biomarkers

The development of anti-CCP antibodies as a more specific marker for RA has reduced the reliance on RF [22]. Anti-CCP has higher specificity for RA and is rarely positive in other conditions [23]. In many cases, the combination of anti-CCP and RF provides the best diagnostic accuracy, particularly in distinguishing RA from other arthritides [24].

3.8 Conclusion

Interpreting RF in RMDs requires a nuanced approach that integrates clinical findings, other laboratory markers and imaging studies. Over-reliance on RF can lead to both overdiagnosis and underdiagnosis, while the pitfalls of false positives and negatives add to the complexity. Clinicians must recognise the limitations of RF and use it as one tool in a broader diagnostic framework. In addition, evolving criteria and the incorporation of more specific markers like anti-CCP provide opportunities to improve diagnostic accuracy and patient care. In the end, the careful and contextual use of RF in clinical practice remains a valuable, though imperfect, element in the rheumatologist's armamentarium.

References

1. Pelechas E, Kaltsonoudis E, Voulgari PV, Drosos AA. Autoimmune rheumatic diseases: pathophysiology and laboratory tests. In: Illustrated handbook of rheumatic and musculo-skeletal diseases. Cham: Springer; 2023. https://doi.org/10.1007/978-3-031-47379-1_2.
2. Wilson D. Rheumatoid factors in patients with rheumatoid arthritis. Can Fam Physician. 2006;52:180–1.
3. Kumar A, Vasdev V, Patnaik SK, Bhatt S, Singh R, Bhayana A, et al. The diagnostic utility of rheumatoid factor and anticitrullinated protein antibody for rheumatoid arthritis in the Indian population. Med J Armed Forces India. 2020;78:S69–74. https://doi.org/10.1016/j.mjafi.2020.04.007.
4. Witte T, Hartung K, Sachse C, Matthias T, Fricke M, Kalden JR, et al. Rheumatoid factors in systemic lupus erythematosus: association with clinical and laboratory parameters. SLE study group. Rheumatol Int. 2000;19:107–11. https://doi.org/10.1007/s002960050112.
5. Fayyaz A, Kurien BT, Scofield RH. Autoantibodies in Sjögren's syndrome. Rheum Dis Clin N Am. 2016;42:419–34. https://doi.org/10.1016/j.rdc.2016.03.002.
6. Mimura Y, Ihn H, Jinnin M, Asano Y, Yamane K, Tamaki K. Rheumatoid factor isotypes in mixed connective tissue disease. Clin Rheumatol. 2006;25:572–4. https://doi.org/10.1007/s10067-005-0185-y.
7. Codes-Méndez H, Jeria S, Park HS, Moya P, Magallares-López B, Moltó E, et al. Clinical and serological profiles in cryoglobulinemia: analysis of isotypes and etiologies. J Clin Med. 2024;13:6069. https://doi.org/10.3390/jcm13206069.
8. Wielosz E, Majdan M, Dryglewska M, Zwolak R. Anti-CCP antibodies and rheumatoid factors in systemic sclerosis: prevalence and relationships with joint manifestations. Adv Clin Exp Med. 2018;27:1253–7. https://doi.org/10.17219/acem/69921.
9. Reyes-Avilés E, Kostadinova L, Rusterholtz A, Cruz-Lebrón A, Falck-Ytter Y, Anthony DD. Presence of Rheumatoid factor during chronic HCV infection is associate with expansion of mature activated memory B-cells that are hypo-responsive to b-cell receptor stimulation and persist during the early stage of IFN Free therapy. PLoS One. 2015;10:e0144629.
10. Starshinova A, Malkova A, Zinchencko Y, Kudryavtsev I, Serebriakova M, Akisheva T, et al. Identification of autoimmune markers in pulmonary tuberculosis. Front Immunol. 2023;13:1059714. https://doi.org/10.3389/fimmu.2022.1059714.
11. Peechakara B, Kadam A, Mewada M, Nakrani A. Infective endocarditis masquerading as rheumatoid arthritis. Cureus. 2019;11:e5626. https://doi.org/10.7759/cureus.5626.
12. Boots AMH, Maier AB, Stinissen P, Masson P, Lories RJ, De Keyser F. The influence of ageing on the development and management of rheumatoid arthritis. Nat Rev Rheumatol. 2013;9:604–13. https://doi.org/10.1038/nrrheum.2013.92.

13. Paroli M, Sirinian MI. When autoantibodies are missing: the challenge of seronegative rheumatoid arthritis. Antibodies (Basel). 2023;12:69. https://doi.org/10.3390/antib12040069.
14. Nordberg LB, Lillegraven S, Aga AB, Sexton J, Olsen IC, Lie E, et al. Comparing the disease course of patients with seronegative and seropositive rheumatoid arthritis fulfilling the 2010 ACR/EULAR classification criteria in a treat-to-target setting: 2-year data from the ARCTIC trial. RMD Open. 2018;4:e000752. https://doi.org/10.1136/rmdopen-2018-000752.
15. Handa R. Rheumatoid factor and rheumatoid arthritis. J Clin Orthop Trauma. 2019;10:629–30. https://doi.org/10.1016/j.jcot.2019.03.007.
16. Pelechas E, Kaltsonoudis E, Voulgari PV, Drosos AA. Rheumatoid arthritis. In: Illustrated handbook of rheumatic and musculo-skeletal diseases. Cham: Springer; 2023. https://doi.org/10.1007/978-3-031-47379-1_5.
17. Oliveira VDRS, Reis APMG, Brenol CV, Pereira IA, Bonfiglioli KR, Pereira LR, et al. High-titer rheumatoid factor is associated with worse clinical outcomes and higher needs for advanced therapies in rheumatoid arthritis under real-life conditions. Rheumatol Ther. 2024; https://doi.org/10.1007/s40744-024-00730-w.
18. Van der Vaart TW, Heerschop LL, Bouma BJ, Freudenburt W, Bonten MJM, Prins JM, et al. Value of diagnosing immunological phenomena in patients with suspected endocarditis. Infection. 2023;51:705–13. https://doi.org/10.1007/s15010-022-01954-0.
19. Falkenburg WJJ, von Richthofen HJ, Koers J, Weykamp C, Schreurs MWJ, Bakker-Jonges LE, et al. Clinically relevant discrepancies between different rheumatoid factor assays. Clin Chem Lab Med. 2018;56:1749–58. https://doi.org/10.1515/cclm-2017-0988.
20. Arnett FV, Edworthy SM, Bloch DA, McShane DJ, Fries JF, Cooper NS, et al. The American Rheumatism Association 1987 revised criteria for the classification of rheumatoid arthritis. Arthritis Rheum. 1988;31:315–24. https://doi.org/10.1012/art.1780310302.
21. Aletaha D, Neogi T, Silman AJ, Funovits J, Felson DT, Bingham CO, et al. 2010 Rheumatoid arthritis classification criteria: an American College of Rheumatology/Europena League Against Rheumatism collaborative initiative. Arthritis Rheum. 2010;62:2569–81. https://doi.org/10.1002/art.27584.
22. Braschi E, Shojania K, Allan GM. Anti-CCP: a truly helpful rheumatoid arthritis test? Can Fam Physician. 2016;62:234.
23. Vannini A, Cheung K, Fusconi M, Stammen-Vogelzangs J, Drenth JPH, Dall-Aglio AC, et al. Anti-cyclic citrullinated peptide positivity in non-rheumatoid arthritis disease samples: citrulline-dependent or not? Ann Rheum Dis. 2006;66:511–6. https://doi.org/10.1136/ard.2006.058933.
24. Lee AN, Beck CE, Hall M. Rheumatoid factor and anti-CCP autoantibodies in rheumatoid arthritis: a review. Clin Lab Sci. 2008;21:15–8.

Pitfalls of Interpreting Antinuclear Antibodies in Rheumatic Diseases

4

Abbreviations

ACA	Anti-centromere antibodies
ACPA	Anti-citrullinated peptide antibody
AIH	Autoimmune hepatitis
ANA	Antinuclear antibodies
AS	Ankylosing spondylitis
CTD	Connective tissue disease
DM	Dermatomyositis
DNA	Deoxyribonucleic acid
ELISA	Enzyme-linked immunosorbent assays
MCTD	Mixed connective tissue disease
PM	Polymyositis
RA	Rheumatoid arthritis
RMDs	Rheumatic diseases
RNA	Ribonucleic acid
SLE	Systemic lupus erythematosus
SS	Sjögren's syndrome
SScl	Systemic sclerosis
TNFi	Tumour necrosis factor alpha inhibitors

4.1 Understanding Antinuclear Antibodies

ANAs are autoantibodies directed against nuclear antigens, including DNA, RNA, histones and other nuclear proteins [1]. They are detected through immunofluorescence or ELISA and can present a range of staining patterns that may suggest different autoimmune conditions. While ANAs are most commonly associated with

E. Pelechas et al., *Pitfalls in Rheumatology*,
https://doi.org/10.1007/978-3-031-98671-0_4

SLE, they are also found in other autoimmune diseases such as SS, SScl, MCTD and AIH. However, their presence is not always indicative of disease, and they can be found in healthy individuals, particularly the elderly. This duality is at the core of interpretive challenges [2]. In Table 4.1 are summarised all possible reasons of a positive ANA test with the known mechanisms so far.

Table 4.1 Conditions that antinuclear antibodies may be positive

Category	Condition	Mechanism of ANA positivity
Autoimmune diseases	Systemic lupus erythematosus	Autoimmune dysregulation leading to production of autoantibodies against nuclear antigens
	Sjögren's syndrome	Chronic B-cell activation and autoantibody production targeting nuclear components
	Systemic sclerosis	Immune activation against nuclear and cytoplasmic antigens
	Mixed connective tissue disease	Overlapping features of autoimmune diseases with autoantibody production against U1-RNP and other nuclear components
	Rheumatoid arthritis	Secondary autoimmune phenomena involving nuclear antigens
	Polymyositis dermatomyositis	Autoimmune targeting of nuclear and cytoplasmic components
	Autoimmune hepatitis	Immune dysregulation and attack on hepatocytes with nuclear involvement
	Hashimoto's thyroiditis—Grave's disease	Cross-reactivity of immune response involving nuclear antigens
	Primary biliary cirrhosis	Autoantibodies targeting mitochondrial and nuclear antigens
Infectious diseases	Hepatitis C	Chronic immune stimulation and cross-reactivity with nuclear antigens
	Hepatitis B	Persistent immune activation affecting nuclear structures
	Epstein–Barr virus	Immune dysregulation and cross-reactivity with nuclear components
	HIV	Chronic immune activation leading to polyclonal antibody production
Other diseases	Malignancies (lymphoma, leukaemia)	Dysregulated immune response and autoantibody production
	Interstitial pulmonary fibrosis	Immune dysregulation with nuclear component involvement
	Idiopathic thrombocytopaenic purpura	Autoimmune activity involving nuclear antigens
	Inflammatory bowel disease	Secondary autoimmune phaenomena involving nuclear structures
Drug-induced	Drug-induced lupus	Certain medications (hydralazine, procainamide and others) induce immune response targeting nuclear antigens
Healthy individuals	Mostly elderly	Age-related immune system changes and mild autoimmune activity

4.2 Ubiquity of Positive Antinuclear Antibodies

One of the most significant challenges in interpreting ANA results is their high prevalence in the general population. Estimates suggest that around 20–30% of healthy individuals have detectable ANAs, particularly at low titres. This can lead to diagnostic confusion and the risk of overdiagnosing autoimmune diseases in patients who may simply have incidental ANA positivity [3].

Low Titres in Healthy Individuals Low titres of ANA (typically 1:80) are often clinically insignificant, particularly in the absence of symptoms. ANA positivity at these low levels can be a normal finding, especially in elderly individuals, where the prevalence of positive ANA results increases with age [4]. In these cases, ANA positivity can result in unnecessary further testing, patient anxiety and even inappropriate treatment if not carefully interpreted in the clinical context.

Drug-Induced ANAs Certain medications, such as hydralazine, procainamide and isoniazid, and also medications that are used for the treatment of autoimmune diseases such as TNFi, can induce ANA production without causing a significant autoimmune disease. This drug-induced ANA phenomenon can be misinterpreted as evidence of systemic autoimmune disease, leading to confusion, especially if clinicians are unaware of the patient's medication history [5].

4.3 Over-Reliance on Antinuclear Antibody Positivity for Diagnosis

ANA positivity is a useful clue in the diagnosis of autoimmune diseases, but relying too heavily on it as a diagnostic tool can lead to both over- and underdiagnosis. Many clinicians outside of rheumatology may overestimate the significance of ANA results, especially when they are unaware of the various diseases associated with ANAs or the context in which these antibodies should be interpreted [6].

Not Specific for Any One Disease While ANAs are a hallmark of SLE, they are not specific to this disease. ANA positivity can occur in a variety of conditions, including SScl, SS and even non-RMDs like autoimmune thyroiditis or chronic infections [7]. The presence of ANAs alone cannot confirm a specific diagnosis without a thorough evaluation of the patient's clinical history, clinical presentation and other laboratory findings [8].

False Security in a Negative ANA Conversely, a negative ANA test does not rule out autoimmune disease. In some patients with SLE, particularly those with predominantly cutaneous manifestations or other specific subtypes, ANA testing may be negative [9]. Additionally, certain autoimmune conditions such as PM, DM and AS may occur without ANA positivity. Clinicians who rely too heavily on ANA results may delay or miss important diagnoses.

4.4 Misinterpretation of Antinuclear Antibody Patterns

ANA testing often includes an assessment of the staining pattern observed in immunofluorescence, which can offer clues about the type of autoimmune disease present. However, interpreting these patterns is complex, and mistakes can easily be made if the clinical context is not considered.

Non-specific Patterns Common ANA staining patterns, such as speckled or homogeneous, are found in many diseases and are not specific to any one condition. For example, a homogeneous pattern is often associated with SLE but can also occur in other CTDs or even in healthy individuals. Similarly, a speckled pattern can be seen in SLE, SS or MCTD, making it difficult to draw definitive conclusions without further testing [10].

Rare Patterns May Be Missed Some ANA patterns, such as the nucleolar or centromere patterns, are more specific to particular diseases like SScl or limited scleroderma [11]. However, these patterns may be overlooked or misinterpreted by laboratories not specialised in autoimmune testing or if they use non-standard protocols and techniques for autoantibody detection, leading to a missed diagnosis or a delay in recognising the specific disease.

4.5 Antinuclear Antibody Titre Interpretation

The titre of ANA, which reflects the concentration of antibodies in the serum, can also present challenges in interpretation.

High Titres Are Not Always Indicative of Disease Although higher titres of ANA (>1:320) are more likely to be associated with autoimmune diseases, they are not an absolute indicator. Some healthy individuals, especially the elderly, can have high ANA titres without any clinical evidence of disease [12]. Conversely, patients with autoimmune disease may have low ANA titres, making it difficult to use titre alone to distinguish between disease and health.

Inconsistent Titre Correlation with Disease Activity In many autoimmune diseases, ANA titres do not correlate well with the disease activity [13]. For example, in SLE, patients may have persistently high ANA titres even during periods of remission. This can lead to confusion if clinicians assume that changes in ANA titres reflect changes in disease activity. Instead, other markers of disease activity, such as complement levels (C3, C4), anti-dsDNA [14], as well as other laboratory markers, e.g. white blood cell count, platelet count, proteinuria or urinary sediment and various clinical symptoms, should be used to assess disease progression or the response to treatment.

4.6 Evolution of Diagnostic Criteria and Tests

As new diagnostic tools and criteria for autoimmune diseases evolve, the role of ANA testing has changed. Many newer classification criteria for diseases like SLE or SScl incorporate additional antibodies or clinical criteria that go beyond ANA testing [15].

Importance of Specific Autoantibodies In addition to ANAs, more specific autoantibodies, such as anti-dsDNA, anti-Sm [16], anti-Ro/SSA and anti-La/SSB and others, are often more diagnostic, and in some instances almost pathognomonic for certain diseases. For example, anti-dsDNA and anti-Sm antibodies are highly specific for SLE, and their presence can confirm the diagnosis in a patient with clinical symptoms. In SScl, the presence of ACA or anti-Scl-70 (topoisomerase) antibodies [17] is more diagnostic than ANA alone. Table 4.2 shows a summary of ANA-positive diseases that may present with specific autoantibodies. The ANA pattern is also included.

Table 4.2 Autoimmune diseases with positive antinuclear antibodies and their specific autoantibodies

Disease	ANA pattern	Specific autoantibodies	Complement levels
Systemic lupus erythematosus	Homogeneous, peripheral, speckled	Anti-dsDNA, Anti-Sm, Anti-RNP	Decreased C3 and/or C4 during active disease
Sjögren's syndrome	Speckled	Anti-Ro/SSA, Anti-La/SSB	Normal or slightly decreased
Systemic sclerosis	Centromere, nucleolar, speckled	Anti-Scl-70, Anti-centromere, Anti-RNA Polymerase III	Normal or slightly decreased
Mixed connective tissue disease	Speckled	Anti-U1-RNP	Normal or decreased
Polymyositis—Dermatomyositis	Speckled	Anti-Jo-1	Normal
Autoimmune hepatitis	Homogeneous	Anti-SMA, Anti-LKM1	Normal or slightly decreased
Primary biliary cirrhosis	Speckled, homogeneous	Anti-AMA	Normal
Hashimoto's thyroiditis	Speckled	Anti-TPO, Anti-Tg	Normal
Grave's disease	Speckled	TRAb	Normal
Drug-induced lupus	Homogeneous, speckled	Anti-histone	Normal or slightly decreased
Antiphospholipid syndrome	Speckled	Anti-cardiolipin, Anti-β2-GPI, lupus anticoagulant	Normal

Incorporating Newer Biomarkers As research continues to identify new biomarkers in autoimmune diseases, the over-reliance on ANA testing may diminish. Biomarkers such as ACPA in RA and interferon signatures in SLE are increasingly being integrated into diagnostic and prognostic models [18]. Clinicians must stay up to date with these advances to avoid placing too much weight on ANA results.

4.7 Conclusion

Interpreting ANA results in RMDs is a nuanced process that requires careful consideration of the clinical context, the patient's history and other laboratory findings. While ANA positivity is an important clue in diagnosing autoimmune diseases, it is neither specific nor exclusive to these conditions. Misinterpretation of ANA titres, patterns and their clinical significance can lead to both over- and underdiagnosis, with potentially harmful consequences for patient care. In the evolving landscape of autoimmune diagnostics, ANA testing should be used as part of a broader diagnostic approach. The integration of more specific autoantibodies, disease-specific biomarkers and clinical criteria is essential for accurate diagnosis and management. Clinicians must remain vigilant to the pitfalls associated with ANA testing, recognising its limitations and ensuring that patients receive appropriate and timely care based on a comprehensive evaluation.

References

1. Pelechas E, Kaltsonoudis E, Voulgari PV, Drosos AA. Autoimmune rheumatic diseases: pathophysiology and laboratory tests. In: Illustrated handbook of rheumatic and musculo-skeletal diseases. Cham: Springer; 2023. https://doi.org/10.1007/978-3-031-47379-1_2.
2. Kraev K, Hristov B, Uchikov P, Kraeva M, Basheva-Kraeva Y, Valova S, Koleva-Ivanova M, et al. Comprehensive exploration of antinuclear antibodies (ANA): unveiling clinical significance, associations with cancer, and the nuances of differential diagnosis in positive ANA patients. Diagnostics (Basel). 2024;14:320. https://doi.org/10.3390/diagnostics14030320.
3. Grygiel-Górniak B, Rogacka N, Puszczewicz M. Antinuclear antibodies in healthy people and non-rheumatic diseases—diagnostic and clinical implications. Reumatologia. 2018;56:243–8. https://doi.org/10.5114/reum.2018.77976.
4. Dinse GE, Parks CG, Weinberg CR, Co CA, Wilkerson J, Zeldin DC, et al. Increasing prevalence of antinuclear antibodies in the United States. Arthritis Rheumatol. 2020;72:1026–35. https://doi.org/10.1002/art.41214.
5. Alarcón-Segovia D. Drug-induced antinuclear antibodies and lupus syndromes. Drugs. 1976;12:69–77. https://doi.org/10.2165/00003495-197612010-00003.
6. Kumar Y, Bhatia A, Minz RW. Antinuclear antibodies and their detection methods in diagnosis of connective tissue diseases: a journey revisited. Diagn Pathol. 2009;4:1. https://doi.org/10.1186/1746-1596-4-1.
7. Zanussi JT, Zhao J, Weil WQ, Karakos G, Chung CP, Feng Q, et al. Clinical diagnoses associated with a positive antinuclear antibody test in patients with and without autoimmune disease. BMC Rheumatol. 2023;7:24. https://doi.org/10.1186/s41927-023-00349-4.
8. Vlachoyiannopoulos PG, Tzavara V, Dafni U, Spanos E, Moutsopoulos HM. Clinical features and evolution of antinuclear antibody positive individuals in a rheumatology outpatient clinic. J Rheumatol. 1998;25:886–91.

9. Tarazi M, Gaffney RG, Kushner CJ, Chakka S, Werth VP. Cutaneous lupus erythematosus patients with a negative antinuclear antibody meeting the American College of Rheumatology and/or systemic lupus international collaborating clinics criteria fos systemic lupus erythematosus. Arthritis Care Res (Hoboken). 2019;71:1404–9. https://doi.org/10.1002/acr.23916.
10. Damoiseaux J, con Mühlen CA, Garcia-De La Torre I, Carballo OG, Cruvinel WM, Francescantonio PLC, Fritzler MJ, et al. International consensus on ANA patterns (ICAP): the bumpy road towars a consensus on reportin ANA results. Auto Immun Highlights. 2016;7:1. https://doi.org/10.1007/s13317-016-0075-0.
11. Ho KT, Reveille JD. The clinical relevance of autoantibodies in scleroderma. Arthritis Res Ther. 2003;5:80–93. https://doi.org/10.1186/ar628.
12. Xavier RM, Yamauchi Y, Nakamura M, Tanigawa Y, Ishikura H, Tsunematsu T, et al. Antinuclear antibodies in healthy aging people: a prospective study. Mech Ageing Dev. 1995;78:145–54. https://doi.org/10.1016/0047-6374(94)01532-q.
13. Ostrov BE. Reliability and reproducibility of antinuclear antibody testing in pediatric rheumatology practice. Front Med (Lausanne). 2023;9:1071115. https://doi.org/10.3389/fmed.2022.1071115.
14. Giles BM, Boackle SA. Linding complement and anti-dsDNA antibodies in the pathogenesis of systemic lupus erythematosus. Immunol Res. 2013;55:10–21. https://doi.org/10.1007/s12026-012-8345-z.
15. Aringer M, Costenbader KH, Daikh DI, Brinks R, Mosca M, Ramsey-Goldman R, et al. 2019 EULAR/ACR classification criteria for systemic lupus erythematosus. Arthritis Rheumatol. 2019;71:1400–12. https://doi.org/10.1002/art.40930.
16. Van Beers JJBC, Schreurs MWJ. Anti-Sm antibodies in the classification criteria of systemic lupus erythematosus. J Transl Autoimmun. 2022;5:100155. https://doi.org/10.1016/j.jtauto.2022.100155.
17. Basu D, Reveille JD. Anti-Scl-70. Autoimmunity. 2005;38:65–72. https://doi.org/10.1080/08916930400022947.
18. Fenton KA, Pedersen. Advanced methods and novel biomarkers in autoimmune diseases—a review of the recent years progress in systemic lupus erythematosus. Front Med (Lausanne). 2023;10:1183535. https://doi.org/10.3389/fmed.2023.1183535.

5 Pitfalls in Interpreting Antiphospholipid Antibodies in Rheumatic Diseases

Abbreviations

aCL	Anticardiolipin antibodies
ANA	Antinuclear antibodies
anti-dsDNA	Anti-double-stranded DNA
anti-β2-GPI	Anti-beta-2 glycoprotein I antibodies
aPL	Antiphospholipid antibodies
APS	Antiphospholipid syndrome
aPTT	Activated partial thromboplastin time
dRVVT	Dilute Russell viper venom time
LA	Lupus anticoagulant
SLE	Systemic lupus erythematosus
SS	Sjögren's syndrome

Recognising that each type of aPL has different implications for diagnosis and management is critical. Misidentifying the type of antibody can lead to misdiagnosis of APS or inadequate patient management. aPLs include several specific types [1]:

LA: a type of aPL that interferes with the phospholipid-dependent clotting tests
aCL: antibodies directed against cardiolipin, a phospholipid component
Anti-β2-GPI: antibodies directed against the beta-2 glycoprotein I, a cofactor for aCL antibodies [2]

E. Pelechas et al., *Pitfalls in Rheumatology*,
https://doi.org/10.1007/978-3-031-98671-0_5

5.1 Timing of Testing and Clinical Context

aPLs may fluctuate over time and can be transient, particularly in patients with infections, certain drugs or other acute illnesses [3].

How to Avoid This Pitfall (a) *Test in a stable clinical context*: it is recommended to test for aPL when patients are stable and not experiencing acute illnesses, as transient aPL can occur in these settings; (b) *repeat testing*: if aPLs are detected during an acute phase, consider repeating the tests after a resolution of the acute condition to confirm persistent positivity [4]. In cases where anticoagulant therapy is being administered, a temporary discontinuation is recommended, followed by testing for LA. The three-step procedure using two testing systems dRVVT and aPTT has essentially remained unchanged [5].

5.2 Distinguishing Between Persistent and Transient Antibodies

The criteria for APS require the presence of aPL on two or more occasions at least 12 weeks apart at a medium/high titre (99th percentile) [6].

How to Avoid This Pitfall (a) *Assess persistence*: clinicians should document the timing of antibody testing to ensure that the antibodies are persistent. A single positive result without follow-up and in the absence of a clinical event is insufficient for diagnosis; (b) *educate on the criteria*: both clinicians and patients must understand the need for repeated testing to confirm the diagnosis, which can help prevent unnecessary anxiety or mismanagement based on isolated test results [7].

5.3 Interference from Other Conditions

Various conditions can lead to the production of antiphospholipid antibodies, including infections [8], malignancies [9] and other autoimmune diseases such as SLE [10] and SS. In Table 5.1, a list with all known possible conditions that may induce positive antiphospholipid antibodies with a proposed mechanism is presented.

How to Avoid This Pitfall (a) *Consider the clinical context*: when interpreting aPL, always take into account the patient's clinical picture. Elevated aPL levels in the absence of APS symptoms or history may be attributable to other conditions; (b) *use a comprehensive approach*: clinicians should integrate clinical, serological and historical data when evaluating aPL, rather than relying solely on serology [11].

Table 5.1 Conditions that may cause positive antiphospholipid antibodies

Category	Condition	Mechanism
Autoimmune diseases	Antiphospholipid syndrome	Primary or secondary autoimmune production of aPL
	Systemic lupus erythematosus	Immune dysregulation leading to production of autoantibodies
	Rheumatoid arthritis	Secondary immune activation
	Sjögren's syndrome	Chronic autoimmune activity
Infectious diseases	Syphilis	Cross-reactivity due to infection-induced immune activation
	Hepatitis C, Hepatitis B, HIV	Immune stimulation by chronic virus infection
	SARS-CoV-2	Due to molecular mimicry, the S1 and S2 glycoprotein subunits of the SARS-CoV-2 viral S protein form a phospholipid-like epitope that induces the formation of aPL
	Tuberculosis	Granulomatous inflammation inducing antibody production
	Epstein–Barr virus	Viral-driven immune activation
Malignancies	Lymphoma, Leukaemia	Dysregulated immune system in malignancies
	Solid tumours (lung, ovarian)	Paraneoplastic antibody production
Medications	Hydralazine, Procainamide, Phenothiazines, haloperidol, clozapine and others	Various mechanisms such as drug-induced immune activation, production of autoantibodies as an adverse reaction or immunostimulatory reasons
Other chronic conditions	Chronic liver disease	Immune dysregulation in chronic inflammation
	Chronic kidney disease	Uraemia-associated immune activation
Transient positivity	Post-infection, post-vaccination	Temporary immune response or immune-stimulation from vaccine antigens
	Pregnancy	Hormonal and immune changes
Healthy individuals	No underlying disease	Subclinical immune activity or laboratory mistake

5.4 Understanding Assay Limitations

The assays used to detect aPL can vary in sensitivity and specificity, and the presence of false positives or false negatives is a significant concern, particularly with aCL [12].

How to Avoid This Pitfall (a) *Use standardised tests*: employ laboratory tests that follow established guidelines and standards. The use of different assays can lead to discrepancies in results [12]; (b) *interpret results cautiously*: understand the limitations of the specific assays used. False positives can occur in conditions like infections, malignancies and even during pregnancy [13].

5.5 Role of Confounding Factors

Certain medications, particularly anticoagulants, can affect the interpretation for laboratory results [14].

How to Avoid This Pitfall (a) *Consider medication effects*: for example, patients on anticoagulants may have altered results in LA testing. Adjusting for medication effects is crucial for accurate interpretation; (b) *communicate with laboratories*: engage with laboratory staff to clarify how medications may influence specific assays and inform them in case the patient's sample contains any of them.

5.6 Misinterpretation of Clinical Symptoms

Not all patients with positive aPL will develop APS or experience thrombosis. Misinterpretation of clinical symptoms can lead to overtreatment or unnecessary anxiety [11].

How to Avoid This Pitfall (a) *Evaluate clinical significance*: a positive aPL result does not equate to the presence of APS. It is essential to assess the full clinical pic ture, including history and symptoms; (b) *educate patients*: provide clear information to patients about the meaning of positive aPL results, ensuring they understand that not all positive indicate a diagnosis of APS or necessitate aggressive treatment.

5.7 Lack of Awareness of Other Antibodies

Some patients with APS may have coexisting autoimmune conditions and additional antibodies, such as ANA or anti-dsDNA antibodies, which may complicate interpretation [15].

How to Avoid This Pitfall (a) *Perform a comprehensive autoantibody profile*: testing for other autoantibodies can provide a more complete picture of the patient's autoimmune status and help clarify the diagnosis; (b) *recognise overlapping conditions*: be aware that conditions such as SLE [15] can coexist with APS, and managing these overlapping conditions requires a nuanced approach.

5.8 Conclusion

The interpretation of aPLs is full of potential pitfalls that can significantly impact diagnosis and management. Awareness of the limitations of assays, the clinical context of testing and the need for persistent positivity is essential to avoid misdiagnosis and unnecessary interventions. By understanding these pitfalls, clinicians can provide better care for patients at risk for or suffering from APS, ultimately improving patient outcomes.

References

1. Pelechas E, Kaltsonoudis E, Voulgari PV, Drosos AA. Autoimmune rheumatic diseases: pathophysiology and laboratory tests. In: Illustrated handbook of rheumatic and musculo-skeletal diseases. Cham: Springer; 2023. https://doi.org/10.1007/978-3-031-47379-1_2.
2. Petri M. Antiphospholipid syndrome. Transl Res. 2020;225:70–81. https://doi.org/10.1016/j.trsl.2020.04.006.
3. Nakayama T, Akahoshi M, Irino K, Kimoto Y, Arinobu Y, Niiro H, et al. Transient antiphospholipid syndrome associated with primary cytomegalovirus infection: a case report and literature review. Case Rep Rheumatol. 2014;2014:271548. https://doi.org/10.1155/2014/271548.
4. Vandevelde A, Devreese KMJ. Laboratory diagnosis of antiphospholipid syndrome: insights and hindrances. J Clin Med. 2022;11:2164. https://doi.org/10.3390/jcm11082164.
5. Devreese KMJ, de Groot PG, de Laat B, Erkan D, Favaloro EJ, Mackie I, et al. Guidance from the scientific and standardization committee for lupus anticoagulant/antiphospholipid antibodies of the international society on thrombosis and haemostasis: update of the guidelines for lupus anticoagulant detection and interpretation. J Thromb Haemost. 2020;18:2828–39. https://doi.org/10.1111/jth.15047.
6. Barbhaiya M, Zuily S, Naden R, Hendry A, Manneville F, Amigo MC, et al. The 2023 ACR/EULAR antiphospholipid syndrome classification criteria. Arthritis Rheumatol. 2023;75:1687–702. https://doi.org/10.1002/art.42624.
7. Qrtel TL. Antiphospholipid syndrome laboratory testing and diagnostic strategies. Am J Hematol. 2012;87:S75–81. https://doi.org/10.1002/ajh.23196.
8. Shoenfeld Y, Blank M, Cervera R, Font J, Raschi E, Meroni PL. Infectious origin of the antiphospholipid syndrome. Ann Rheum Dis. 2006;65:2–6. https://doi.org/10.1136/ard.2005.045443.
9. Gómez-Puerta J, Cervera R, Espinosa G, Aguiló S, Bucciarelli S, Ramos-Casals M, et al. Antiphospholipid antibodies associated with malignancies: clinical and pathological and pathological characteristics of 120 patients. Semin Arthritis Rheum. 2006;35:322–32. https://doi.org/10.1016/j.semarthrit.2005.07.003.
10. Kokosi M, Lams B, Agarwal S. Systemic lupus erythematosus and antiphospholipid antibody syndrome. Clin Chest Med. 2019;40:519–29. https://doi.org/10.1016/j.ccm.2019.06.001.
11. Grygiel-Górniak B, Mazurkiewicz Ł. Positive antiphospholipid antibodies: observation or treatment? J Thromb Thrombolysis. 2023;56:301–14. https://doi.org/10.1007/s11239-023-02834-6.
12. Meroni PL, Borghi MO. Antiphospholipid antibody assays in 2021: looking for a predictive value in addition to a diagnostic one. Front Immunol. 2021;12:726820. https://doi.org/10.3389/fimmu.2021.726820.
13. Mallhi RS, Kushwaha N, Chatterjee T, Philip J. Antiphospholipid syndrome: a diagnostic challenge. Med J Armed Forces India. 2016;72:S31–6. https://doi.org/10.1016/j.mjafi.2016.05.001.
14. Tripodi A, Scalambrino E, Clerici M, Peyvandi F. Laboratory diagnosis of antiphospholipid syndrome in anticoagulated patients. Biomedicine. 2023;11:1760. https://doi.org/10.3390/biomedicines11061760.
15. Ferro D, Pittoni V, Quintarelli C, Basili S, Saliola M, Caroselli C, et al. Coexistence of antiphospholipid antibodies and endothelial perturbation in systemic lupus erythematosus patients with ongoing prothrombotic state. Circulation. 1997;95:1425–32. https://doi.org/10.1161/01.cir.95.6.1425.

Pitfalls in the Management of Corticosteroids in Rheumatic Diseases

6

Abbreviations

ACTH	Adrenocorticotropic hormone
bDMARDs	Biologic DMARDs
BMD	Bone mineral density
CS	Corticosteroids
CS	Cyclophosphamide
csDMARDs	Conventional synthetic DMARDs
DMARDs	Disease-modifying anti-rheumatic drugs
GCA	Giant cell arteritis
HCQ	Hydroxychloroquine
i.v.	Intravenous
IGRA	Interferon-gamma release assay
IL	Interleukin
JAKi	Janus kinase inhibitors
LEF	Leflunomide
LN	Lupus nephritis
MMF	Mycophenolate mofetil
MTX	Methotrexate
PJP	Pneumocystis jirovecii pneumonia
PM	Polymyositis
PROs	Patient-reported outcomes
PsA	Psoriatic arthritis
QoL	Quality of life
RA	Rheumatoid arthritis
RMDs	Rheumatic diseases
RTX	Rituximab
SLE	Systemic lupus erythematosus

E. Pelechas et al., *Pitfalls in Rheumatology*,
https://doi.org/10.1007/978-3-031-98671-0_6

TB	Tuberculosis
TNFi	Tumour necrosis factor α inhibitors
tsDMARDs	Targeted synthetic DMARDs

6.1 Over-Reliance on Corticosteroids for Long-Term Management

A common pitfall is over-reliance on CS as a long-term treatment rather than as a bridging therapy until other DMARDs become effective. While CS can provide rapid symptom relief [1, 2], chronic use, even at the minimum dose, may lead to numerous adverse effects, including osteoporosis, diabetes, hypertension, weight gain, skin thinning and an increased risk of infections [3, 4].

How to Avoid This Pitfall (a) *Limit long-term use*: CS should be used as a short-term solution for controlling acute flares and as a bridge to more sustainable therapies, such as DMARDs [5]; (b) *initiate steroid-sparing therapies early*: early introduction of csDMARDs (MTX, HCQ and LEF) or bDMARDs (TNFi and IL-inhibitors) and tsDMARDs (JAKi) can reduce dependence on CS [6]; (c) *taper when possible*: once disease control is achieved with other therapies, CS should be tapered to the lowest possible dose or ideally discontinued. Tapering must be done gradually to avoid rebound inflammation or adrenal insufficiency [7].

6.2 Inadequate Dosing During Acute Flares

Another pitfall is underdosing CS during severe disease flares. Some clinicians may prescribe low doses of CS even in cases of severe systemic inflammation, risking inadequate control of disease and irreversible organ damage. For example, in conditions like GCA or severe LN, where the recommended dose of CS is 0.5–1.0 mg/kg body weight of prednisone (or an equivalent CS), or pulse CS therapy in cases of imminent organ-threatening involvement, failure to prescribe high enough doses can lead to complications such as vision loss or kidney failure, respectively [8, 9].

How to Avoid This Pitfall (a) *Use appropriate high-dose therapy in acute flares*: in severe, life-threatening situation like LN, PM, or vasculitis, high-dose CS, meaning 1 mg/kg/day of prednisone or i.v. methylprednisolone pulse therapy, should be initiated promptly [10, 11]; (b) *tailor dosing to disease severity*: the dose of CS should match the severity of the disease flare. Lower doses are appropriate for milder disease, but high doses or i.v. administration may be required for organ-threatening manifestations. In Table 6.1, a summary of the dosing of CS for induction and maintenance therapy in various autoimmune conditions is presented.

Table 6.1 Summary of CS dosing for induction and maintenance therapy in various autoimmune conditions

Condition	Induction therapy	Maintenance therapy
Lupus nephritis	High-dose prednisone: 0.5–1 mg/kg/day (up to 60 mg/day)	Gradual taper over 6–12 months to 5–10 mg/day or less
	Pulse methylprednisolone: 500–1000 mg i.v. daily for 3 days	
ANCA-associated vasculitis (with kidney involvement)	High-dose prednisone: 12.5–25 mg/day	Taper by 1 mg every 1–2 months to 5–10 mg/day, then taper slower over 1–2 years
	Pulse methylprednisolone: 500–1000 mg i.v. daily for 3 days	
Giant cell arteritis	High-dose prednisone: 40–60 mg/day	Taper to 10 mg/day over 4–6 months, then taper by 1 mg/month to discontinue over 1–2 years
	Pulse methylprednisolone: 500–1000 mg i.v. daily for 3 days (in case of vision loss or severe disease)	
IgG4-Related disease	Moderate-dose prednisone: 30–40 mg/day	Taper to 5–10 mg/day over 3–6 months and maintain for 1–2 years (depending on relapse risk)
Polymyalgia rheumatica	Moderate-dose prednisone: 12.5–25 mg/day	Taper by 1 mg every 1–2 months to 5–10 mg/day, then taper slower (over 1–2 years)

Clinicians should keep in mind that tapering schedules depend on the disease activity, risk of relapse and side effects of CS, and many of these conditions also involve the use of combination therapy with immunosuppressants such as RTX, CS, MMF and MTX; (c) *frequent reassessment*: in cases of severe disease flares, reassess the patient frequently to ensure that the CS dose is adequate and adjust the dose as needed to control inflammation.

6.3 Failure to Implement Proper Tapering Schedules

Tapering CS too rapidly or too slowly can both lead to problems. Rapid tapering can result in disease flare-ups whereas abrupt discontinuation to adrenal insufficiency [12], while overly slow tapering may result in prolonged exposure to unnecessary CS toxicity. Determining the correct tapering schedule should be individualised and requires careful consideration of disease activity, underlying treatment response and patient factors.

How to Avoid This Pitfall (a) *Monitor disease activity*: tapering should be individualised based on disease control. Monitoring disease activity through clinical assessment, biomarkers and PROs can guide safe tapering. For instance, in GCA, tapering should be slow and carefully monitored to avoid relapse [13]. Furthermore, in cases where there are laboratory and/or clinical signs of relapse and it is feasible, a csDMARD should be added. However, in more resistant cases, evaluation for the initiation of a biologic agent such as an IL-6 inhibitor or the recently approved JAK inhibitor upadacitinib should be considered [14, 15]; (b) *gradual tapering at low doses*: once CS doses are reduced to physiological levels (<7.5 mg/day of prednisone or analogues), tapering should be slower to prevent adrenal insufficiency. Patients on long-term CS may need months to taper completely; (c) *adrenal function testing*: in patients on prolonged high-dose CS, consider testing adrenal function before discontinuing therapy to assess for adrenal insufficiency [16].

6.4 Ignoring the Side Effects of Long-Term Corticosteroid Therapy

CS doses are associated with numerous side effects, including osteoporosis, hypertension, hyperglycaemia, cataracts, glaucoma, weight gain and an increased risk of infections. Prolonged use of even low doses of CS can lead to these adverse effects. Ignoring the risks or failing to provide prophylactic treatment for side effects can significantly impact patient QoL. In Table 6.2, a summary of the CS side effects categorised by the affected system is presented.

How to Avoid This Pitfall (a) *Screen and prevent osteoporosis*: osteoporosis is one of the most common side effects of long-term CS use. All patients on long-term CS should receive adequate calcium and vitamin D supplementation, and bisphosphonates should be considered in high-risk individuals or in those who by definition are expected to receive high doses for a prolonged period of time, as is the case in vasculitides or other conditions involving major organ involvement. BMD testing should be performed regularly [17]; (b) *monitor blood pressure and glucose*: CS can exacerbate hypertension and cause or worsen diabetes. Regular monitoring of blood pressure and blood glucose levels is essential, and antihypertensive or hypoglycaemic medications should be adjusted as needed [18, 19]; (c) *regular eye exams*: patients on long-term CS should have regular ophthalmologic evaluations to screen for cataracts and glaucoma [20]; (d) *vaccination and infection prevention*: long-term CS use increases susceptibility to infections. Patients should be up to date on vaccinations, particularly pneumococcal and influenza vaccines. In certain cases, prophylaxis for opportunistic infections, such as PJP, should be considered [21]. Finally, in cases requiring high-dose and prolonged CS therapy, performing a Mantoux test and/or IGRA should be considered to avoid the risk of reactivation of latent TB.

Table 6.2 Summary of the CS side effects

System	Side effects	Mechanism
Endocrine	Weight gain	Increased appetite, fat redistribution
	Hyperglycaemia, diabetes mellitus	Increased gluconeogenesis and insulin resistance
	Dyslipidaemia	Altered lipid metabolism
	Adrenal suppression	Negative feedback on hypothalamic-pituitary-adrenal axis
	Cushingoid appearance (moon face, buffalo hump)	Chronic high cortisol levels
	Growth suppression in children	Inhibition of growth hormone activity
Musculoskeletal	Osteoporosis	Inhibition of bone formation and calcium absorption
	Myopathy (proximal muscle wasting)	Protein catabolism
	Avascular necrosis (mainly of the femoral head)	Impaired blood supply to bones
Cardiovascular	Hypertension	Sodium and water retention, increased vascular sensitivity to catecholamines
	Increased risk of atherosclerosis and thrombosis	Metabolic effects and endothelial dysfunction
Dermatologic	Skin thinning, bruising	Reduced collagen synthesis
	Skin striae	Skin atrophy and loss of elasticity
	Delayed wound healing	Impaired fibroblast function
	Acne, hirsutism	Hormonal effects
Immune system	Increased risk of infections and reactivation of latent infections	Suppression of cell-mediated and humoral immunity. Reduced immune surveillance
Neuropsychiatric	Mood changes, insomnia, depression, cognitive impairment	Central nervous system effects cortisol's stimulatory effects, altered neurotransmitter activity
Ophthalmologic	Cataracts (posterior subcapsular), glaucoma	Impaired lens metabolism and increased intraocular pressure
Reproductive	Menstrual irregularities	Suppression of gonadotropin secretion
Haematologic	Leukocytosis	Demargination of neutrophils

6.5 Failure to Recognise Corticosteroid-Related Adrenal Insufficiency

Prolonged CS use suppresses the HPA axis, which can lead to adrenal insufficiency if CS is withdrawn too quickly or abruptly. Symptoms of adrenal insufficiency are non-specific and may include fatigue, hypotension, nausea and weakness, which may be mistaken for a flare of the underlying disease or other conditions [22].

How to Avoid This Pitfall (a) *Taper CS gradually*: to prevent adrenal insufficiency, CS should be tapered slowly, particularly at low doses. Patient who have been on CS for more than a few weeks may need months to completely taper off; (b) *monitor for symptoms of adrenal insufficiency*: patients should be educated about the symptoms of adrenal insufficiency, and clinicians should have a high index of suspicion for this condition in patients with prolonged CS use who report non-specific symptoms like fatigue or dizziness during tapering; (c) *consider adrenal function testing*: in patients at risk for adrenal insufficiency, morning serum cortisol or ACTH stimulation tests can be used to assess adrenal function before tapering CS completely [23].

6.6 Inappropriate Use of Intramuscular or Depot Corticosteroids

Depot CS injections such as triamcinolone may be used in certain situations to provide long-term symptom relief, particularly in patients with poor adherence to oral medications. However, depot steroids can cause prolonged systemic exposure to CS, increasing the risk of side effects such as osteoporosis, diabetes and adrenal suppression. Moreover, once administered, depot CS cannot be quickly tapered or stopped, making them potentially a risky choice in some patients [24].

How to Avoid This Pitfall (a) *Consider the risks before using depot steroids*: the decision to use depot steroids should be made carefully, considering the patient's overall health, risk factors for CS toxicity and the need for flexibility in tapering. Moreover, if there are signs of infection, never use depot CS; (b) *reserve for select situations*: depot CS may be appropriate for pateints with compliance issues or for those who require long-term symptom control with minimal medical follow-up. However, they should generally not be used as first-line therapy; (c) *monitor for side effects*: patients receiving depot CS should be closely monitored for side effects, particularly in terms of bone health, glucose control and signs of adrenal insufficiency [24].

6.7 Overuse of Corticosteroids in Diseases Amenable to Other Therapies

In diseases like RA, SLE and PsA, CS are often overused when more effective, steroid-sparing treatments such as cs/b/tsDMARDs are available. Failure to transition to these therapies can result in unnecessary CS exposure and an increased burden of side effects [13].

How to Avoid This Pitfall (a) *Emphasize early use of DMARDs: in diseases like RA and SLE, the primary goal should be to reduce CS use by transitioning to DMARDs (such as MTX, TNFi, JAKi, HCQ and belimumab) as quickly as possible*; (b) *regularly reassess treatment*: patients on chronic CS should be reassessed frequently to determine if their disease can be controlled with alternative therapies. Early and aggressive treatment of the underlying disease can often minimise the need for CS [13].

6.8 Conclusion

CS are essential in managing many RMDs, but they come with significant risks, particularly when used long-term or at high doses. The pitfalls in CS management, including over-reliance on CS, failure to taper appropriately and underestimating side effects, can lead to significant patient morbidity. By recognising these pitfalls and implementing strategies to minimise CS exposure, clinicians can optimise outcomes for patients while minimising the adverse effects associated with CS therapy.

References

1. Van Ouwerkerk L, Vershueren P, Boers M, Emery P, de Jong PHP, Landewé RB, et al. Initial glucocorticoid bridging in rheumatoid arthritis: does it affect glucocorticoid use over time? Ann Rheum Dis. 2024;83:65–71. https://doi.org/10.1136/ard-2023-224270.
2. Pelechas E, Drosos AA. State-of-the-art glucocorticoid-targeted drug therapies for the treatment of rheumatoid arthritis. Expert Opin Pharmacother. 2022;23:703–11. https://doi.org/10.1080/14656566.2022.2049238.
3. Pelechas E, Kaltsonoudis E, Voulgari PV, Drosos AA. Adverse drug reactions in rheumatology. In: Illustrated handbook of rheumatic and musculo-skeletal diseases. Cham: Springer; 2023. https://doi.org/10.1007/978-3-031-47379-1_19.
4. Gensler LS. Glucocorticoids. Neurohospitalist. 2013;3:92–7. https://doi.org/10.1177/1941874412458678.
5. Prior JA, Roddy E, Solis-Trapala I, Cornwall N, Jinks C, Abhishek A, et al. How do clinicians prescribe bridging glucocorticoids in people starting or escalating disease-modifying anti-rheumatic drugs for rheumatoid arthritis: a service evaluation survey. Rheumatol Adv Pract. 2023;15:rkad102. https://doi.org/10.1093/rap/rkad102.
6. Nell VPK, Machold KP, Eberl G, Stamm TA, Uffmann M, Smolen JS. Benefit of very early referral and very early therapy with disease-modifying anti-rheumatic drugs in patients with early rheumatoid arthritis. Rheumatology (Oxford). 2004;43:906–14. https://doi.org/10.1093/rheumatology/keh199.
7. Priya G, Laway BA, Ayyagari M, Gupta M, Bhat GHK, Dutta D. The glucocorticoid taper: a primer for the clinicians. Indian J Endocrinol Metab. 2024;28:350–62. https://doi.org/10.4103/ijem.ijem_410_23.
8. Ponte C, Rodrigues AF, O'Neill L, Lugmani RA. Giant cell arteritis: current treatment and management. World J Clin Cases. 2015;3:484–94. https://doi.org/10.12998/wjcc.v3.i6.484.
9. Mejía-Vilet J, Ayoub I. The use of glucocorticoids in lupus nephritis: new pathways for an old drug. Front Med (Lausanne). 2021;8:622225. https://doi.org/10.3389/fmed.2021.622225.
10. Choy EH, Isenberg DA. Treatment of dermatomyositis and polymyositis. Rheumatology (Oxford). 2002;41:7–13. https://doi.org/10.1093/rheumatology/41.1.7.
11. Walsh M, Merkel PA, Peh CA, Szpirt WM, Puéchal X, Fujimoto S, et al. Plasma exchange and glucocorticoids in severe ANCA-associated vasculitis. N Engl J Med. 2020;382:622–31. https://doi.org/10.1056/NEJMoa1893537.
12. Prete A, Bancos I. Glucocorticoid induced adrenal insufficiency. BMJ. 2021;374:n1380. https://doi.org/10.1136/bmj.n1380.

13. Muratore F, Marvisi C, Castrignanó P, Croci S, Bonacini M, Boiardi L, et al. Effectiveness and safety of a 26-week taper regimen of glucocorticoid in GCA patients: results from a prospective cohort study. Semin Arthritis Rheum. 2024;64:152351. https://doi.org/10.1016/j.semarthrit.2023.152351.
14. Stone JH, Han J, Aringer M, Blockmans D, Brouwer E, Cid MC, et al., GiACTA investigators. Long-term effect of tocilizumab in patients with giant cell arteritis: open-label extension phase of the Giant Cell Arteritis Actemra (GiACTA) trial. Lancet Rheumatol. 2021;3:e328–36. https://doi.org/10.1016/S2665-9913(21)00038-2.
15. Blockmans D, Penn SK, Setty AR, Schmidt WA, Rubbert-Roth A, Hauge EM, et al. A phase 3 trial of upadacitinib for giant-cell arteritis. N Engl J Med. 2025; https://doi.org/10.1056/NEJMoa2413449.
16. Pelewicz K, Miśkiewicz P. Glucocorticoid withdrawal—an overview on when and how to diagnose adrenal insufficiency in clinical practice. Diagnostics (Basel). 2021;11:728. https://doi.org/10.3390/diagnostics11040728.
17. Laurent MR, Goemaere S, Verroken C, Bergmann P, Body JJ, Bruyère O, et al. Prevention and treatment of glucocorticoid-induced osteoporosis in adults: consensus recommendations form the Belgian bone club. Front Endocrinol (Lausanne). 2022;13:908727. https://doi.org/10.3389/fendo.2022.908727.
18. Hattori T, Murase T, Iwase E, Takahashi K, Ohtake M, Tsuboi K, et al. Glucocorticoid-induced hypertension and cardiac injury: effects of mineralocorticoid and glucocorticoid receptor antagonism. Nagoya J Med Sci. 2013;75:81–2.
19. Shah P, Kalra S, Yadav Y, Deka N, Lathia T, Jagan J, et al. Management of glucocorticoid-induced hyperglycemia. Diabetes Metab Syndr Obes. 2022;15:1577–88. https://doi.org/10.2147/DMSO.S330253.
20. Dibas A, Yorio T. Glucocorticoid therapy and ocular hypertension. Eur J Pharmacol. 2016;787:57–71. https://doi.org/10.1016/j.ejphar.2016.06.018.
21. Fardet L, Petersen I, Nazzareth I. Common infections in patients prescribed systemic glucocorticoids in primary care: a population-based cohort study. PLoS Med. 2016;13:e1002024. https://doi.org/10.1371/journal.pmed.1002024.
22. Torpy DJ, Lim WT. Glucocorticoid-induced adrenal suppression: physiological basis and strategies foo glucocorticoid weaning. Med J Aust. 2023;219:444–7. https://doi.org/10.5694/mja2.52140.
23. Beuschlein F, Else T, Bancos I, Hahner S, Hamidi O, van Hulsteijn L, et al. European Society of Endocrinology and Endocrine Society joint clinical guideline: diagnosis and therapy of glucocorticoid-induced adrenal insufficiency. Eur J Endrocrinol. 2024;190:G25–51. https://doi.org/10.1093/ejendo/lvae029.
24. Stout A, Friedly J, Standaert C. Systemic absorption and side effects of locally injected glucocorgicoids. PM R. 2019;11:409–19. https://doi.org/10.1002/pmrj.12042.

Pitfalls in the Management of Drugs in Rheumatology

7

Abbreviations

AS	Ankylosing spondylitis
AZA	Azathioprine
bDMARDs	Biologic DMARDs
CS	Corticosteroids
csDMARDs	Conventional synthetic disease-modifying anti-rheumatic drugs
FBC	Full blood count
HBV	Hepatitis B virus
HCQ	Hydroxychloroquine
HCV	Hepatitis C virus
HZV	Herpes zoster virus
i.v.	Intravenous
JAKi	Janus kinase inhibitors
LDA	Low disease activity
LEF	Leflunomide
LFTs	Liver function tests
MTX	Methotrexate
NSAIDs	Non-steroidal anti-inflammatory drugs
OTC	Over-the-counter
p.o.	Per os
PsA	Psoriatic arthritis
QoL	Quality of life
RA	Rheumatoid arthritis
RMDs	Rheumatic diseases
s.c.	Subcutaneous
SLE	Systemic lupus erythematosus

E. Pelechas et al., *Pitfalls in Rheumatology*,
https://doi.org/10.1007/978-3-031-98671-0_7

T2T	Treat-to-target
TB	Tuberculosis
tsDMARDs	Targeted synthetic DMARDs

7.1 Delayed or Inadequate Use of DMARDs

One of the most significant challenges in rheumatology is the delayed initiation of underuse of DMARDs. This often occurs due to hesitance or due to insufficient training and inability to properly inform the patient about the safety and efficacy of the medications on the part of the clinician or patient concerns about side effects, cost or complex administration methods. In diseases like RA, SLE and AS, early and aggressive treatment with DMARDs is critical to preventing irreversible joint damage and systemic complications [1].

Consequences (a) *Disease progression*: delayed treatment can result in progressive joint destruction, organ damage and disability in conditions like RA, PsA and SLE; (b) *inadequate symptom control*: patients may suffer from chronic pain, stiffness and fatigue, significantly impacting their QoL.

Strategy (a) *T2T*: use a T2T approach with regular assessments of disease activity to adjust treatment as needed. Early initiation of DMARDs is essential for patients with moderate-to-severe disease [2]; (b) *patient education*: educate patients about the importance of early treatment to prevent long-term damage, addressing concerns about side effects or administration. For the different categories of DMARDs, discuss options like s.c. injections, i.v. infusions or p.o. administration to match patient preferences [3]; (c) *shared decision-making*: engage patients in shared decision-making to help them weigh the risks and benefits of treatment, ensuring they are active participants in their care plan [4].

7.2 Over-Reliance on Corticosteroids (See Also Chap. 6)

CS, such as prednisone, are often used to rapidly control inflammation as well as for the management of other life-threatening conditions, such as involvement of target organs in RMDs [5]. However, long-term or excessive reliance on CS can lead to a range of serious complications, including osteoporosis, diabetes, hypertension, adrenal suppression and increased risk of infections. In many cases, CS are used as bridging therapy when DMARD treatment initiation takes place or as on-top treatment on DMARDs for disease flares.

Consequences (a) *CS dependence*: patients may become dependent on CS for symptom relief, leading to prolonged use and increased risk of serious side effects; (b) *delayed DMARD use*: over-reliance on CS may delay the introduction or escalation of more appropriate therapies, such as DMARDs (cs, b or ts); (c) *delayed referral: or inadequate knowledge of the efficacy and safety on newer DMARDs may also lead to a delay in initiating the appropriate pharmacological treatment.*

Strategy (a) *Tapering and minimisation*: use the lowest effective CS dose for the shortest possible duration. Establish a clear plan for tapering CS as soon as disease control is achieved through other therapies; (b) *CS-sparing agents*: prioritise the use of CS-sparing agents, such as MTX and AZA, to reduce the reliance on CS [6]; (c) *bone health monitoring*: in patients requiring long-term CS therapy, use calcium, vitamin D and bisphosphonates to prevent osteoporosis. Regularly assess bone density and consider fracture prevention strategies; (d) *choice of immunomodulatory therapy*: personalise DMARD therapy based on age, comorbidities and other factors that may potentially increase the risk of adverse effects. Use any available prognostic factors to guide a more targeted treatment approach, which enhances the likelihood of achieving the therapeutic goal—remission, or alternatively, LDA.

7.3 Inadequate Monitoring of Drug Toxicities

Many drugs used in rheumatology, such as MTX, LEF, HCQ and other categories of DMARDs, have potential for significant toxicity [7]. MTX can cause liver damage, LEF can lead to hepatotoxicity and hypertension, both in leukopenia/thrombocytopenia, and HCQ can result in retinal toxicity. Failure to monitor patients regularly for these toxicities can result in serious and sometimes irreversible harm. In Table 7.1, a list of the most common toxicities is presented along with the appropriate monitoring.

Consequences (a) *Organ damage*: without regular monitoring, patients on MTX or LEF may develop liver damage, while HCQ use can lead to irreversible vision loss; (b) *increased risk of infections*: patients on immunosuppressive drugs, including b and tsDMARDs, are at increased risk of infections, including opportunistic infections such as TB and fungal infections.

Strategy (a) *Regular laboratory monitoring*: for drugs like MTX, LEF and AZA, regularly check LFTs, FBC and renal function. Adjust dosing based on toxicity levels and patient risk factors [8]; (b) *ophthalmologic screening*: patients on HCQ should have baseline and future ophthalmologic screening according to their treating physician's guidance to detect early signs of retinal toxicity [9]; (c) *infection screening*: before initiating bDMARDs or tsDMARDs (JAKi), screen for latent infections such as TB, HBV and HCV. Repeat TB screening periodically in high-risk patients and monitor for signs of infections throughout therapy; (d) *dose reduction*: in patients who have achieved the therapeutic target over the long term, dose adjustment (reduction) should be considered to avoid unnecessary cumulative immunosuppression.

Table 7.1 Most common drug toxicities and monitoring

Drug	Most common toxicities	Monitoring
Methotrexate	Gastrointestinal (nausea, vomiting, stomatitis), hepatotoxicity, myelosuppression	FBC, LFTs, renal function
Leflunomide	Hepatotoxicity, diarrhoea	FBC, LFTs, renal function
Cyclosporine	Nephrotoxicity, hypertension	Renal function, blood pressure
Azathioprine	Myelosuppression, gastrointestinal (nausea, vomiting)	FBC, LFTs
Hydroxychloroquine	Retinal toxicity, gastrointestinal (nausea, abdominal pain), headache	Regular ophthalmologic exams
TNF inhibitors	Increased risk of infections, injection site reactions	TB screening, infection surveillance
IL-6 inhibitors	Infections, hyperlipidaemia, injection site reactions, haematopoiesis disturbances	Infection monitoring, lipid profile, FBC
IL-17 inhibitors	Infections, injection site reactions	Infection monitoring
IL-23 inhibitors	Infections, injection site reactions	Infection monitoring
JAK inhibitors	Infections including herpes zoster, thrombosis	Infection monitoring, cardiovascular examination
Rituximab	Infusion reactions, hypogammaglobulinaemia	Pre-medication, monitor during infusion, immunoglobulin levels
Cyclophosphamide	Myelosuppression, haemorrhagic cystitis	FBC, hydration, MESNA use
Mycophenolate mofctil	Gastrointestinal (diarrhoea, nausea, abdominal pain)	FBC, LFTs

7.4 Infection Risk and Immunosuppression

Immunosuppressive drugs, including CS, csDMARDs, bDMARDs [10] and tsDMARDs [11], increase the risk of infections, particularly opportunistic infections. Infections are a leading cause of morbidity and mortality in patients with rheumatologic diseases, especially in those receiving combination therapies and in cases of uncontrolled disease (significant disease activity). Failure to take appropriate preventive measures can lead to serious infections.

Consequences (a) *Severe infections*: immunosuppressive therapies can increase the risk of bacterial, viral and fungal infections, leading to complications such as pneumonia, sepsis and reactivation of latent infections like TB; (b) *infection-related morbidity and mortality*: serious infections can result in hospitalisation, long-term health issues or death in immunosuppressed patients.

Strategy (a) *Pretreatment screening*: before starting biologics, JAK inhibitors or other potent immunosuppressants, screen patients for latent infections, including

TB [12] and HBV/HCV. Screen for and vaccinate against infections like HZV and pneumococcal disease when appropriate; (b) *vaccination*: ensure that patients are up-to-date on their vaccinations before starting immunosuppressive therapy. Vaccinate for influenza, pneumococcal infection, hepatitis and HZV, but avoid live vaccines in patients on significant immunosuppression [13]; (c) *prophylaxis and vigilance*: consider antimicrobial prophylaxis in high-risk patients. Educate patients about the signs of infections and encourage them to seek prompt medical attention if they develop symptoms like fever, cough or shortness of breath [14]. Regular monitoring should include, among others, FBC and urinalysis for the early detection of signs suggestive of infection or findings that predispose to infection, such as cytopenias.

7.5 Polypharmacy and Drug Interactions

Patients with RMDs often have multiple comorbidities, leading to polypharmacy [15]. The use of multiple medications increases the risk of drug interactions, which can reduce drug efficacy or increase toxicity. For example, NSAIDs may interact with antihypertensive drugs, reducing blood pressure control, while MTX may have increased toxicity when combined with other hepatotoxic agents such as statins.

Consequences (a) *Adverse drug reactions*: polypharmacy increases the risk of adverse drug reactions, which can lead to hospitalisations, reduced QoL or permanent organ damage; (b) *reduced treatment efficacy*: drug interactions may interfere with the efficacy of rheumatologic therapies, leading to inadequate disease control [16].

Strategy (a) *Medication review*: conduct regular reviews of the patient's medication list, including OTC drugs and supplements, to identify potential interactions. Use drug interaction checkers and consult pharmacists when needed; (b) *simplify regimens*; when possible, simplify medication regimens to reduce the risk of interactions and improve patient adherence; (c) *monitor for interactions*: be vigilant about potential interactions, especially when adding new medications. Given that patients with rheumatic diseases have an increased cardiovascular risk of hepatotoxicity, particularly when co-administered with MTX, LEF or other drugs with hepatic metabolism, monitor for signs of toxicity or treatment failure and adjust therapy as needed.

7.6 Inconsistent Patient Adherence to Treatment

Non-adherence to treatment is a common issue in patients with chronic diseases, including RMDs. Factors such as fear of side effects, complexity of the medication regimen, cost or lack of understanding of the importance of long-term therapy can lead to poor adherence. In DMARD therapy, missed doses or improper administration techniques can result in suboptimal outcomes [17].

Consequences (a) *Flare-ups and disease progression*: non-adherence to DMARDs or other therapies can result in disease flare-ups, progression of joint damage or organ involvement in diseases like SLE; (b) *increased healthcare costs*: poor adherence often leads to increased healthcare utilisation, including emergency room visits, hospitalisations and the need for more intensive therapy; (c) *reduced QoL*: decreased work productivity, absenteeism and disability pensions.

Strategy (a) *Patient education*: educate patients about the importance of medication adherence, the expected benefits of therapy and the potential consequences of non-adherence. Address fears about side effects and provide reassurance where appropriate; (b) *simplify regimens*: where possible, simplify treatment regimens to make adherence easier, such as reducing dosing frequency or switching to combination therapies; (c) *adherence support*: use tools such as reminder systems, adherence apps or pillboxes. Encourage regular follow-ups to discuss any challenges the patient may be facing with their medication [18]; (d) *medication substitution*: consider switching medication even in cases of mild but bothersome symptoms related to its use, as these are long-term treatments and the risk of non-adherence becomes highly likely.

7.7 Conclusion

The effective management of rheumatology drugs involves navigating numerous pitfalls, including delayed treatment initiation, over-reliance on CS, inadequate monitoring of toxicities, non-adherence to treatment and infection risks. By adopting a proactive approach that includes regular monitoring, patient education and a focus on early and aggressive treatment, clinicians can minimise these pitfalls and improve patient outcomes.

References

1. Kedra J, Granger B, Emilie S, Gaujoux-Viala C, Rat AC, Combe B, et al. Time to initiation of biologic disease-modifying antirheumatic drugs in the French cohort ESPOIR. Joint Bone Spine. 2021;88:105060. https://doi.org/10.1016/j.jbspin.2020.07.009.
2. Smolen JS, Breedveld FC, Burmester GR, Bykerk V, Dougados M, Emery P, et al. Treating rheumatoid arthritis to target: 2014 update of the recommendations of an international task force. Ann Rheum Dis. 2016;75:3–15. https://doi.org/10.1136/annrheumdis-2015-207524.
3. Riemsma R, Taal E, Kirwan JR, Rasker JJ. Patient education programmes for adults with rheumatoid arthritis. BMJ. 2002;325:558–9. https://doi.org/10.1136/bmj.325.7364.558.

4. Morrison T, Foster E, Dougherty J, Barton J. Shared decision making in rheumatology: a scoping review. Semin Arthritis Rheum. 2022;56:152041. https://doi.org/10.1016/j.semarthrit.2022.152041.
5. Doumen M, Pazmino S, Bertrand D, Westhovens R, Verschueren P. Glucocorticoids in rheumatoid arthritis: balancing benefits and harm by leveraging the therapeutic window of opportunity. Joint Bone Spine. 2023;90:105491. https://doi.org/10.1016/j.jbspin.2022.105491.
6. Vinicki JP, Cusa A, Domingo D, Zamora JLV, Magri S, Brigante A, et al. Effectiveness of methotrexate and leflunomide as corticoid-sparing drugs in patients with polymyalgia rheumatica. Rheumatol Adv Pract. 2024;8:rkae033. https://doi.org/10.1093/rap/rkae033.
7. Sun J, Dai S, Zhang L, Feng Y, Yu X, Zhang Z. Investigating the safety and compliance of using csDMARDs in rheumatoid arthritis treatment through face-to-face interviews: a cross-sectional study in China. Clin Rheumatol. 2020;40:1789–98. https://doi.org/10.1007/s10067-020-05458.
8. Rigby WFC, Lampl K, Low JM, Furst DE. Review of routine laboratory monitoring for patients with rheumatoid arthritis receiving biologic or nonbiologic DMARDs. Int J Rheumatol. 2017;2017:9614241. https://doi.org/10.1155/2017/9614241.
9. Geamãnu A, Popa-Cherecheanu A, Marinescu B, Geamãnu CD, Voinea LM. Retinal toxicity associated with chronic exposure to hydroxychloroquine and its ocular screening. Review. J Med Life. 2014;7:322–6.
10. Quartuccio L, Zabotti A, Del Zotto S, Zanier L, De Vita S, Valent F. Risk of serious infection among patients receiving biologics for chronic inflammatory diseases. Usefulness of administrative data. J Adv Res. 2018;15:87–93. https://doi.org/10.1016/j.jare.2018/09.003.
11. Adas MA, Alveyn E, Cook E, Dey M, Galloway JB, Beckman K. The infection risks of JAK inhibition. Expert Rev Clin Immunol. 2021;18:253–61. https://doi.org/10.1080/1744666X.2022.2014323.
12. Pradhan S, Madke B, Neema S, Kabra P, Singh AL, Yadav S. Screening of latent tuberculous infection (LTBI) before starting anti-tumor necrosis factor therapy in patients with psoriasis: a primer for clinical dermatologist. Indian J Dermatol. 2021;66:501–7. https://doi.org/10.4103/ijd.IJD_649_16.
13. Chat VS, Ellebrecht CT, Kingston P, Gondo G, Bell S, Cordoro KM, et al. Vaccination recommendations for adults receiving biologics and oral therapies for psoriasis and psoriatic arthritis. Delphi consensus form the medical board of the National Psoriasis Foundation. J Am Acad Dermatol. 2024;90:1170–81. https://doi.org/10.1016/j.jaad.2023.12.070.
14. Zangi HA, Ndosi M, Adams J, Andersen L, Bode C, Boström C, et al. EULAR recommendations for patient education for people with inflammatory arthritis. Ann Rheum Dis. 2015;74:954–62. https://doi.org/10.1136/annrheumdis-2014-206807.
15. Gomides APM, Albuquerque CP, Santos ABV, Amorim RBC, Bértolo MB, Júnior PL, et al. High levels of polypharmacy in rheumatoid arthritis—a challenge not covered by current management recommendations: data from a large real-life study. J Pharm Pract. 2021;34:365–71. https://doi.org/10.1177/0897190019869158.
16. Pflugbeil S, Böckl K, Pongratz R, Leitner M, Graninger W, Ortner A. Drug interactions in the treatment of rheumatoid arthritis and psoriatic arthritis. Rheumatol Int. 2020;40:511–21. https://doi.org/10.1007/s00296-020-04526-3.
17. Harrold LR, Andrade SE. Medication adherence of patients with selected rheumatic conditions: a systematic review of the literature. Semin Arthritis Rheum. 2008;38:396–402. https://doi.org/10.1016/j.semarthrit.2008.01.011.
18. Marengo MF, Suarez-Almazor ME. Improving treatment adherence in patients with rheumatoid arthritis: what are the options? Int J Clin Rheumatol. 2015;10:345–56. https://doi.org/10.2217/ijr.15.39.

8 Pitfalls in the Differential Diagnosis of Rheumatic Diseases and Rheumatic Mimickers

Abbreviations

ACE	Angiotensin-converting enzyme
ANA	Anti-nuclear antibodies
anti-CCP	Anti-cyclic citrullinated peptide
AS	Ankylosing spondylitis
CRP	C-reactive protein
CS	Corticosteroids
CSF	Cerebrospinal fluid
DIL	Drug-induced lupus
DM	Dermatomyositis
DMARD	Disease-modifying anti-rheumatic drug
ESR	Erythrocyte sedimentation rate
HBV	Hepatitis B virus
HCV	Hepatitis C virus
HIV	Human immunodeficiency virus
IA	Inflammatory arthritis
MRI	Magnetic resonance imaging
MSK	Musculoskeletal
MSKUS	Musculoskeletal ultrasound
OA	Osteoarthritis
PM	Polymyositis
PMR	Polymyalgia rheumatica
PsA	Psoriatic arthritis
RA	Rheumatoid arthritis
RF	Rheumatoid factor
RMDs	Rheumatic diseases
SLE	Systemic lupus erythematosus

E. Pelechas et al., *Pitfalls in Rheumatology*,
https://doi.org/10.1007/978-3-031-98671-0_8

SS	Sjögren's syndrome
SScl	Systemic sclerosis
TB	Tuberculosis
TSH	Thyroid-stimulating hormone

8.1 Assuming Inflammatory Symptoms Always Indicate Rheumatic Disease

One of the most common pitfalls is assuming that symptoms like joint pain, swelling, or stiffness automatically suggest an RMD. In reality, many non-RMD conditions, including infections, malignancies and metabolic disorders, can present with similar symptoms. For instance, septic arthritis, reactive arthritis, malignancy-related arthritis [1] and even hyperthyroidism [2] can mimic inflammatory joint diseases such as RA or SLE.

How to Avoid This Pitfall (a) *Consider a broad differential*: always think beyond rheumatic causes when evaluating inflammatory symptoms. Infectious, neoplastic or metabolic causes should be included in the differential, especially in atypical presentations or when systemic symptoms like fever, weight loss or night sweats are prominent; (b) *use specific diagnostic tests*: utilise appropriate tests to rule out non-RMD conditions. For example, joint aspiration and culture are essential in ruling out septic arthritis, while imaging or biopsy may be needed to exclude malignancy in patients with unexplained systemic symptoms; (c) *assess the duration of symptoms*: in cases of acute-onset arthritis with pronounced symptoms, beyond crystal-induced arthritis, one should also consider and rule out infectious arthritis.

8.2 Misinterpreting Serologic Tests in Isolation

Autoantibody tests, such as RF, anti-CCP and ANA, are often used to support the diagnosis of RMDs. However, relying on these tests in isolation without clinical correlation can lead to misdiagnosis. For example, RF can be positive in chronic infections, malignancies and even in healthy individuals, especially the elderly. Similarly, a positive ANA test is non-specific and can be seen in many non-RMD conditions, including viral infections and chronic liver disease.

How to Avoid This Pitfall (a) *Interpret serology in the appropriate clinical context*: always interpret autoantibody results in conjunction with the clinical picture. For example, a positive ANA should only be considered meaningful in the context of symptoms consistent with SLE or another RMD [3]; (b) *understand the limitations of serology*: be aware that many autoantibodies lack specificity and may be present in healthy individuals or those with non-RMDs [4]. Positive test results should prompt further evaluation, but never dictate self-diagnosis.

8.3 Overlooking Infection as a Cause of Rheumatic Symptoms

Infections are a common and important mimicker of RMDs. Bacterial, viral and fungal infections can present with joint pain, swelling and systemic symptoms like fever and fatigue, closely resembling conditions such as RA or vasculitis [5]. For instance, parvovirus B19, HBV, HCV, HIV and Lyme disease are notable infections that can mimic RMDs.

How to Avoid This Pitfall (a) *Consider infectious aetiologies*: always include infection in the differential diagnosis, particularly in patients with acute onset of symptoms, fever or a history of travel or exposure risks; (b) *order appropriate infectious workup*: for patients presenting with joint pain and systemic symptoms, consider tests for viral, bacterial and, in some cases, fungal infections (such as HBV, Lyme serology and histoplasmosis in endemic areas, respectively); (c) *avoid premature immunosuppression*: starting immunosuppressive therapy in patients with undiagnosed infection can have devastating consequences. In cases where infection is suspected, delay CS or DMARD therapy until infection is definitively ruled out; (d) *do not rush to start treatment*: even in a patient who meets criteria for an RMD, if there is suspicion of infection, it should be ruled out with appropriate laboratory testing, and immunosuppressive therapy should be delayed until infection in definitively excluded.

8.4 Failure to Recognise Malignancy-Associated Rheumatic Syndromes

Malignancies can present with MSK or systemic symptoms that mimic RMDs [6]. For example, paraneoplastic syndromes such as HOA [7] or DM [8] may precede the diagnosis of cancer. Additionally, some cancers, such as lymphomas and leukemias, can present with inflammatory arthritis or vasculitis-like syndromes [9].

How to Avoid This Pitfall (a) *Be aware of red flags for malignancy*: symptoms such as unexplained weight loss, night sweats, anaemia, lack of response or even an unexpected response to typical rheumatologic treatment should raise suspicion for an underlying malignancy; (b) *order age-appropriate cancer screening*: in patients with new-onset rheumatic symptoms and red flags, consider cancer screening, including imaging and laboratory tests, as part of the initial evaluation; (c) *biopsy when necessary*: in cases of suspected malignancy or paraneoplastic syndromes, tissue biopsy or bone marrow evaluation may be necessary for diagnosis [10].

8.5 Mistaking Degenerative Conditions for Inflammatory Rheumatic Diseases

Degenerative joint diseases like OA can mimic RMDs, especially when patients present with pain, stiffness and swelling. In some cases, OA may cause synovitis, joint effusion or even an elevated ESR or CRP, leading to confusion with disease like RA or PsA [11, 12]. Conversely, early-stage IA may present with minimal signs of inflammation, leading to misdiagnosis as OA.

How to Avoid This Pitfall (a) *Differentiate between inflammatory and degenerative features*: IA often presents with morning stiffness lasting >30 min, multiple joints involved symmetrically and systemic features such as fatigue [13]. OA typically causes stiffness lasting <30 min and is more localised to weight-bearing joints [14]; (b) *use imaging to clarify diagnosis*: in cases where the diagnosis is unclear, imaging such as X-rays or MSKUS can help distinguish OA from IA [15]. The former can present with joint space narrowing and osteophyte formation, whereas the latter can present with synovitis and erosions; (c) *consider laboratory testing*: while not always definitive, serologic testing such as RF and anti-CCP can help differentiate RA from OA in patients with overlapping symptoms.

8.6 Overlooking Drug-Induced Rheumatic Syndromes

Certain medications can induce symptoms that closely mimic RMDs. For instance, hydralazine and procainamide can cause DIL [16], while checkpoint inhibitors used in cancer therapy can trigger IA or more rarely vasculitis [17]. Additionally, some antibiotics, statins and anticonvulsants can cause drug-induced myopathies that may be mistaken for PM or DM [18].

How to Avoid This Pitfall (a) *Review the patient's medication history*: always take a thorough medication history, including recent changes or additions. Consider the possibility of drug-induced rheumatic syndromes when new symptoms arise after starting a medication; (b) *consider drug discontinuation*: in suspected cases of drug-induced rheumatic disease, consider discontinuing the offending agent or do a dose modification where this is feasible and observe for symptom resolution before making a definitive diagnosis of an RMD by initiating long-term immunosuppressive therapy.

8.7 Misinterpreting Fibromyalgia and Other Non-inflammatory, Psychologically Mediated Pain Syndromes as Rheumatic Disease

Fibromyalgia, a common pain syndrome, is often confused with inflammatory RMDs due to the presence of widespread pain, fatigue and stiffness. However, fibromyalgia is a non-inflammatory condition and should not be treated with immunosuppressive therapy. Misdiagnosis can lead to unnecessary treatments, potential harm from medications and worsening patient outcomes. On the other hand, fibromyalgia often coexists with RMDs, and in such cases, careful assessment of the underlying RMD is essential (based on monitoring indices) in order to avoid unnecessary immunosuppressive therapy and its potential consequences.

How to Avoid This Pitfall (a) *Recognise the features of fibromyalgia*: fibromyalgia typically presents with widespread pain, fatigue and non-restorative sleep, without objective signs of inflammation such as joint swelling or synovitis. Patients often report tenderness in specific trigger points on physical examination which you should be aware of and take into consideration [19]; (b) *use clinical judgement*: ESR and CRP levels are typically normal in fibromyalgia [20]. Additionally, autoantibody tests such as RF and ANA are often negative, though they may be positive in low titres incidentally. Consider the overall clinical picture rather than relying solely on lab tests.

8.8 Misdiagnosing Rheumatic Conditions as Psychiatric or Functional Disorders

Patients with systemic RMDs, such as SLE or vasculitis, can present with non-specific symptoms like fatigue, weakness or neuropsychiatric manifestations such as depression, anxiety and cognitive dysfunction. These symptoms may be mistakenly attributed to psychiatric or functional disorders, leading to delays in diagnosis and treatment [21].

How to Avoid This Pitfall (a) *Consider systemic disease in the presence of unexplained symptoms*: in patients with unexplained fatigue, mood changes or cognitive impairment, particularly in the presence of multisystem involvement affecting, for example, skin, kidneys and joints, consider an underlying RMD like SLE or vasculitis; (b) *use specific testing for systemic involvement*: autoantibody testing, complement levels and imaging such as brain MRI for neuropsychiatric SLE or elevated inflammatory markers in the case of vasculitis can help distinguish between RMD and functional or psychiatric disorders [22].

8.9 Conclusion

The differential diagnosis of RMDs is full of challenges, given the broad spectrum of symptoms and the presence of numerous mimickers. Clinicians must maintain a high index of suspicion for both RMDs and their mimics, integrate clinical findings with laboratory and imaging data and remain vigilant for atypical presentations and/or coexisting conditions. A careful and systematic approach can reduce diagnostic errors, ensuring appropriate treatment and better outcomes for patients. In Table 8.1, a summary of all the potential rheumatic mimickers is presented with some key findings that may help differentiating them from true RMDs.

Table 8.1 Rheumatic mimickers and key findings that help to differentiate them from true RMDs

Category	Condition	Rheumatic disease mimicked	Key findings for differentiation
Infectious diseases	Tuberculosis	RA, vasculitis	Chronic fever, weight loss, granulomas, positive TB test
	Lyme disease	RA, SLE	Erythema migrans, history of tick bite, positive Lyme serology
	Viral arthritis	RA	Acute onset, self-limited, associated viral symptoms
	HIV	SLE, PM	Constitutional symptoms, immunodeficiency
	Endocarditis	Vasculitis	Fever, heart murmur, blood cultures
Malignancies	Lymphoma	SLE, SS	Lymphadenopathy, night sweats, abnormal peripheral smear
	Leukemia	RA, vasculitis	Pancytopaenia, blasts in blood or marrow
	Paraneoplastic syndromes	PM, DM	Underlying malignancy, atypical age for RMD
	Solid tumours (e.g. lung)	Vasculitis	Positive imaging, tumour markers
Endocrine disorders	Hypothyroidism	Fibromyalgia, myositis	High TSH, fatigue, weight gain, bradycardia
	Hyperthyroidism	RA, PMR	Low TSH, tachycardia, tremors
	Diabetes-related cheiroarthropathy	SScl	Glycaemic history, thickened hand skin without SScl signs
Neurological disorders	Multiple sclerosis	SLE, vasculitis	MRI with demyelinating lesions, CSF oligoclonal bands
	Cerebrovascular event (ischaemic or haemorrhagic)	Vasculitis	Imaging confirmation, acute onset
	Neuropathy (diabetic, alcoholic)	Vasculitis, SS	History of diabetes or alcohol use, nerve conduction studies
Haematological disorders	Haemophilia	Haemarthrosis in RA	Bleeding diathesis, prolonged clotting times
	Thrombotic thrombocytopaenic purpura	Vasculitis	Low platelets, schistocytes on blood smear

(continued)

Table 8.1 (continued)

Category	Condition	Rheumatic disease mimicked	Key findings for differentiation
Genetic disorders	Ehlers–Danlos syndrome	Joint hypermobility syndrome	Hyperextensible skin, positive family history
	Marfan syndrome	AS	Tall stature, aortic involvement, lens dislocation
	Bertolotti syndrome	AS	Non-inflammatory low back pain, imaging studies
Psychiatric disorders	Somatisation, conversion disorder	Fibromyalgia, myositis	Inconsistent findings, psychiatric history
Degenerative diseases	Osteoarthritis	RA, PMR	Non-inflammatory synovial fluid, absence of systemic signs
	Spinal stenosis	AS	Neurogenic claudication, imaging findings
Metabolic disorders	Gout	Septic arthritis, RA	Monosodium urate crystals in synovial fluid, acute onset, imaging studies
	Pseudogout (CCPD)	Septic arthritis, RA	Calcium pyrophosphate crystals in synovial fluid, imaging studies
	Haemochromatosis	RA	Iron overload, family history
Drug-induced syndromes	Drug-induced lupus	SLE	Resolves after drug discontinuation, anti-histone antibodies
	CS withdrawal	PMR	History of steroid use, rapid symptom onset
Other conditions	Fibromyalgia	RA, SLE, PMR	Widespread pain, normal inflammatory markers
	Sarcoidosis	SLE, RA, vasculitis	Bilateral hilar lymphadenopathy, elevated ACE levels
	Vitamin D deficiency	Myopathy, fibromyalgia	Low serum vitamin D, non-inflammatory findings

References

1. Bojinca V, Janta I. Rheumatic diseases and malignancies. Maedica (Bucur). 2012;7:364–71.
2. Tagoe CE, Zezon A, Khattri S. Rheumatic manifestations of autoimmune thyroid disease: the other autoimmune disease. J Rheumatol. 2012;39:1125–9. https://doi.org/10.3899/jrheum.120022.
3. Satoh M, Vánquez-Del Mercado M, Chan EKL. Clinical interpretation of antinuclear antibody tests in systemic rheumatic diseases. Mod Rheumatol. 2009;19:219–28. https://doi.org/10.1007/s10165-009-0155-3.

4. Rönnelid J, Turesson C, Kastbom A. Autoantibodies in rheumatoid arthritis—laboratory and clinical perspectives. Front Immunol. 2021;12:685312. https://doi.org/10.3389/fimmun.2021.685312.
5. Sharma V, Sharma A. Infectious mimics of rheumatoid arthritis. Best Pract Res Clin Rheumatol. 2022;36:101736. https://doi.org/10.1016/j.berh.2021.101736.
6. Jacobson AF. Musculoskeletal pain as an indicator of occult malignancy. Yield of bone scintigraphy. Arch Intern Med. 1997;157:105–9.
7. Martínez-Lavín M. Hypertrophic osteoarthropathy. Best Pract Res Clin Rheumatol. 2020;34:101507. https://doi.org/10.1016/j.berh.2020.101507.
8. Orton C, Topham C, Madigan LM. Paraneoplastic dermatomyositis. Am J Med. 2022;135:969–71. https://doi.org/10.1016/j.amjmed.2022.01.016.
9. Bornstein G, Furie N, Perel N, Ben-Zvi I, Grossman C. Hematological malignancies mimicking rheumatic syndromes: case series and review of the literature. Rheumatol Int. 2018;38:1743–9. https://doi.org/10.1007/s00296-018-4107-0.
10. Sing BSM, Wan SA, Cheong YK, Chuah SL, The CL, Jobli AT. Arthritis as an initial presentation of malignancy: two case reports. J Med Case Rep. 2021;15:94. https://doi.org/10.1186/s13256-020-02642-z.
11. Kepp FH, Huber FA, Wurnig MC, Mannil M, Kaniewska M, Guglielmi R, et al. Differentiation of inflammatory from degenerative changes in the sacroiliac joints my machine learning supported texture analysis. Eur J Radiol. 2021;140:109755. https://doi.org/10.1016/j.ejrad.2021.109755.
12. Kaeley GS, Bakewell C, Deodhar A. The importance of ultrasound in identifying and differentiating patients with early inflammatory arthritis: a narrative review. Arthritis Res Ther. 2020;22:1. https://doi.org/10.1186/s13075-019-2050-4.
13. Wasserman AM. Diagnosis and management of rheumatoid arthritis. Am Fam Physician. 2011;84:1245–52.
14. Abramoff B, Caldera FE. Osteoarthritis: pathology, diagnosis, and treatment options. Med Clin North Am. 2020;104:293–311. https://doi.org/10.1016/j.mcna.2019.10.007.
15. Wenham CYJ, Grainger AJ, Conaghan PG. The role of imaging modalities in the diagnosis, differential diagnosis and clinical assessment of peripheral joint osteoarthritis. Osteoarthr Cartil. 2014;22:1692–702. https://doi.org/10.1016/j.joca.2014.06.005.
16. He Y, Sawalha AH. Drug-induced lupus erythematosus: an update on drugs and mechanisms. Curr Opin Rheumatol. 2018;30:490–7. https://doi.org/10.1097/BOR.0000000000000522.
17. Gediz F, Kobak S. Immune checkpoint inhibitors-related rheumatic diseases: what rheumatologist should know? Curr Rheumatol Rev. 2019;15:201–8. https://doi.org/10.2174/1573397115666190119094736.
18. Miernik S, Matusiewicz A, Olesińka M. Drug-induced myopathies: a comprehensive review and update. Biomedicine. 2024;12:987. https://doi.org/10.3390/biomedicines12050987.
19. Friend R, Bennett RM. Distinguishing fibromyalgia form rheumatoid arthritis and systemic lupus in clinical questionnaires: an analysis of the revised fibromyalgia impact questionnaire (FIQR): and its variant, the symptom impact questionnaire (SIQR), along with pain locations. Arthritis Res Ther. 2011;13:R58. https://doi.org/10.1186/ar3311.
20. Galvez-Sánchez CM, Paso GA. Diagnostic criteria for fibromyalgia: critical review and future perspectives. J Clin Med. 2020;9:1219. https://doi.org/10.3390/jcm9041219.
21. Meszaros ZS, Perl A, Faraone SV. Psychiatric symptoms in systemic lupus erythematosus: a systematic review. J Clin Psychiatry. 2012;73:993–1001. https://doi.org/10.4088/JCP.11r07425.
22. Petri M, Nagibuddin M, Carson KA, Wallace D, Weisman MH, Holliday S, et al. Brain magnetic resonance imaging in newly diagnosed systemic lupus erythematosus. J Rheumatol. 2008;35:2348–54. https://doi.org/10.3899/jrheum.071010.

9 Pitfalls in Rheumatoid Arthritis

Abbreviations

bDMARDs	Biologic DMARDs
CCP	Cyclic citrullinated peptide
CS	Corticosteroids
csDMARDs	Conventional synthetic disease-modifying anti-rheumatic drugs
CVD	Cardiovascular disease
GI	Gastrointestinal
IL-6	Interleukin-6
ILD	Interstitial lung disease
JAKi	Janus kinase inhibitors
LDA	Low disease activity
LEF	Leflunomide
LFTs	Liver function tests
MRI	Magnetic resonance imaging
MTX	Methotrexate
OA	Osteoarthritis
PFTs	Pulmonary function tests
PsA	Psoriatic arthritis
PUK	Peripheral ulcerative keratopathy
QoL	Quality of life
RA	Rheumatoid arthritis
RF	Rheumatoid factor
SLE	Systemic lupus erythematosus
TB	Tuberculosis
TNFi	Tumour necrosis factor-alpha inhibitors
tsDMARDs	Targeted synthetic DMARDs
US	Ultrasound

E. Pelechas et al., *Pitfalls in Rheumatology*,
https://doi.org/10.1007/978-3-031-98671-0_9

9.1 Delayed Diagnosis

One of the earliest and most significant pitfalls in RA management is delayed diagnosis. RA symptoms often start subtly and may be mistaken for other conditions, such as OA or SLE or crystal arthropathies. Patients may present with non-specific symptoms like fatigue, minor joint stiffness or low-grade fever before joint inflammation becomes overt. In some cases, joint pain might even be intermittent, leading to a delay in seeking medical attention [1, 2].

Consequences of Delayed Diagnosis (a) *Joint damage*: without early treatment, irreversible joint damage can occur within the first few months of the disease onset [3]. In Fig. 9.1, a 55-year-old patient with untreated RA is shown; (b) *systemic involvement*: RA can affect organs beyond the joints, such as the lungs, heart and eyes [4]. Delaying treatment increases the risk of complications like ILD or cardiovascular issues [5]; (c) *reduced treatment response*: early aggressive therapy is linked to better long-term outcomes [6]. Delaying diagnosis reduces the window for effective intervention, making it harder to achieve disease remission.

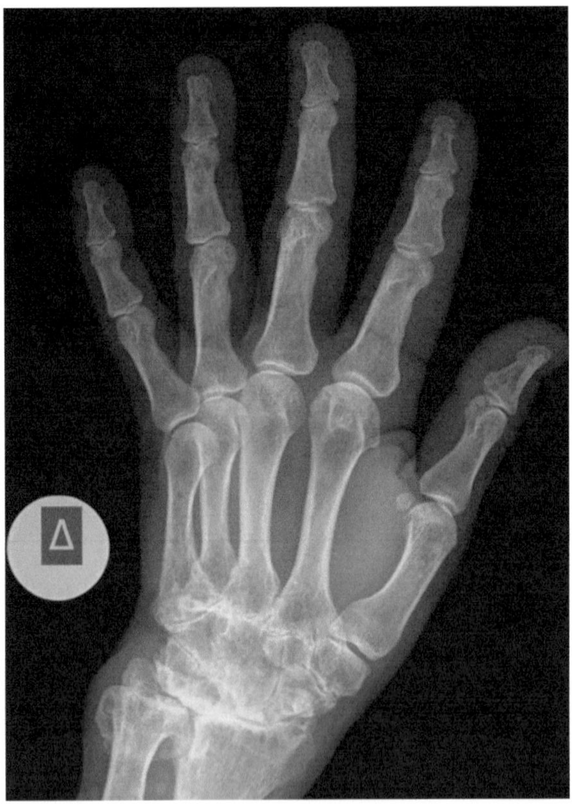

Fig. 9.1 Hand X-ray with total ankylosis of the wrist due to delayed diagnosis and treatment in a 55-year-old female with RA

Overcoming This Pitfall Public awareness campaigns and better screening tools in primary care settings can help promote early detection. Additionally, healthcare providers should maintain a high index of suspicion when patients, particularly women aged 40–60, present with joint pain or stiffness.

9.2 Misdiagnosis and Overdiagnosis

The diagnostic criteria for RA can overlap with other inflammatory diseases, and distinguishing RA from conditions like SLE, PsA or fibromyalgia is often challenging. Blood markers like RF and anti-CCP are useful but not definitive. A patient can have RA with negative markers (seronegative RA) or have positive markers without clinical RA [7].

Risk of Misdiagnosis (a) *Inappropriate* treatment: misdiagnosing RA can lead to the inappropriate use of immunosuppressive therapies, which may expose patients to unnecessary side effects without benefit [8]; (b) *progression of the true disease*: in cases of misdiagnosed RA with another condition, patients are left untreated for the actual condition, which could worsen while receiving incorrect therapy [9].

Overcoming This Pitfall Employing diagnostic tools such as imaging (X-rays, US or MRI) and consulting rheumatology specialists early in the diagnostic process can help refine the diagnosis. Always have in mind that a patient with arthritis can be easily screened with conventional X-rays [10, 11] (Fig. 9.2). A detailed clinical history, careful examination and ongoing re-evaluation over time are essential.

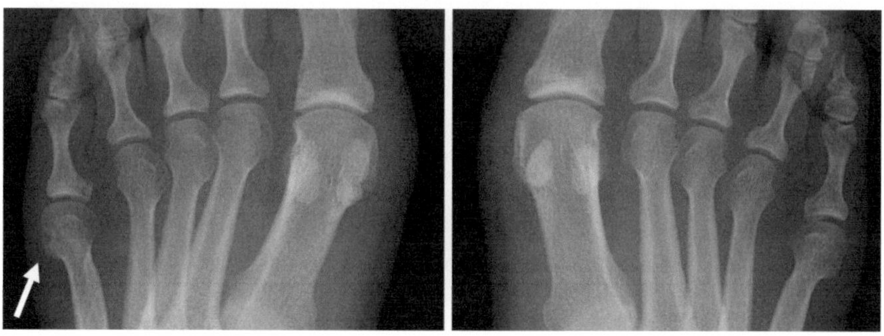

Fig. 9.2 Feet X-ray in a 40-year-old female with morning stiffness lasting >30 min and no findings on hand X-ray. The white arrow points a small erosion of the fifth metatarsal head of the right foot

9.3 Suboptimal Treatment Strategies

RA treatment has dramatically evolved, with csDMARDs like MTX, LEF, bDMARDs (e.g. TNFi and IL-6i) and tsDMARDs (JAKi) significantly improving patient outcomes. However, not all patients receive optimal treatment for various reasons, including physician hesitance, comorbidities, patient non-compliance and socioeconomic factors [12].

Pitfalls in Treatment (a) *Undertreatment*: some clinicians may undertreat RA, especially in elderly patients or those with mild symptoms, fearing side effects. This "wait and see" approach can allow the disease to progress, causing joint erosion and systemic complications, often losing the "window of opportunity" period for treatment [13]; (b) *overtreatment*: on the flip side, aggressive treatment without proper monitoring can lead to complications, particularly from the long-term use of CS or bDMARDs. These medications increase the risk of infections, osteoporosis and other adverse effects, some of them being more rare, if not managed carefully [14, 15]; (c) *lack of personalised treatment*: RA is a heterogeneous disease, and what works for one patient may not work for another. Failure to individualise therapy can result in suboptimal control and an increased risk of complications and side effects from the treatment.

Overcoming This Pitfall Rheumatologists should aim for early and aggressive treatment strategies, titrating medications to minimise disease activity while carefully monitoring for side effects. Furthermore, dose reduction of medications in cases of long-term disease remission should be pursued to minimise cumulative exposure and reduce the risk of adverse effects. Sharing decision-making with patients is critical, ensuring they understand the risks and benefits of therapy and encouraging adherence. Regular follow-ups and using a treat-to-target approach aiming for remission or LDA are essential.

9.4 Medication Side Effects and Toxicity

RA medications, though highly effective, come with their own set of challenges. MTX, for example, is a cornerstone of RA treatment [16] but carries risks such as liver toxicity, bone marrow suppression and GI disturbances. On the other hand, bDMARDs, while revolutionary in controlling inflammation, increase the risk of infections, including TB and opportunistic pathogens [17]. JAKi appear to increase the risk of thromboembolic events and malignancy risks [18].

Pitfalls Related to Medication Toxicity (a) *Inadequate monitoring*: regular monitoring of blood counts, LFTs and screening for latent infections is essential but often overlooked. Inadequate follow-up may allow preventable side effects to go unnoticed until they cause serious harm; (b) *patient non-adherence*: fear of side effects can lead to poor adherence, where patients reduce their medication dosage or stop taking it entirely, increasing the risk of disease flares and joint destruction [19]; (c) *medication adjustment*: in cases of prolonged remission or in the presence of coexisting conditions, failure to appropriately titrate the dose (either increasing or decreasing) may lead to unnecessary overtreatment on one hand and potentially harmful undertreatment on the other.

Overcoming This Pitfall Regular laboratory monitoring and patient education are crucial to managing these risks. Rheumatologists should communicate clearly about the importance of adherence while addressing concerns over side effects. Additionally, preventive measures like vaccinating against influenza, pneumococcus and eventually herpes zoster, as well as screening for TB and hepatitis, can mitigate the risks associated mostly with bDMARDs and tsDMARDs [20]. Finally, in all immunosuppressed patients, the importance of early initiation of antibiotic therapy in the event of an infection and the immediate discontinuation of immunosuppression should be emphasized, due to the increased risk of complications they face.

9.5 Extra-articular Manifestations

RA is not confined to the joints. It can affect multiple organ systems, leading to complications such as CVD, pulmonary fibrosis, vasculitis, eye involvement (Fig. 9.3) and rheumatoid nodules. Many clinicians and patients may focus exclusively on joint symptoms, overlooking the broader systemic implications of the disease [21].

Pitfalls of Ignoring Extra-articular Disease (a) *CVD risk*: RA patients have a significantly increased risk of CVD, which is a leading cause of mortality in this population. Chronic inflammation accelerates atherosclerosis, but this risk is often underappreciated [22]; (b) *pulmonary complications*: ILD is a serious complication in RA and can progress to respiratory failure [23]. Symptoms may be subtle and easily missed without vigilant monitoring. Figure 9.4 shows a 79-year-old patient with a rheumatoid nodule and reticulonodular interstitial findings on a chest X-ray.

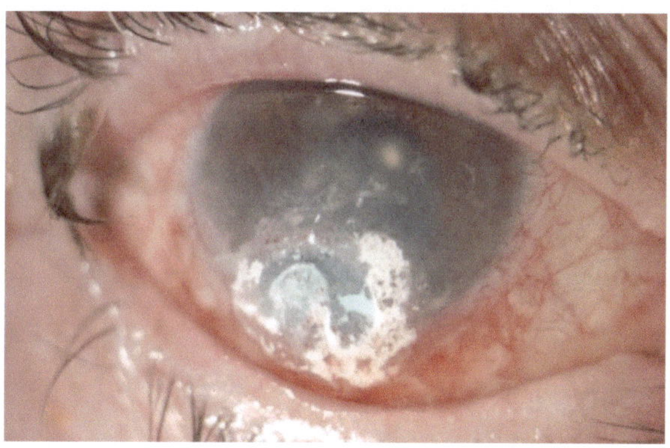

Fig. 9.3 PUK in a patient with RA. Thinning of the peripheral cornea and perforation. Therapeutic application of cyanoacrylate corneal glue has been performed

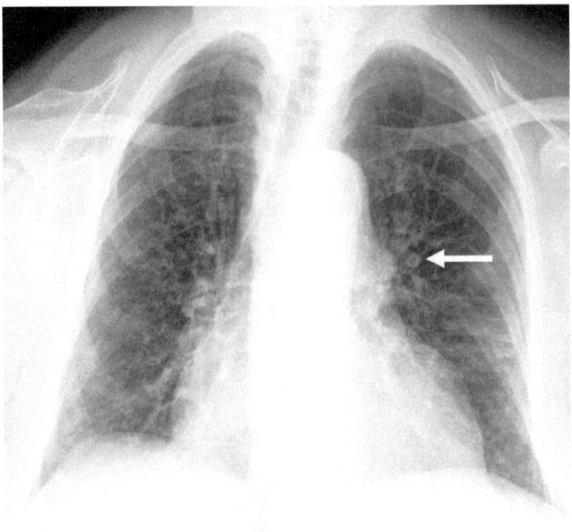

Fig. 9.4 Chest X-ray of a 79-year-old patient with a rheumatoid nodule (white arrow) and reticulonodular opacities (confirmed by CT scanning)

Overcoming This Pitfall A multidisciplinary approach is essential in managing RA. Collaboration with cardiologists, pulmonologists and other specialists is necessary to address systemic manifestations. Clinicians should assess cardiovascular risk factors (cholesterol levels, smoking habits, etc.) regularly and monitor for lung symptoms, using appropriate imaging of PFTs when needed. Finally, adequate control of inflammation should be pursued, as it is directly linked to the increased cardiovascular risk in RA.

9.6 Psychosocial Factors and Mental Health

RA is a life-altering disease that affects patients physically, emotionally and socially. Depression, anxiety and fatigue are common comorbidities that often go unaddressed in the clinical setting, yet they have a profound impact on a patient's quality of life and treatment adherence [24].

Pitfalls Related to Mental Health (a) *Under-recognised depression and anxiety*: mental health issues are frequently underdiagnosed and untreated in RA patients, despite their high prevalence. Depression can exacerbate pain perception and reduce the likelihood of successful disease management; (b) *social isolation and work disability*: the physical limitations caused by RA can lead to reduced mobility, social withdrawal and difficulty maintaining employment, all of which contribute to the psychological burden [25].

Overcoming This Pitfall Incorporating mental health screenings into routine RA care is essential. Cognitive–behavioural therapy, social support and medications like anti-depressants can improve the emotional well-being of RA patients. Moreover, addressing fatigue through lifestyle modifications, exercise and medication adjustments can significantly enhance overall functioning and QoL [26].

9.7 Conclusion

Managing RA is fraught with potential pitfalls that can hinder effective treatment and worsen outcomes if not proactively addressed. Early and accurate diagnosis, vigilant monitoring for medication side effects and a holistic approach that considers both joint and extra-articular symptoms are essential for optimising care. Additionally, integrating regular exercise, mental health and psychosocial support into the treatment plan can improve adherence, reduce disability and enhance the overall quality of life for RA patients. By recognising and navigating these pitfalls, healthcare providers and patients can work together to control the disease and minimise its long-term impact.

References

1. Taylor PC. Update on the diagnosis and management of early rheumatoid arthritis. Clin Med (Lond). 2020;20:561–4. https://doi.org/10.7861/clinmed.2020.0727.
2. Pelechas E, Kaltsonoudis E, Voulgari PV, Drosos AA. Rheumatoid arthritis. In: Illustrated handbook of rheumatic and musculo-skeletal diseases. Cham: Springer; 2023. https://doi.org/10.1007/978-3-031-47379-1_5.
3. Drosos AA, Pelechas E, Voulgari PV. Treatment strategies are more important than drugs in the management of rheumatoid arthritis. Clin Rheumatol. 2020;39:1363–8. https://doi.org/10.1007/s10067-020-05001-x.
4. Wu D, Luo Y, Li T, Zhao X, Lv T, Fang G, et al. Systemic complications of rheumatoid arthritis: focus on pathogenesis and treatment. Front Immunol. 2022;13:1051082. https://doi.org/10.3389/fimmu.2022.1051082.
5. Drosos AA, Venetsanopoulou AA, Pelechas E, Voulgari PV. Exploring cardiovascular risk factors and atherosclerosis in rheumatoid arthritis. Eur J Intern Med. 2024;128:1–9. https://doi.org/10.1016/j.ejim.2024.07.016.
6. Resman-Targoff BH, Cicero M. Aggressive treatment of early rheumatoid arthritis: recognizing the window of opportunity and treating to target goals. Am J Manag Care. 2010;16:S249–58.
7. Van Delft MAM, Huizinga TWJ. An overview of autoantibodies in rheumatoid arthritis. J Autoimmun. 2020;110:102392. https://doi.org/10.1016/j.jaut.2019.102392.
8. Drosos AA, Pelechas E, Voulgari PV. A patient with symmetrical polyarthritis. The value of conventional radiography for a correct diagnosis. Rheumatol Ther. 2022;9:771–9. https://doi.org/10.1007/s40744-022-00426-z.
9. Agelii ML, Hafström I, Svensson B, Ajeganova S, Forslind K, Andersson M, et al. Misdiagnosis of rheumatoid arthritis in a long-term cohort of early arthritis based on the ACR-1987 classification criteria. Open Access Rheumatol. 2022;14:187–94. https://doi.org/10.2147/OARRR.S372724.
10. Drosos AA, Pelechas E, Voulgari PV. Radiological findings of the cervical spine in rheumatoid arthritis: what a rheumatologist should know. Curr Rheumatol Rep. 2020;22:19. https://doi.org/10.1007/s11926-020-00894-8.

11. Drosos AA, Pelechas E, Voulgari PV. Conventional radiography of the hands and wrists in rheumatoid arthritis. What a rheumatologist should know and how to interpret the radiological findings. Rheumatol Int. 2019;39:1331–41. https://doi.org/10.1007/s00296-019-04326-4.
12. Gavigan K, Nowell WB, Serna MS, Stark JL, Yassine M, Curtis JR. Barriers to treatment optimization and achievement of patient' goals: perspectives from people living with rheumatoid arthritis enrolled in the ArthritisPower registry. Arthritis Res Ther. 2020;22:4. https://doi.org/10.1186/s13075-019-2076-7.
13. Burgers LE, Raza K, van der Helm-van MA. Window of opportunity in rheumatoid arthritis—definitions and supporting evidence: from old to new perspectives. RMD Open. 2019;5:e000870. https://doi.org/10.1136/rmdopen-2018-000870.
14. Skalkou A, Pelechas E, Voulgari PV, Drosos AA. TNF-induced lupus. A case-based review. Curr Rheumatol Rev. 2022;18:72–82. https://doi.org/10.2174/1573397117666211102094330.
15. Pelechas E, Memi T, Markatseli TE, Voulgari PV, Drosos AA. Adalimumab-induced myasthenia gravis: case-based review. Rheumatol Int. 2020;40:1891–4. https://doi.org/10.1007/s00296-020-04587-4.
16. Weinblatt ME. Methotrexate in rheumatoid arthritis: a quarter century of development. Trans Am Clin Climatol Assoc. 2013;124:16–25.
17. Singh JA, Cameron C, Noorbaloochi S, Cullis T, Tucker M, Christensen R, et al. Risk of serious infection in biological treatment of patients with rheumatoid arthritis: a systematic review and meta-analysis. Lancet. 2015;386:258–65. https://doi.org/10.1016/S0140-6736(14)61704-9.
18. Molander V, Bower H, Frisell T, Delcoigne B, Di Giuseppe D, Askling J. Venous thromboembolism with JAK inhibitors and other immune-modulatory drugs: a Swedish comparative safety study among patients with rheumatoid arthritis. Ann Rheum Dis. 2023;82:189–97. https://doi.org/10.1136/ard-20220223050.
19. Marengo M, Suarez-Almazor ME. Improving treatment adherence in patients with rheumatoid arthritis: what are the options? Int J Clin Rheumatol. 2015;10:345–56. https://doi.org/10.2217/ijr.15.39.
20. Bass AR, Chakravarty E, Akl EA, Bingham CO, Calabrese L, Cappelli L, et al. American College of Rheumatology guideline for vaccinations in patients with rheumatic and musculoskeletal diseases. Arthritis Care Res (Hoboken). 2022;2023(75):449–64. https://doi.org/10.1002/acr.25045.
21. Kim JW, Suh CH. Systemic manifestations and complications in patients with rheumatoid arthritis. J Clin Med. 2020;9:2008. https://doi.org/10.3390/jcm9062008.
22. Venetsanopoulou AI, Pelechas E, Voulgari PV, Drosos AA. The lipid paradox in rheumatoid arthritis: the dark horse of the augmented cardiovascular risk. Rheumatol Int. 2020;40:1181–91. https://doi.org/10.1007/s00296-020-04616-2.
23. Bendstrup E, Møller J, Kronborg-White S, Prior TS, Hyldgaard C. Interstitial lung disease in rheumatoid arthritis remains a challenge for clinicians. J Clin Med. 2019;21:2038. https://doi.org/10.3390/jcm8122038.
24. Ionescu CE, Popescu CC, Agache M, Dinache G, Codreanu C. Depression in rheumatoid arthritis: a narrative review-diagnostic challenges, pathogenic mechanisms and effects. Medicina (Kaunas). 2022;58:1637. https://doi.org/10.3390/medicina58111637.
25. Bay LT, Ellingsen T, Giraldi A, Graugaard C, Nielsen DS. "To be lonely in your own loneliness": the interplay between self-perceived loneliness and rheumatoid arthritis in everyday life: a qualitative study. Musculoskeletal Care. 2020;18:450–8. https://doi.org/10.1002/msc.1480.
26. Chehade L, Jaafar ZA, Masri DE, Zmerly H, Kreidieh D, Tannir H, et al. Lifestyle modification in rheumatoid arthritis: dietary and physical activity recommendations based on evidence. Curr Rheumatol Rev. 2019;15:209–14. https://doi.org/10.2174/1573397115666190121135940.

Pitfalls in Psoriatic Arthritis

10

Abbreviations

AS	Ankylosing spondylitis
bDMARDs	Biologic DMARDs
CS	Corticosteroids
csDMARDs	Conventional synthetic DMARDs
CVD	Cardiovascular disease
DMARDs	Disease-modifying anti-rheumatic drugs
IL-17i	Interleukin-17 inhibitors
JAKi	Janus kinase inhibitors
LDA	Low disease activity
MRI	Magnetic resonance imaging
MTX	Methotrexate
OA	Osteoarthritis
PEST	Psoriasis epidemiology screening tool
PsA	Psoriatic arthritis
QoL	Quality of life
RA	Rheumatoid arthritis
RMDs	Rheumatic diseases
TNFi	Tumour necrosis factor alpha inhibitors
tsDMARDs	Targeted synthetic DMARDs
US	Ultrasound

E. Pelechas et al., *Pitfalls in Rheumatology*,
https://doi.org/10.1007/978-3-031-98671-0_10

10.1 Delayed or Missed Diagnosis

One of the most significant pitfalls in PsA management is delayed or missed diagnosis [1]. PsA can develop years after the onset of psoriasis, but many patients with skin involvement do not connect their joint symptoms to the underlying psoriatic disease. Furthermore, PsA can be confused with other forms of arthritis, including RA, AS, OA, trauma or gout, as the joint involvement may mimic these conditions [2]. In Fig. 10.1, a 27-year-old male with skin psoriasis presented to an orthopaedic doctor with foot pain, and he attributed the findings to old trauma.

Consequences of Delayed Diagnosis (a) *Joint damage*: without early intervention, PsA can lead to permanent joint damage and deformities. Bone erosion and destruction of cartilage can occur rapidly in untreated patients with devastating results that may need surgical interventions in order to get fixed [3]; (b) *reduced treatment efficacy*: delayed diagnosis often correlates with delayed treatment initiation, leading to a diminished response to therapy and lower chances of achieving remission.

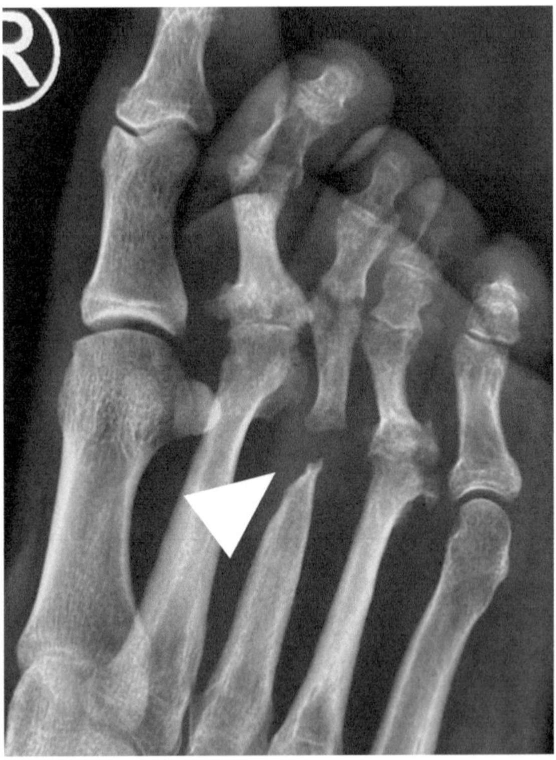

Fig. 10.1 Foot X-ray showing a characteristic lesion of PsA named "licked candy stick" appearance with total resorption of the third metatarsophalangeal bone (white arrowhead)

Overcoming This Pitfall Dermatologists and primary care physicians should be vigilant in screening psoriasis patients for joint symptoms. Simple screening tools, such as the PEST tool, can help identify those at risk. Early referral to a rheumatologist when joint pain, stiffness or swelling is present is essential for timely diagnosis [4].

10.2 Misdiagnosis

PsA can present in various forms, leading to diagnostic confusion with other RMDs or other degenerative arthritides. The clinical overlap between PsA and conditions like RA, AS or gout complicates the diagnostic process. Furthermore, PsA can sometimes appear in patients with small or without obvious skin lesions, making diagnosis even more elusive [5].

Pitfalls in Misdiagnosis (a) *Inappropriate treatment*: a misdiagnosis can lead to improper treatment choices. For example, CS, which are commonly used in RA with good results, can trigger severe flares of skin psoriasis in PsA patients [6]; (b) *uncontrolled disease*: if PsA is treated as a different type of arthritis, the skin and nail involvement may not be adequately addressed, leading to worsening symptoms or a lack of overall disease control.

Overcoming This Pitfall Careful clinical evaluation is critical, with a focus on the presence of psoriasis, dactylitis or nail changes, all of which strongly suggest PsA. Imaging modalities such as MRI and US can help differentiate PsA from other arthritic conditions by showing characteristic features like enthesitis or joint erosions [7]. In Fig. 10.2, MRI of a PsA patient with heel pain is shown that revealed a full-length thickening of the Achilles tendon.

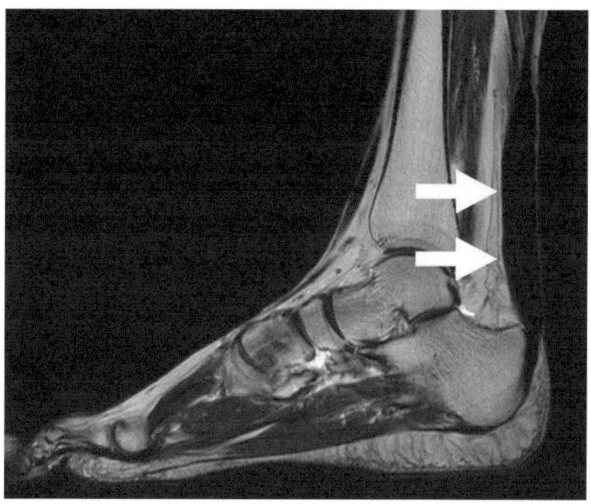

Fig. 10.2 MRI image in sagittal plane with fusiform thickening (white arrows) in full length of the Achilles tendon

10.3 Heterogeneous Disease Presentation

PsA has a wide variety of clinical manifestations, making it a challenging disease to fully assess and treat. The disease can affect peripheral joints, the spine (axial PsA), the entheses and even the fingers and toes in the form of dactylitis. In rare cases, uveitis in a patient with psoriasis may lead the treating clinician to systemic treatment (Fig. 10.3). Each of these domains requires specific therapeutic considerations [8].

Challenges of Heterogeneous Presentation (a) *Suboptimal treatment*: some treatments may work well for one aspect of PsA but fail to address other domains of the disease. For example, a medication that improves peripheral arthritis may not adequately control axial symptoms or enthesitis; (b) *overlooking certain symptoms*: patients and physicians may focus more, on certain symptoms, such as joint pain, while underestimating the impact of enthesitis, dactylitis or skin disease [9].

Overcoming This Pitfall A comprehensive approach to treatment that addresses all aspects of PsA is essential. Rheumatologists should assess patients for symptoms in multiple domains, including skin, nails, joints and entheses, to ensure that the chosen treatment addresses the full spectrum of the disease. Regular follow-ups and multidisciplinary care involving dermatologists are also crucial [9].

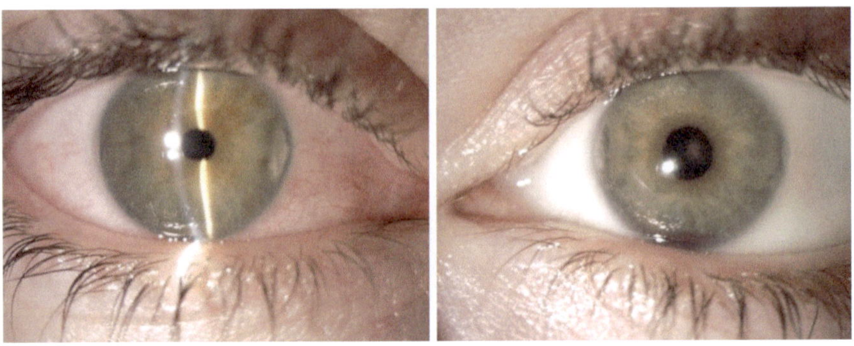

Fig. 10.3 Uveitis in the right eye with a healthy left eye. Perilimbal injection, conjunctival redness, and sphincter pupillae spasm and anisocoria due to inflammation can be also seen

10.4 Inadequate Control of Skin Disease

While joint symptoms are often the focus in PsA, skin involvement remains a central feature of the disease. Many patients have significant psoriasis (Fig. 10.4), which can be resistant to treatment. Inadequate control of skin lesions not only impacts QoL but also increases the risk of long-term complications like metabolic syndrome and CVD [10].

Pitfalls in Treating Skin Disease (a) *Underappreciation of psoriasis*: rheumatologists may focus on joint symptoms and undertreat the skin disease, especially if the psoriasis is not severe; (b) *choosing ineffective therapies*: some medications are better suited for joint disease but may not adequately control psoriasis (conversely, certain medications are more effective for the skin but not as effective for the joints), leading to a disconnect between joint and skin symptom management [11].

Overcoming This Pitfall Choosing DMARDs that target both joint and skin involvement is crucial for managing PsA comprehensively. TNFi, IL-17i, IL-23i and JAKi have shown efficacy in treating both psoriasis and arthritis. Regular assessment of skin and nail symptoms should be incorporated into routine care to ensure full disease control [12].

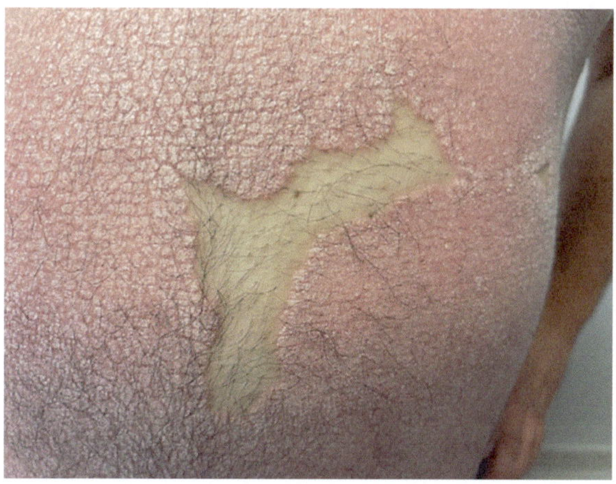

Fig. 10.4 Severe skin involvement in a young patient with psoriasis, treated with topical ointments and lotions by his dermatologist!

10.5 Medication Toxicity and Side Effects

Managing PsA often requires the use of potent immunosuppressive drugs, including traditional csDMARDs like MTX, and bDMARDs such as TNFi, IL-17i or IL-23i as well as the newer tsDMARDs (JAKi). However, these medications come with significant risks (some less and others more), including infections, liver toxicity and increased cancer risk [13, 14].

Pitfalls in Managing Medication Toxicity (a) *Inadequate monitoring*: insufficient monitoring of liver function, blood counts and infection risk can lead to serious complications from all kinds of DMARDs; (b) *CS overuse*: while CS can be useful for acute flares, long-term use is associated with numerous complications, including osteoporosis, diabetes and CVD, and can worsen skin psoriasis; (c) *overtreatment*: in cases of remission, efforts should be made to taper therapy in order to avoid unnecessary cumulative immunosuppression, which increases the risk of treatment-related complications [15].

Overcoming This Pitfall Close monitoring of patients on systemic therapies is essential. Regular blood tests, infection screening, vaccinations and early recognition of adverse effects can prevent serious complications. Physicians should also limit CS use to the shortest duration possible and employ steroid-sparing strategies, using all kinds of DMARDs as a long-term approach. Finally, individualising pharmacologic treatment based on the patient's age and comorbidities will also contribute to reducing medication-related toxicity.

10.6 Cardiovascular and Metabolic Complications

PsA, like psoriasis, is associated with a higher risk of CVD and metabolic syndrome, including obesity, diabetes and hyperlipidaemia. Chronic systemic inflammation contributes to this increased risk, and the traditional focus on skin and joint symptoms may overshadow the need for cardiovascular risk management [16].

Pitfalls of Ignoring Cardiovascular Risks (a) *Increased morbidity and mortality*: failure to address the cardiovascular risks in PsA patients can lead to preventable complications, including heart attacks and strokes; (b) *overlooked risk factors*: physicians may not routinely assess or manage the underlying cardiovascular risk factors in PsA patients, such as hypertension, obesity and insulin resistance.

Overcoming This Pitfall A multidisciplinary approach to PsA management that includes cardiovascular risk assessment is essential [17]. Rheumatologists should work closely with primary care physicians or cardiologists to monitor and treat comorbidities like hypertension, diabetes and dyslipidaemia. Lifestyle interventions, such as weight management, regular exercise and smoking cessation, should also be emphasized as part of the treatment plan [18].

10.7 Impact on Mental Health

PsA is not just a physical disease. It also has a profound impact on mental health. Patients with PsA are at a higher risk for depression, anxiety and reduced QoL, partly due to the visible nature of skin disease and chronic pain and disability associated with joint involvement [19].

Pitfalls Related to Mental Health (a) *Under-recognition of mental health issues*: depression and anxiety are frequently underdiagnosed in PsA patients, even though they significantly contribute to disability and poor treatment adherence; (b) *social isolation*: PsA can lead to embarrassment due to visible psoriasis, as well as physical limitations due to joint pain and stiffness, resulting in social withdrawal and reduced participation in everyday activities.

Overcoming This Pitfall Screening for mental health issues should be a routine part of PsA management [20]. Cognitive–behavioural therapy, counselling or medication may be necessary to address depression and anxiety [21]. Additionally, managing skin disease aggressively can improve body image and confidence, enhancing overall well-being.

10.8 Conclusion

PsA is a complex and multifaceted disease with several potential pitfalls in its diagnosis and management. Delayed or missed diagnosis, suboptimal treatment of its diverse manifestations and the challenges of medication toxicity all pose significant barriers to effective care, Additionally, the increased cardiovascular risk, mental health impact and heterogeneity of PsA require a multidisciplinary and personalised approach to ensure that all aspects of the disease are addressed. By being aware of these pitfalls and adopting a proactive, comprehensive approach, clinicians can improve outcomes and QoL for patients with PsA.

References

1. Haroon M, Gallagher P, FitzGerald O. Diagnostic delay of more than 6 months contributes to poor radiographic and functional outcome in psoriatic arthritis. Ann Rheum Dis. 2015;74:1045–50. https://doi.org/10.1136/annrheumdis-2013-204858.
2. Pelechas E, Kaltsonoudis E, Voulgari PV, Drosos AA. Psoriatic arthritis. In: Illustrated handbook of rheumatic and musculo-skeletal diseases. Cham: Springer; 2023. https://doi.org/10.1007/978-3-031-47379-1_9.
3. Karmacharya P, Wright K, Achenbach SJ, Bekele D, Crowson CS, Ogdie A, et al. Diagnostic delay in psoriatic arthritis: a population-based study. J Rheumatol. 2021;48:1410–6. https://doi.org/10.3899/jrheum.201199.
4. Mease PJ, Palmer JB, Hur P, Strober BE, Lebwohl M, Karki C, et al. Utilization of the validated psoriasis epidemiology screening tool to identify signs and symptoms of psoriatic arthritis among those with psoriasis: a cross-sectional analysis from the US-based Corrona Prosiasis Registry. J Eur Acad Dermatol Venereol. 2019;33:886–92. https://doi.org/10.1111/jdv.15443.

5. Floris A, Mugheddu C, Sichi L, Dessì M, Anedda J, Frau A, et al. The challenging differentiation of psoriatic arthritis from other arthropathies and nonspecific arthralgias in patients with psoriasis: results of a cross-sectional rheumatologic assessment of a large dermatologic cohort. J Clin Med. 2023;12:6090. https://doi.org/10.3390/jcm12188690.
6. Vincken NLA, Balak DMW, Knulst AC, Welsing PMJ, van Laar JM. Systemic glucocorticoid use and the occurrence of flares in psoriatic arthritis and psoriasis: a systematic review. Rheumatology (Oxford). 2022;61:4232–44. https://doi.org/10.1093/rheumatology/keac129.
7. Pelechas E, Kaltsonoudis E, Voulgari PV, Drosos AA. Musculoskeletal ultrasound in rheumatology. In: Illustrated handbook of rheumatic and musculo-skeletal diseases. Cham: Springer; 2023. https://doi.org/10.1007/978-3-031-47379-1_4.
8. Soriano ER, Coates LC, Kavanaugh A. GRAPPA 2021 treatment recommendations for psoriatic arthritis. J Rheumatol. 2023;50:31–2. https://doi.org/10.3899/jrheum.2023-0522.
9. Coates LC, Soriano ER, Corp N, Bertheussen H, Duffin KC, Campanholo CB, et al. Group for research and assessment of psoriasis and psoriatic arthritis (GRAPPA): updated treatment recommendations for psoriatic arthritis 2021. Nat Rev Rheumatol. 2022;18:465–79. https://doi.org/10.1038/s41584-022-00798-0.
10. Zhu TY, Li EK, Tam LS. Cardiovascular risk in patients with psoriatic arthritis. In J Rheumatol. 2012;2012:714321. https://doi.org/10.1155/2012/714321.
11. Pelechas E, Memi T, Voulgari PV, Drosos AA. A case of recalcitrant psoriatic arthritis to TNF inhibitors improved after administration of secukinumab, an IL-17A inhibitor. Rheumatol Ther. 2017;4:509–13. https://doi.org/10.1007/s40744-017-0084-0.
12. Pelechas E, Kaltsonoudis E, Migkos MP, Koletsos N, Karagianni PG, Drosos AA, Voulgari PV. State of the art review on the treatment of psoriatic disease. Mediterr J Rheumatol. 2024;35:66–72. https://doi.org/10.31138/mjr.040123.sot.
13. Bastard L, Claudepierre P, Penso L, Sbidian E, Vegas LP. Risk of serious infection associated with different classes of targeted therapies used in psoriatic arthtitis: a nationwide cohort study from the French health insurance database (SNDS). RMD Open. 2024;10:e003865. https://doi.org/10.1136/rmdopen-2023-003865.
14. Luo X, Deng C, Fei Y, Zhang W, Li Y, Zhang X, et al. Malignancy development risk in psoriatic arthritis patients undergoing treatment: a systematic review and meta-analysis. Semin Arthritis Rheum. 2019;48:626–31.
15. Gossec L, Kerschbaumer A, Ferreira RJO, Aletaha D, Baraliakos X, Bertheussen H, et al. EULAR recommendations for the management of psoriatic arthritis with pharmacological therapies: 2023 update. Ann Rheum Dis. 2024;83:706–19. https://doi.org/10.1136/ard-2024-225531.
16. Gupta S, Syrimi Z, Hughes DM, Zhao SS. Comorbidities in psoriatic arthritis: a systematic review and meta-analysis. Rheumatol Int. 2021;41:275–84. https://doi.org/10.1007/s00296-020-04775-2.
17. Zheng YX, Zheng M. A multidisciplinary team for the diagnosis and management of psoriatic arthritis. Chin Med J. 2021;134:1387–9. https://doi.org/10.1097/CM9.0000000000001588.
18. Betteridge N, Boehncke WH, Bundy C, Gossec L, Gratacós J, Augustin M. Promoting patient-centred care in psoriatic arthritis: a multidisciplinary European perspective on improving the patient experience. J Eur Acad Dermatol Venereol. 2015;30:576–85. https://doi.org/10.1111/jdv.133306.
19. Mathew A, Chandran V. Depression in psoriatic arthritis: dimensional aspects and link with systemic inflammation. Rheumatol Ther. 2020;7:287–300. https://doi.org/10.1007/s40744-020-00207-6.
20. Frede N, Hiestand S, Schauer F, Endres D, van Elst LT, Zeisbrich M, et al. Psoriasis and psoriatic arthritis have a major impact on quality of life and depressive symptoms: a cross-sectional study of 300 patients. Rheumatol Ther. 2023;10:1655–68. https://doi.org/10.1007/s40744-023-00602-9.
21. Batko B. Patient-centered care in psoriatic arthritis—a perspective on inflammation, disease activity, and psychosocial factors. J Clin Med. 2020;9:3103. https://doi.org/10.3390/jcm9103103.

Pitfalls in Ankylosing Spondylitis

11

Abbreviations

AS	Ankylosing spondylitis
ASAS	Assessment of spondyloarthritis international society
bDMARDs	Biologic DMARDs
CVD	Cardiovascular
DMARDs	Disease-modifying anti-rheumatic drugs
GI	Gastrointestinal
HLA	Human leucocyte antigen
IBD	Inflammatory bowel disease
IL-17i	Interleukin 17 inhibitors
JAKi	Janus kinase inhibitors
LBP	Low back pain
LDA	Low disease activity
MRI	Magnetic resonance imaging
NSAIDs	Non-steroidal anti-inflammatory drugs
QoL	Quality of life
ROM	Range of motion
SI	Sacroiliac
SpA	Spondyloarthritis
T2T	Treat-to-target
TB	Tuberculosis
TNFi	Tumour necrosis factor alpha inhibitors
tsDMARDs	Targeted synthetic DMARDs

E. Pelechas et al., *Pitfalls in Rheumatology*,
https://doi.org/10.1007/978-3-031-98671-0_11

11.1 Delayed Diagnosis

One of the most significant and common pitfalls in AS is delayed diagnosis [1]. The symptoms of AS often begin subtly, with LBP and stiffness, and are frequently mistaken for mechanical back pain, muscle strain or degenerative disc disease [2]. Furthermore, since AS usually affects younger adults (often males in their 20s or 30s), there is a tendency to attribute their symptoms to activity-related injuries or poor posture rather than an underlying systemic disease.

Consequences of Delayed Diagnosis (a) *Permanent structural damage*: the delay in diagnosis often leads to ongoing inflammation, causing progressive spinal damage, bone formation and fusion of vertebrae (Fig. 11.1) and sacroiliac joints (see Fig. 12.2a). This can lead to decreased spinal mobility and chronic pain [3]; (b) *reduced treatment response*: delayed intervention reduces the likelihood of achieving optimal disease control and can limit the effectiveness of available treatment in halting disease progression; (c) *decreased quality of life*: persistent symptoms without a diagnosis often result in decreased physical activity, social isolation and poor mental health [4].

Overcoming This Pitfall Educating primary care physicians and physical therapists about the hallmark features of AS, such as morning stiffness that improves with activity, alternating buttock pain and the presence of inflammatory markers, is crucial. Early referral to a rheumatologist for imaging and testing, including SI joint MRI and HLA-B27 genetic testing, can significantly reduce diagnostic delays [5].

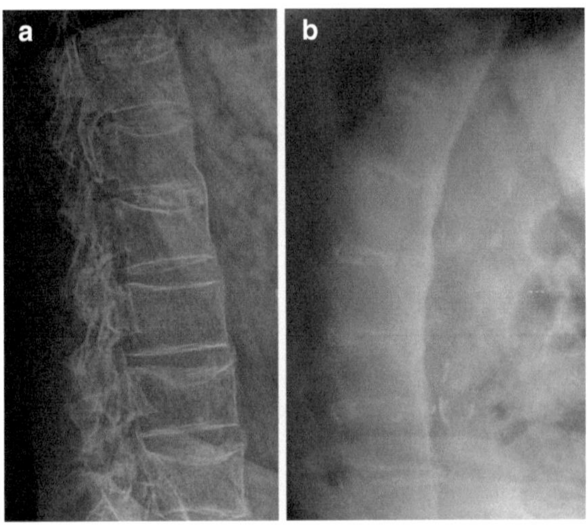

Fig. 11.1 (**a**) Fine ossification of the anterior longitudinal ligament and (**b**) complete fusion of the vertebrae in two different stages of patients with a delayed diagnosis of ankylosing spondylitis

11.2 Misdiagnosis

Due to the overlapping symptoms of AS with other conditions that cause back pain, misdiagnosis is another common pitfall. Mechanical back pain, degenerative arthritis, fibromyalgia, congenital disorders of the spine and even herniated discs can mimic the symptoms of AS. Additionally, AS can occur without classic radiographic findings early in the disease course, leading to an incorrect diagnosis or prolonged uncertainty [6, 7].

Consequences of Misdiagnosis (a) *Inappropriate treatment*: patients may receive inappropriate therapies, such as over-reliance on opioids or muscle relaxants, which do not address the underlying inflammatory process. Worse, some treatments may exacerbate the disease or its symptoms [8]; (b) *worsening disease activity*: misdiagnosed patients may experience ongoing inflammation and structural damage due to the lack of appropriate anti-inflammatory treatments like NSAIDs or treatments with DMARDs.

Overcoming This Pitfall Diagnostic tools such as MRI can detect SI joint inflammation early in the disease, even when X-rays show no abnormalities [9]. Clinicians should have a high index of suspicion for AS in young patients with chronic back pain, especially if the pain improves with activity and worsens with rest. Utilising criteria such as the ASAS classification can also help guide diagnosis [10].

11.3 Underappreciation of Extra-Spinal Manifestations

Although AS primarily affects the spine and SI joints, it can also present with extra-spinal manifestations such as uveitis, enthesitis, peripheral arthritis and IBD (Fig. 11.2). Overlooking these features can lead to an incomplete understanding of the patient's disease and suboptimal treatment [11].

Pitfalls of Overlooking Extra-Spinal Involvement (a) *Inadequate treatment*: patients with significant extra-spinal symptoms may require specific treatments, such as bDMARDs, that target both spinal and non-spinal inflammation. Focusing solely on spinal symptoms may result in undertreatment [12]; (b) *complication form untreated disease*: uveitis, a common manifestation of AS, can lead to blindness if not properly managed. Similarly, untreated IBD can lead to serious GI complications [13]. Furthermore, a delayed recognition and intervention in enthesitis may lead to tendon rupture and significant disability.

Overcoming This Pitfall A thorough assessment of patients should include screening for uveitis, enthesitis (especially heel pain) and GI symptoms. Collaboration with ophthalmologists and gastroenterologists may be required for

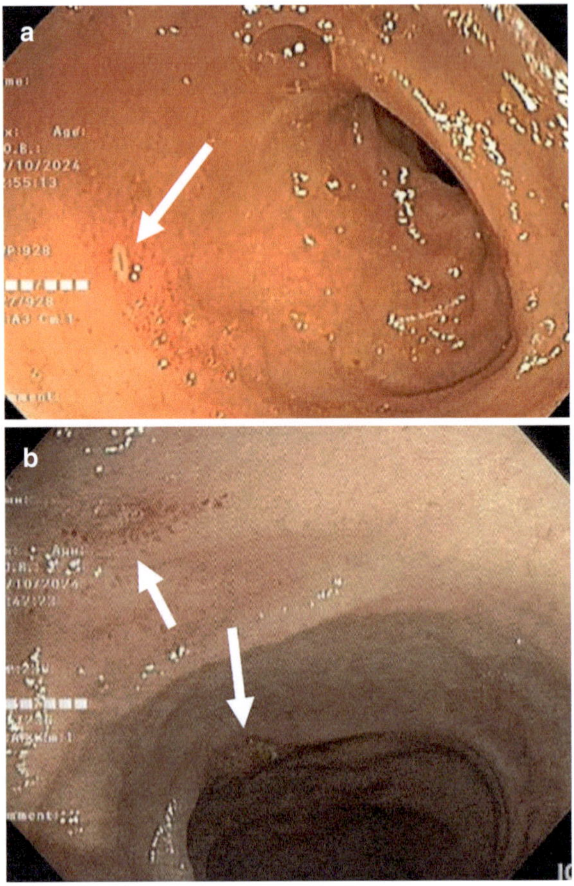

Fig. 11.2 Aphthous ulcers in the terminal ileum in a patient diagnosed with ankylosing spondylitis. The findings are typical for Crohn's disease

comprehensive management. Treating AS with bDMARDs or tsDMARDs that target the underlying inflammatory pathways, such as TNFi, IL-17i or JAKi, can also improve extra-articular symptoms [14].

11.4 Suboptimal Treatment Choices

The treatment of AS has evolved with the advent of biologic therapies, especially TNF inhibitors and IL-17 inhibitors, which have revolutionised care. However, there are still unmet needs and pitfalls related to suboptimal treatment choices [15]. These include over-reliance on NSAIDs, inadequate use of b and tsDMARDs or failure to escalate treatment when needed.

Pitfalls in Treatment Choices (a) *Over-reliance on NSAIDs*: while NSAIDs are the first-line treatment for AS, they may not be sufficient to control disease activity in many patients. Long-term NSAID use can also lead to GI, renal and cardiovascular side effects [16]; (b) *inadequate use of b and tsDMARDs*: some physicians may hesitate to start DMARDs due to concerns about side effects or cost, despite the strong evidence for their safety and effectiveness in controlling disease progression; (c) *failure to escalate therapy*: some patients with moderate to severe disease or with significant disease activity are not treated aggressively enough, leading to uncontrolled symptoms and long-term complications [17].

Overcoming This Pitfall Physicians should follow a T2T approach in AS management, aiming for remission or alternatively for LDA. Early initiation of bDMARDs, particularly in patients with high disease activity or extra-articular manifestations, should be considered to prevent long-term structural damage [18]. Additionally, patient education about the benefits of biologic therapy is crucial to improve adherence [19].

11.5 Medication Side Effects and Toxicity

Although DMARDs have transformed the management of AS, they come with their own risks, including infections, malignancies and rare adverse events like demyelination [20]. NSAIDs, which are commonly used, can cause GI ulcers, hypertension and renal impairment if used long-term.

Pitfalls of Medication Toxicity (a) *Infections*: patients on DMARD therapies, especially TNFi, are at increased risk of serious infections, including TB, which can complicate treatment; (b) *long-term NSAID use*: chronic use of NSAIDs without appropriate monitoring can lead to GI bleeding, kidney damage and cardiovascular events; (c) *poor patient adherence*: fear of side effects may cause patients to stop taking medications or reduce their dose, leading to disease flares and worsening outcomes; (d) *non-individualised treatment*: therapy that is not tailored to the specific needs of the disease—both in terms of drug selection and dosing—may lead to overtreatment or undertreatment.

Overcoming This Pitfall Before starting bDMARDs or tsDMARDs therapy, patients should undergo screening for TB and other infections [21]. Regular follow-up visits are necessary to monitor for side effects, and patients should be educated about the importance of medication adherence and the risks of untreated disease. For those on long-term NSAIDs, regular GI and renal function monitoring as well as blood pressure monitoring should be part of routine care.

11.6 Underappreciation of the Psychological Impact

Like other chronic inflammatory diseases, AS can have a significant psychological impact on patients. Chronic pain, limited mobility and the fear of permanent disability can lead to depression, anxiety and a diminished QoL. However, the psychological aspect of AS is often overlooked, leading to unaddressed mental health issues [22].

Pitfalls in Mental Health Management (a) *Undiagnosed depression and anxiety*: the psychological burden of AS is frequently underdiagnosed and untreated, which can worsen physical symptoms and reduce treatment adherence; (b) *social isolation*: chronic pain and reduced mobility can cause patients to withdraw from social activities, leading to loneliness and further mental health decline; (c) *fibromyalgia*: patients with unrecognised depression may confuse the symptoms of the disease with those of depression, potentially leading to overtreatment of AS or unnecessary changes in medication.

Overcoming This Pitfall Routine mental health screening should be incorporated into the care of AS patients. Referrals to mental health professionals, including psychologists, can help address issues like depression and anxiety. Additionally, encouraging physical activity and participation in social or support groups can improve mental well-being [23].

11.7 Neglecting Physical Therapy and Exercise

Physical therapy and exercise are essential components of AS management, but they are often underutilised or not emphasized enough. Maintaining spinal mobility and posture through regular exercise can prevent deformities, reduce pain and improve overall function. However, some patients, due to pain or lack of guidance, may not engage in the necessary exercises [24].

Pitfalls Related to Inadequate Physical Therapy (a) *Loss of spinal mobility*: without regular exercise, AS patients can lose spinal mobility and flexibility, leading to the classic stooped posture associated with severe AS; (b) *increased pain and disability*: lack of exercise can lead to muscle deconditioning, which exacerbates pain and stiffness, creating a vicious circle of inactivity and worsening symptoms; (c) *emotional impact*: non-adherence to exercise programs may negatively affect the emotional well-being of patients with AS.

Overcoming This Pitfall Physicians should work closely with physical therapists to develop tailored exercise programmes for AS patients. These programmes should focus on posture, spinal extension and flexibility exercises. Patients should be encouraged to remain active and engage in low-impact activities like swimming, yoga or cycling, which can help preserve joint mobility without exacerbating pain [25, 26]. In Table 11.1, a summary of the consequences of neglecting exercise in AS is presented.

Table 11.1 Consequences of neglecting exercise in ankylosing spondylitis

Category	Consequence	Description	Impact on patient
Musculoskeletal	Increased spinal stiffness	Progression of ankylosis and loss of spinal mobility	Difficulty performing daily activities
	Decreased joint ROM	Contractures and reduced flexibility in peripheral joints	Impaired physical function
	Muscle weakness	Disuse atrophy of supporting muscles	Increased risk of falls and reduced posture stability
	Postural deformities	Worsening kyphosis and stooped posture	Chronic pain, breathing difficulties, and body image issues
	Osteoporosis and fractures	Inactivity reducing bone density	Increased risk of vertebral and peripheral fractures
Cardiopulmonary	Restrictive lung disease	Reduced chest expansion and pulmonary capacity	Dyspnoea, reduced exercise tolerance
	Deconditioning	Decline in cardiovascular fitness	Increased fatigue and risk of CVD
Pain management	Increased pain and stiffness	Prolonged inactivity exacerbating inflammation and rigidity	Reduced QoL
	Higher dependence on medications	Reliance on analgesics and NSAIDs for symptom control	Increased risk of medication side effects
Functional	Reduced independence	Difficulty in performing self-care tasks	Increased reliance on caregivers or assistive devices
	Loss of work and productivity	Physical limitations affecting occupational performance	Economic strain and reduced self-esteem
Psychological	Depression and anxiety	Isolation and frustration from progressive disability	Worsening mental health and reduced social interactions
	Low self-esteem	Negative feelings due to physical decline and dependence	Reduced motivation to engage in rehabilitation
Systemic health	Increased systemic inflammation	Inactivity leading to chronic inflammation	Worsening disease progression and comorbidities
	Weight gain	Sedentary lifestyle causing obesity	Increased strain on joints and higher risk of metabolic syndrome
Disease progression	Accelerated spinal fusion	Lack of movement promoting ossification of spinal ligaments	Permanent disability
	Peripheral joint involvement	Neglecting mobility exercises increasing joint inflammation	Reduced hand and leg functionality

11.8 Conclusion

AS is a complex and chronic disease with numerous pitfalls that can lead to delayed diagnosis with permanent structural damage. When the appropriate treatment is not given in a timely manner or treatment escalation fails, serious side effects may appear or even worsening of the disease activity. Finally, extra-spinal manifestation should be sought, and a multidisciplinary approach is needed. Furthermore, the psychological impact of the disease should not be overlooked as patients may suffer from depression and anxiety.

References

1. Fallahi S, Jamshidi AR. Diagnostic delay in ankylosing spondylitis: related factors and prognostic outcomes. Arch Rheumatol. 2015;31:24–30. https://doi.org/10.5606/ArchRheumatol.2016.5562.
2. Pelechas E, Kaltsonoudis E, Voulgari PV, Drosos AA. Ankylosing spondylitis. In: Illustrated handbook of rheumatic and musculo-skeletal diseases. Cham: Springer; 2023. https://doi.org/10.1007/978-3-031-47379-1_8.
3. Seo MR, Baek HL, Yoon HH, Ryu HJ, Choi HJ, Baek HJ, et al. Delayed diagnosis is linked to worse outcomes and unfavourable treatment responses in patients with axial spondyloarthritis. Clin Rheumatol. 2015;34:1397–405. https://doi.org/10.1007/s10067-014-2768-y.
4. Yi E, Ahuja A, Rajput T, George AT, Park Y. Clinical, economic, and humanistic burden associated with delayed diagnosis of axial spondyloarthritis: a systemic review. Rheumatol Ther. 2020;7:65–87. https://doi.org/10.1007/s40744-020-00194-8.
5. Bennett AN, McGonagle D, O'Connor P, Hensor EMA, Sivera F, Coates LC, et al. Severity of baseline magnetic resonance imaging—evident sacroiliitis and HLA-B27 status in early inflammatory back pain predict radiographically evident ankylosing spondylitis at eight years. Arthritis Rheum. 2008;58:3413–8. https://doi.org/10.1002/art.24024.
6. Mease P, Deodhar A. Differentiating nonradiographic axial spondyloarthritis form its mimics: a narrative review. BMC Musculoskelet Disord. 2022;23:240. https://doi.org/10.1186/s12891-022-05073-7.
7. Pelechas E, Kosta P, Voulgari PV, Drosos AA. Bertolotti syndrome: a not-to-miss cause of chronic low back pain in young adults. Acta Reumatol Port. 2020;45:58–60.
8. Patel P, Hussain H, Fahey J. Delayed diagnosis of ankylosing spondylitis: a missed opportunity? Cureus. 2019;11:e5723. https://doi.org/10.7759/cureus.5723.
9. Østergaard M, Lambert RGW. Imaging in ankylosing spondylitis. Ther Adv Musculoskelet Dis. 2012;4:301–11. https://doi.org/10.1177/1759720X11436240.
10. Rudwaleit M, van der Heijde D, Landewé R, Listing J, Akkoc N, Brandt J, et al. The development of assessment of spondyloarthritis international society classification criteria for axial spondyloarthritis: validation and final selection. Ann Rheum Dis. 2009;68:777–83. https://doi.org/10.1136/ard.2009.108233.
11. Maghraoui AE. Extra-articular manifestations of ankylosing spondylitis: prevalence, characteristics and therapeutic implications. Eur J Intern Med. 2011;22:554–60. https://doi.org/10.1016/j.ejim.2011.06.006.
12. Proft F, Duran TZ, Ghoreschi K, Pleyer U, Siegmung B, Poddubnyy D. Treatment strategies for spondyloarthritis: implementation of precision medicine—or "one size fits all" concept? Autoimmun Rev. 2024;23:103638. https://doi.org/10.1016/j.autrev.2024.103638.

13. Michelena X, Zhao SS, Marco-Pascual C, Almirall M, Collantes-Estevez E, Font-Ugalde P, et al. Diagnostic delay is associated with uveitis and inflammatory bowel disease is AS: a study of extra-musculoskeletal manifestations in SpA. Rheumatology (Oxford). 2024;63:430–5. https://doi.org/10.1093/rheumatology/kead225.
14. Gudu T, Jadon DR. Multidisciplinary working in the management of axial and peripheral spondyloarthritis. Ther Adv Musculoskelet Dis. 2020;12:1759720X20975888. https://doi.org/10.1177/1759720X20975888.
15. Pelechas E, Kaltsonoudis E, Voulgari PV, Drosos AA. Unmet needs in the treatment of ankylosing spondylitis: a long-term observational study from a single university center. Rheumatol Int. 2019;39:663–8. https://doi.org/10.1007/s00296-019-04277-w.
16. Kroon FPB, van der Burg LRA, Ramiro S, Landewé RBM, Buchbinder R, Falzon L, et al. Non-steroidal anti-inflammatory drugs (NSAIDs) for axial spondyloarthritis (ankylosing spondylitis and non-radiographic axial spondyloarthritis). Cochrane Database Syst Rev. 2015;2015:CD010952. https://doi.org/10.1002/14651858.CD010952.pub2.
17. Moon KH, Kim YT. Medical treatment of ankylosing spondylitis. Hip Pelvis. 2014;26:129–35. https://doi.org/10.5371/hp.2014.26.3.129.
18. Aouad K, El-Zorkany B. Treat-to-target in axial spondyloarthritis: are we there yet? Mediterr J Rheumatol. 2022;33:137–41. https://doi.org/10.31138/mjr.33.1.137.
19. Drosos AA, Pelechas E, Venetsanopoulou AI, Voulgari PV. TNFα inhibitors versus newer therapies in spondyloarthritis: where do we stand today? Mediterr J Rheumatol. 2024;35:519–27. https://doi.org/10.31138/mjr.040224.tvn.
20. Kaltsonoudis E, Voulgari PV, Konitsiotis S, Drosos AA. Demyelination and other neurological adverse events after anti-TNF therapy. Autoimmun Rev. 2014;13:54–8. https://doi.org/10.1016/j.autrev.2013.09.002.
21. Maeda T, Connolly M, Thevenet-Morrison K, Levy P, Utell M, Munsiff S, et al. Tuberculosis screening for patients on biologic medications: a single-center experience and society guideline review, Monroe county, New York, 2018-2021. J Clin Tuberc Other Mycobact Dis. 2024;36:100460. https://doi.org/10.1016/j.jctube.2024.100460.
22. Parkinson JT, Foley EM, Jadon DR, Khandaker GM. Depression in patients with spondyloarthritis: prevalence, incidence, risk factors, mechanisms and management. Ther Adv Musculoskelet Dis. 2020;12:1759720X20970028. https://doi.org/10.1177/1759720X20970028.
23. Carbo M, Paap D, van Overbeeke L, Wink F, Bootsma H, Arends S, et al. Higher levels of physical activity are associated with less evasive coping, better physical function and quality of life in patients with axial spondyloarthritis. PLoS One. 2024;19:e0301965. https://doi.org/10.1371/journal.Pone.0301965.
24. Gravaldi LP, Bonetti F, Lezzerini S, De Maio F. Effectiveness of physiotherapy in patients with ankylosing spondylitis: a systematic review and meta-analysis. Healthcare (Basel). 2022;10:132. https://doi.org/10.3390/healthcare10010132.
25. Regnaux JP, Davergne T, Palazzo C, Roren A, Rannou F, Boutron I, et al. Exercise programmes for ankylosing spondylitis. Cochrane Database Syst Rev. 2019;2019:CD011321. https://doi.org/10.1002/14651858.CD011321.pub2.
26. Kaltsonoudis E, Karagianni P, Memi T, Pelechas E. State-of-the-art review on the treatment of axial spondyloarthritis. Med Sci (Basel). 2025;13:32. https://doi.org/10.3390/medsci13010032.

Pitfalls in Diffuse Idiopathic Skeletal Hyperostosis

12

Abbreviations

ALL	Anterior longitudinal ligament
AS	Ankylosing spondylitis
CRP	C-reactive protein
CS	Corticosteroids
CT	Computed tomography
CVD	Cardiovascular disease
DDD	Degenerative disc disease
DEXA	Dual-energy X-ray absorptiometry
DISH	Diffuse idiopathic skeletal hyperostosis
ESR	Erythrocyte sedimentation rate
MRI	Magnetic resonance imaging
MSK	Musculoskeletal
NSAIDs	Non-steroidal anti-inflammatory drugs
OA	Osteoarthritis
QoL	Quality of life
ROM	Range of motion
SI	Sacroiliac
SpA	Spondyloarthropathy

E. Pelechas et al., *Pitfalls in Rheumatology*,
https://doi.org/10.1007/978-3-031-98671-0_12

12.1 Misidentification of DISH as a Degenerative Disc Disease or Ankylosing Spondylitis

DISH can be misdiagnosed as DDD or AS due to overlapping features, particularly spinal stiffness and back pain. However, these conditions have distinct clinical, laboratory, radiographic and pathophysiological differences that require careful evaluation [1].

How to Avoid This Pitfall (a) *Recognise key radiographic features*: the hallmark of DISH is the presence of flowing ossifications along the ALL of at least four contiguous vertebral bodies, most commonly in the thoracic spine (Fig. 12.1). In contrast to AS, which primarily involves the SI joints and can result in vertebral fusion, DISH typically spares the SI joints and involves the peripheral skeleton more than the axial skeleton [2]; (b) *lack of intervertebral disc involvement*: in DISH, there is typically minimal or no disc space narrowing or vertebral body ankylosis, distinguishing it from DDD or AS where these changes are common. The preservation of disc spaces between the ossified areas is a key feature of DISH; (c) *understand the non-inflammatory nature of DISH*: DISH is non-inflammatory, whereas AS is an

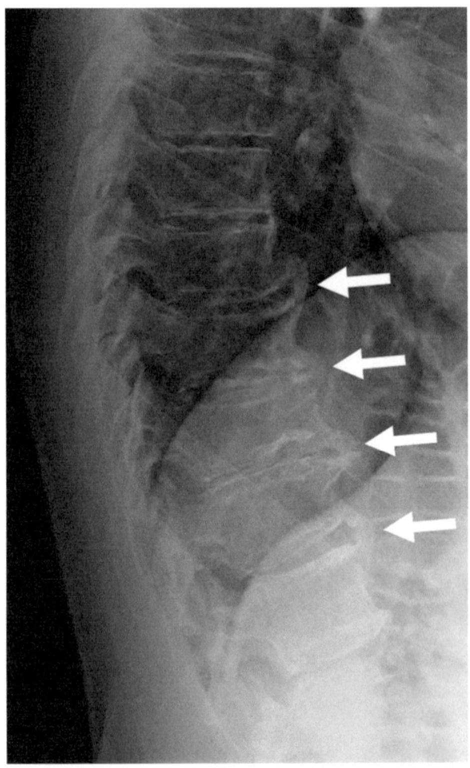

Fig. 12.1 Flowing ossifications along the anterior longitudinal ligament of four contiguous vertebral bodies of the lower thoracic spine

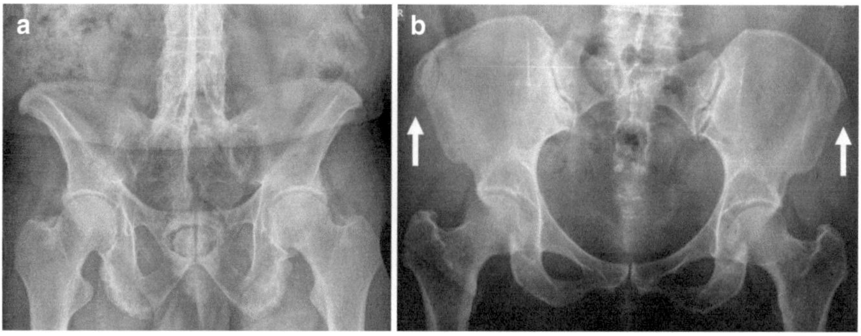

Fig. 12.2 Pelvic X-rays. (**a**) On the left, an AS patient with complete fusion of the SI joints and presence of the so called "bamboo spine". (**b**) On the right, a patient with extra-spinal DISH and normal space of the SI joints (extra-spinal locations of DISH will be presented in the next figures). Light whiskering of the anterior superior iliac spine can be attributed to DISH (white arrows)

inflammatory SpA. A normal ESR or CRP, combined with the absence of sacroiliitis on imaging, supports the diagnosis of DISH over AS [3]; (d) *patterns of stiffness*: stiffness presents with different clinical patterns, with morning stiffness being more prominently associated with AS, whereas the generalised, continuous spinal stiffness is more commonly seen in DISH. In Fig. 12.2a, a complete fusion of the lumbar vertebrae and the sacroiliac joints is presented in a patient with AS. On the other hand, in a DISH patient (Fig. 12.2b), there are no such bone complications.

12.2 Failure to Recognise Extra-Spinal Manifestations

DISH primarily affects the spine, but it also involves the peripheral skeleton and can lead to extra-spinal symptoms. Enthesopathy in areas like the shoulders, hips, elbows, ankles and knees can cause pain, stiffness and functional impairment, yet these manifestations are often overlooked [4] (Fig. 12.3).

How to Avoid This Pitfall (a) *Look for peripheral enthesopathy*: patients with DISH may develop bony spurs and calcifications in the Achilles tendon, plantar fascia, patellar tendons or elbow ligaments. These can cause significant discomfort, leading to impaired mobility, misdiagnosis as other tendinopathies or delayed treatment [5]; (b) *screen for dysphagia*: ossification of the ALL in the cervical spine can cause compression of the oesophagus, leading to dysphagia. This is a quite frequent yet underdiagnosed complication. Always inquire about swallowing difficulties in patients with cervical involvement, particularly in advanced disease stages [6]; (c) *recognise the risk of spinal fractures*: patients with DISH are at higher risk for fractures, particularly in the thoracic and cervical spine, due to the rigidity of the spine from calcified ligaments. Fractures in DISH may occur with minimal trauma and are often unstable, requiring prompt recognition and careful management to prevent neurological injury [7].

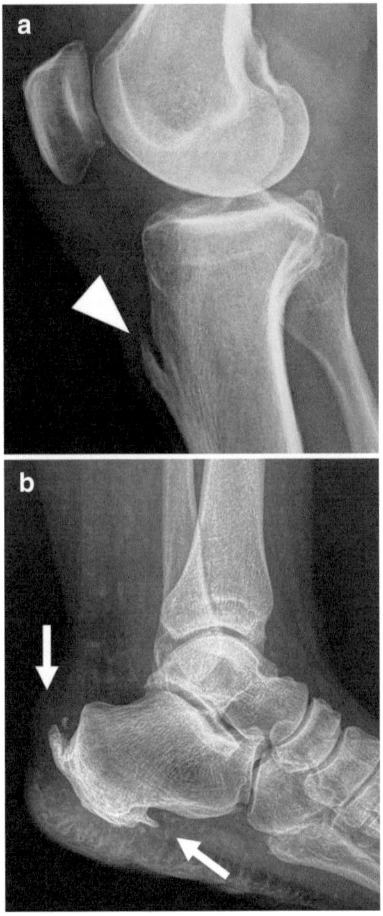

Fig. 12.3 (**a**) Enthesophyte of the tibial tuberosity (arrowhead) and (**b**) enthesopathy of the Achilles tendon and plantar fascia (arrows). Both X-rays are from the same patient in Fig. 12.2b diagnosed as having extra-spinal DISH

12.3 Confusing DISH with Osteoarthritis

Due to the fact that DISH can present with joint pain and stiffness, it may be confused with OA, especially in older adults. However, the pathophysiology and clinical course of these conditions differ significantly.

How to Avoid This Pitfall (a) *Differentiate based on radiographic findings*: DISH is characterised by flowing ligamentous ossification along the spine and extra-spinal entheses, whereas OA primarily involves joint space narrowing, subchondral sclerosis and osteophyte formation. While both conditions may coexist, DISH can cause widespread ossification not seen in typical OA [8]; (b) *recognise distinct patterns of joint involvement*: DISH affects large tendons and ligaments rather than the articular cartilage, which is the primary site of pathology in OA. Joint pain in DISH often stems from enthesopathy rather than from cartilage degeneration, as seen in OA; (c) *assess systemic metabolic risk factors*: DISH is associated with metabolic conditions, such as obesity, type 2 diabetes and hyperlipidaemia, which are less commonly linked to OA. Recognising these associations can help differentiate between the two diseases [9].

12.4 Failure to Identify Metabolic Risk Factors

DISH is often associated with metabolic conditions such as obesity, diabetes and hyperlipidaemia. These factors contribute to the pathogenesis of the disease, and failure to address them can lead to disease progression and poor overall health outcomes.

How to Avoid This Pitfall (a) *Screen for metabolic syndrome*: evaluate patients with DISH for the components of metabolic syndrome, including central obesity, insulin resistance, dyslipidaemia and hypertension. These factors not only contribute to the progression of DISH but also increase the patient's risk for CVD [10]; (b) *incorporate lifestyle and metabolic management into treatment plans*: beyond symptomatic treatment of the MSK symptoms, addressing modifiable risk factors like weight, glucose control and lipid levels can potentially slow the progression of DISH and improve the patient's overall health; (c) *collaborate with endocrinologists*: for patients with significant metabolic abnormalities, involving endocrinologists can help optimise the management of underlying conditions such as diabetes or dyslipidaemia [11]; (d) *incorporation of exercise and/or physiotherapy programmes*: supervised exercise programmes with individually tailored intensity can also help relieve symptoms and potentially slow the progression of radiographic manifestations.

12.5 Overlooking the Impact on Spinal Mobility and Function

Although DISH is often asymptomatic in its early stages, as the disease progresses, it can cause significant spinal stiffness and reduced mobility. However, these symptoms are sometimes dismissed as a normal part of aging or attributed to other conditions like OA or spondylosis.

How to Avoid This Pitfall (a) *Assess for reduced spinal mobility*: in patients with DISH, particularly those with advanced disease, there may be noticeable stiffness and decreased ROM in the thoracic and cervical spine. Assessing spinal flexibility, particularly in the lateral bending and rotational movements, can reveal functional impairment [12]; (b) *evaluate impact on daily living*: DISH can significantly reduce patients' ability to perform daily activities, especially if cervical or thoracic spine stiffness limits their ROM. Ask about difficulties with activities that involve turning, bending or maintaining posture; (c) *physical therapy and mobility training*: incorporating physical therapy early in the management of DISH can help maintain flexibility and improve functional outcomes. Exercises focusing on spinal mobility and overall conditioning are crucial in preventing further disability [13].

12.6 Lack of Awareness of Spinal Fracture Risk

The ossified ligaments in DISH create a stiff, brittle spine that is more prone to fracture with minor trauma, particularly in the thoracic and cervical regions. These fractures are often unstable and can lead to serious complications, including spinal cord injury, if not properly recognised ana managed [14].

How to Avoid This Pitfall (a) *Recognise the heightened fracture risk*: in patients with DISH, particularly those who present after trauma, always consider the possibility of a vertebral fracture, even in cases of minor trauma. These patients are at risk for fractures with relatively low-impact mechanisms, such as falls from standing height; (b) *obtain appropriate imaging*: if a fracture is suspected, plain radiographs may not be sufficient. Consider advanced imaging such as CT or MRI to better visualise fractures, especially if there is neurological involvement [15]; (c) *aggressive fracture management*: due to the instability of fractures in DISH, these injuries often require more aggressive management than typical vertebral fractures. Surgical intervention may be needed in cases of instability or spinal cord involvement; (d) *prevention of fracture risk factors*: regular assessment for coexisting bone loss or osteoporosis is recommended, including DEXA scanning. In cases of abnormal findings, appropriate treatment should be initiated.

12.7 Underestimation of Pain and Functional Impact

Because DISH is often considered a "silent" condition, its potential impact on QoL is sometimes underestimated. While many patients may be asymptomatic, those with significant enthesopathy, spinal stiffness or fracture complications can experience substantial pain and disability.

How to Avoid This Pitfall (a) *Address pain management*: patients with DISH may experience significant pain from enthesopathy or spinal rigidity. Ensuring adequate pain management, including the use of NSAIDs, physical therapy and possibly local CS injections, is essential to maintaining QoL; (b) *monitor for functional decline*: over time, patients with severe DISH may lose spinal flexibility and develop compensatory postures that can impair balance and increase the risk of falls. Early intervention with physical therapy, assistive devices and education about fall prevention is important [16]; (c) *patient education*: patients should be encouraged to follow regular daily exercises being particularly beneficial.

12.8 Conclusion

DISH is often under-recognised or misdiagnosed due to its overlapping symptoms with other rheumatologic and orthopaedic conditions. A thorough understanding of its characteristic radiographic findings, extra-spinal manifestations, metabolic associations and potential complications is crucial for accurate diagnosis and optimal management. By avoiding these common pitfalls, clinicians can provide better care for patients with DISH, helping to prevent complications, manage pain and improve QoL.

References

1. Pelechas E, Kaltsonoudis E, Voulgari PV, Drosos AA. Miscellaneous conditions. In: Illustrated handbook of rheumatic and musculo-skeletal diseases. Cham: Springer; 2023. https://doi.org/10.1007/978-3-031-47379-1_18.
2. Eshed I. Imaging characteristics of diffuse idiopathic skeletal hyperostosis: more than just spinal bony bridges. Diagnostics (Basel). 2023;13:563. https://doi.org/10.3390/diagnostics13030563.
3. Vaishya R, Vijay V, Nwagbara IC, Agarwal AK. Diffuse idiopathic skeletal hyperostosis (DISH)—a common but less known cause of back pain. J Clin Orthop Trauma. 2017;8:191–6. https://doi.org/10.1016/j.jcot.2016.11.006.
4. Mader R, Sarzi-Puttini P, Atzeni F, Olivieri I, Pappone N, Verlaan JJ, et al. Extraspinal manifestations of diffuse idiopathic skeletal hyperostosis. Rheumatology (Oxford). 2009;48:1478–81. https://doi.org/10.1093/rheumatology/kep308.
5. Littlejohn GO, Urowitz MB. Peripheral enthesopathy in diffuse idiopathic skeletal hyperostosis (DISH): a radiologic study. J Rheumatol. 1982;9:568–72.
6. Lee JH, Paeng SH, Pyo SY, Kim ST, Lee WH. Swallowing difficulty in diffuse idiopathic skeletal hyperostosis with metabolic syndrome. Korean J Neurotrauma. 2020;16:90–8. https://doi.org/10.13004/kjnt.2020.16.e4.
7. Okada E, Shimizu K, Kato M, Fukuda K, Kaneko S, Ogawa J, et al. Spinal fractures in patients with diffuse idiopathic skeletal hyperostosis: clinical characteristics by fracture level. J Orthop Sci. 2019;24:393–9. https://doi.org/10.1016/j.jos.2018.10.017.
8. Mader R. Diffuse idiopathic skeletal hyperostosis: a distinct clinical entity. Isr Med Assoc J. 2003;5:506–8.
9. Okada E, Ishihara S, Azuma K, Michikawa T, Suzuki S, Tsuji O, Nori S, et al. Metabolic syndrome is a predisposing factor for diffuse idiopathic skeletal hyperostosis. Neurospine. 2020;18:109–16. https://doi.org/10.14245/ns.2040350.175.
10. Vezyroglou G, Mitropoulos A, Antoniadis C. A metabolic syndrome in diffuse idiopathic skeletal hyperostosis. A controlled study. J Rheumatol. 1996;23:672–6.
11. Mader R, Verlaan JJ, Eshed I, Jacome BA, Puttini PS, Atzeni F, et al. Diffuse idiopathic skeletal hyperostosis (DISH): where we are now and where to go next. RMD Open. 2022;3 https://doi.org/10.1136/rmdopen-2017-000472.
12. Giammalva GR, Maugeri R, Cusimano LM, Sciortino AS, Bonosi L, Brunasso L, et al. Diffuse idiopathic skeletal hyperostosis: a functional enemy of vertebral stability—case series and surgical considerations of craniovertebral junction involvement. J Craniovertebr Junct Spine. 2023;14:274–80. https://doi.org/10.4103/jcvjs.jcvjs_72_73.
13. Al-Herz A, Snip JP, Clark B, Esdaile JM. Exercise therapy for patients with diffuse idiopathic skeletal hyperostosis. Clin Rheumatol. 2008;27:207–10. https://doi.org/10.1007/s10067-007-0693-z.

14. Harlianto NI, Ezzafzafi S, Foppen W, Kuperus JS, van der Horst-Bruinsma IE, de Jong PA, et al. The prevalence of vertebral fractures in diffuse idiopathic skeletal hyperostosis and ankylosing spondylitis: a systematic review and meta-analysis. N Am Spine Soc J. 2024;17:100312. https://doi.org/10.1016/j.xnsj.2024.100312.
15. Mader R, Baraliakos X, Eshed O, Novofastovski I, Bieber A, Verlaan JJ, et al. Imaging of diffuse idiopathic skeletal hyperostosis (DISH). RMD Open. 2020;6:e001151. https://doi.org/10.1136/rmdopen-2019-001151.
16. Mader R. Current therapeutic options in the management of diffuse idiopathic skeletal hyperostosis. Expert Opin Pharmacother. 2005;6:1313–8. https://doi.org/10.1517/14656566.6.8.1313.

Pitfalls in Crystal Arthropathies

13

Abbreviations

CKD	Chronic kidney disease
CPPD	Calcium pyrophosphate deposition
CS	Corticosteroids
CT	Computed tomography
CVD	Cardiovascular disease
GI	Gastrointestinal
IA	Inflammatory arthritis
MTP	Metatarsophalangeal
MUC	Monosodium urate crystals
NSAIDs	Non-steroidal anti-inflammatory drugs
OA	Osteoarthritis
QoL	Quality of life
RA	Rheumatoid arthritis
ULT	Urate-lowering therapy

13.1 Misdiagnosis and Delayed Recognition

Crystal arthropathies, particularly gout, are frequently misdiagnosed because their clinical presentations can overlap with other forms of arthritis, such as septic arthritis, RA or OA. Both gout and CPPD can present with acute, monoarticular inflammation, often mimicking other conditions, which may delay the correct diagnosis [1].

Consequences of Misdiagnosis (a) *Inappropriate treatment*: a missed or delayed diagnosis may lead to inappropriate treatment, such as unnecessary antibiotics in

E. Pelechas et al., *Pitfalls in Rheumatology*,
https://doi.org/10.1007/978-3-031-98671-0_13

the case of presumed septic arthritis or CS in the case of misdiagnosed IA; (b) *uncontrolled disease*: failure to recognise gout or CPPD can result in recurrent attacks of acute inflammation, leading to chronic joint damage over time [2, 3], as well as other organ involvement, such as renal and cardiovascular damage.

Overcoming This Pitfall Clinicians should maintain a high index of suspicion for crystal arthropathies, particularly in patients presenting with acute monoarthritis or recurrent joint inflammation. A definitive diagnosis requires joint aspiration and synovial fluid analysis for crystals. Attention should also be paid to cases where crystal-induced arthritis coexists with other forms of IA and/or OA, especially when the diagnosis of the other type of arthritis precedes it. Gout is confirmed by the presence of negatively birefringent, needle-shaped MUC, while CPPD is characterised by positively birefringent, rhomboid-shaped calcium pyrophosphate crystals. Even when joint aspiration is not possible, a thorough clinical history and imaging (e.g., dual-energy CT for gout) can help differentiate crystal arthropathies from other forms of arthritis [4]. Common sites of CPPD findings with plain X-rays are the triangular fibrocartilage of the wrists (Fig. 13.1a) and knees (Fig. 13.1b), but other sites such as the ligament tissue around the odontoid process of the axis can occur (Fig. 13.1c). The so-called "crowned dens syndrome" is characterised by acute neck pain, stiffness, fever and elevated inflammatory markers and can be attributed to other conditions.

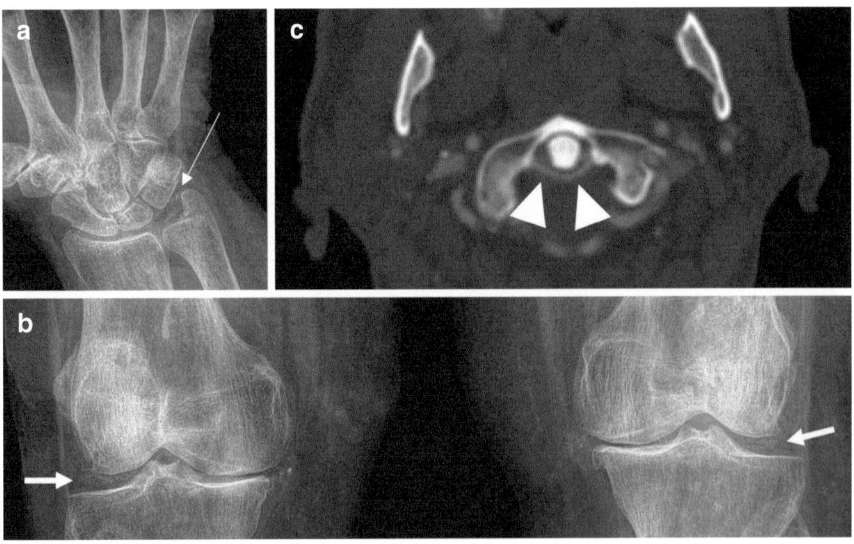

Fig. 13.1 (**a**) CPPD of the triangular fibrocartilage of the wrist (thin arrow), along with (**b**) CPPD of the knees (thick arrows) are the most common sites of X-ray findings termed as chondrocalcinosis. A more rare finding is the (**c**) "crowned dens syndrome" a condition that occurs due to deposition of calcium pyrophosphate in the ligament tissue around the odontoid process of the axis (arrowheads)

13.2 Underestimation of the Prevalence of Atypical Gout

Gout is often thought of as a disease affecting the first MTP joint (podagra), but it can present in various atypical forms. For example, patients may develop gout in the knees, ankles, wrists or even small hand joints, mimicking other forms of arthritis. Additionally, while gout is often seen as a disease of older men, it can occur in the presence of genetic deficiencies in males of any age and in women, especially post-menopausal women. In some cases, tophi may develop and resemble rheumatoid nodules. In Fig. 13.2, some of the findings of gout are presented.

Pitfalls of Atypical Gout Presentation (a) *Misdiagnosis in atypical joints*: when gout presents in less typical locations, such as the knee or wrist, it may be misdiagnosed as RA, CPPD or septic arthritis; (b) *overlooking gout in women*: clinicians may overlook the possibility of gout in women, particularly younger women of those without classic risk factors, leading to delays in diagnosis and treatment [5].

Overcoming This Pitfall Recognise that gout can affect any joint and that it can occur in women and younger individuals [6]. In patients with unexplained acute or chronic arthritis, gout should always be considered, especially if there are known risk factors such as hyperuricemia, renal disease or a history of alcohol use or diuretic therapy. Joint aspiration and crystal analysis remain the gold standard for diagnosis, even in atypical cases [7].

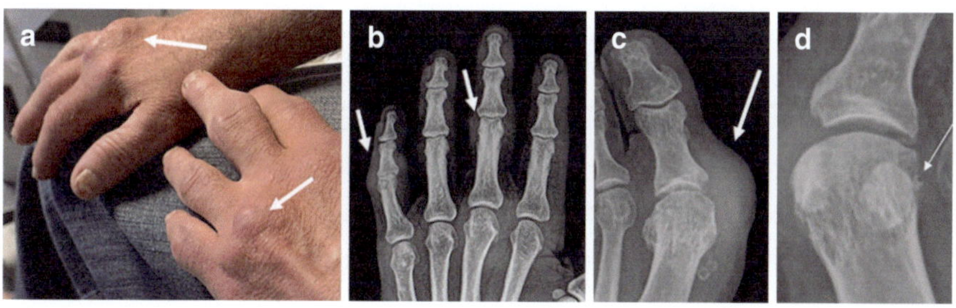

Fig. 13.2 (**a**) Tophi on the dorsal area of both hands (thick arrows). Tophi are pathognomonic for the disease of gout; (**b**, **c**) on plain X-ray the tophi appear as eccentric, juxta-articular soft tissue nodules (thick arrows) as in these X-rays of the hands and feet; (**d**) bony erosions with sclerotic margins and overhanging edges can be also found as in this case. All these photos are from the same patient with a diagnosis of tophaceous gout

13.3 Failure to Treat Hyperuricemia Appropriately in Gout

A major pitfall in the management of gout is the failure to adequately treat hyperuricemia, the underlying cause of urate crystal deposition. Many patients receive treatment for acute gout flares but are not started on ULT to prevent future attacks and long-term complications. Furthermore, some clinicians aim for insufficiently low target serum urate levels, which leads to persistent crystal formation and recurrent flares.

Consequences of Inadequate Uric Acid Management (a) *Recurrent gout flares*: without appropriate ULT, patients are likely to experience repeated acute gout flares, which can become more frequent and severe over time; (b) *tophaceous gout*: chronic untreated hyperuricemia can lead to the development of tophi, which can cause deformities and joint destruction; (c) *increased cardiovascular and renal risks*: chronic hyperuricemia is associated with an increased risk of CVD, CKD, nephrolithiasis and other comorbidities [8].

Overcoming This Pitfall ULT should be initiated in all patients with recurrent gout flares, tophaceous gout or evidence of joint damage. The goal of ULT is to lower serum uric acid levels to less than 6 mg/dL (or less than 5 mg/dL in patients with severe tophaceous disease). Allopurinol is the first-line agent, and febuxostat can be used in patients who cannot tolerate allopurinol. Prophylactic colchicine or NSAIDs should be used during the initiation of ULT to prevent gout flares. Regular monitoring of serum uric acid levels is essential to ensure that the target is achieved and maintained [9]. Finally, in younger patients without classic risk factors for hyperuricemia, it is advisable to investigate the underlying cause and consider genetic testing.

13.4 Mismanagement of Acute Flares

Managing acute flares of gout or CPPD can be challenging, particularly in patients with comorbid conditions such as CKD or CVD, which may limit treatment options. Common pitfalls include the inappropriate use of medications (e.g., NSAIDs in patients with CKD) or inadequate dosing of CS or colchicine [10].

Pitfalls in Treating Acute Flares (a) *Inappropriate use of NSAIDs*: NSAIDs are a mainstay of acute flare management but are contraindicated or risky in patients with kidney disease, heart failure or GI bleeding risks; (b) *underdosing colchicine*: colchicine is effective for acute gout flares, but the traditional high-dose regimen is associated with GI toxicity. On the other hand, undertreatment with low doses may result in ineffective flare control; (c) *delayed or suboptimal use of CS*: CS are highly effective for controlling acute flares, but clinicians may hesitate to use them due to concerns about side effects, particularly in patients with diabetes or hypertension.

Overcoming This Pitfall Acute gout and CPPD flares should be treated promptly with appropriate anti-inflammatory therapy. In patients without contraindications, NSAIDs can be effective. In those with contraindications (e.g., CKD and heart failure), low-dose colchicine or CS should be used instead. The recommended dosing of colchicine for acute gout is 1.2 mg, followed by 0.6 mg after 1 h. For CS, oral prednisone or intra-articular CS injections can be considered based on the severity and number of joints involved. Patients with multiple comorbidities may benefit from a personalised approach, and consultation with a rheumatologist may be helpful in complex cases [11].

13.5 Overlooking CPPD

CPPD, or pseudogout, is often overshadowed by gout and is less frequently diagnosed. It typically affects older adults and presents with acute, monoarticular arthritis, often in large joints such as the knee or wrist. Misdiagnosis as OA, septic arthritis or even RA is common due to the lack of awareness of CPPD as a cause of acute joint inflammation.

Pitfalls of Overlooking CPPD (a) *Misdiagnosis as OA*: chronic CPPD can lead to joint degeneration that mimics OA, especially in the elderly. Misdiagnosis can result in failure to address the inflammatory component of the disease; (b) *underutilisation of synovial fluid analysis*: because CPPD presents similar to other forms of arthritis, clinicians may not perform joint aspiration, leading to missed opportunities for diagnosis [12].

Overcoming This Pitfall CPPD should be considered in any older adult presenting with acute or chronic monoarticular arthritis, particularly in large joints. Joint aspiration and synovial fluid analysis for calcium pyrophosphate crystals is the definitive diagnostic test. Radiographic evidence of chondrocalcinosis can also support the diagnosis. Treatment of CPPD flares involves NSAIDs, colchicine or CS, similar to gout. Chronic CPPD management may involve low-dose colchicine for flare prevention, and patients with recurrent flares may benefit from regular monitoring.

13.6 Failure to Address Comorbidities in Gout Patients

Gout is often associated with multiple comorbidities, including hypertension, diabetes, CKD, obesity and CVD. Focusing solely on managing acute flares without addressing these comorbid conditions can lead to poor long-term outcomes and increased morbidity [13].

Consequences of Ignoring Comorbidities (a) *Worsening cardiovascular and renal disease*: untreated hyperuricemia and recurrent gout flares can exacerbate underlying cardiovascular and renal conditions, increasing the risk of heart disease and progression of kidney disease [14]; (b) *poor gout control*: conditions such as obesity, diabetes and alcohol use can contribute to increased serum uric acid levels, making it more difficult to control gout without addressing these underlying factors [15]; (c) *treatment modification*: modification, where feasible, of medications that increase uric acid levels, such as diuretic therapy.

Overcoming This Pitfall A holistic approach to managing gout should include not only ULT but also treatment of associated comorbidities. Lifestyle modifications such as weight loss, dietary changes (e.g., reducing purine intake and alcohol consumption) and optimising blood pressure and glucose control can help reduce serum uric acid levels and improve overall health outcomes. In patients with CKD, medication choices for both gout and comorbid conditions should be tailored to minimise nephrotoxicity and cardiovascular risk [16].

13.7 Conclusion

Crystal arthropathies, including gout and CPPD, pose diagnostic and management challenges due to their diverse clinical presentations, associated comorbidities and the complexities of treatment. Avoiding the common pitfalls (such as misdiagnosis, inadequate treatment of hyperuricemia and failure to address comorbidities) requires a thorough understanding of the disease process and a patient-centred, multidisciplinary approach to care. Early recognition, prompt and appropriate treatment of acute flares and long-term management of hyperuricemia and associated comorbid conditions can improve patient outcomes and QoL.

References

1. Pelechas E, Kaltsonoudis E, Voulgari PV, Drosos AA. Crystal arthropathies. In: Illustrated handbook of rheumatic and musculo-skeletal diseases. Cham: Springer; 2023.
2. Singh JA. Are the days of missed or delayed diagnosis of gout over? Nat Rev Rheumatol. 2019;15:578–80. https://doi.org/10.1038/s41584.
3. Fuller A, Cai K, Filippou G, Pascart T, Diaz-Torne C, Hensey O, et al. Experience and impact of crystal pyrophosphate deposition (CPPD) from a patient and caregiver perspective: a qualitative exploration from the OMERACT CPPD Working Group. Semin Arthritis Rheum. 2021;51:655–60. https://doi.org/10.1016/j.semarthrit.2021.04.010.
4. Mandl P, D'Agostino MA, Navarro-Compán V, Geßi I, Sakellariou G, Abhishek A, et al. 2023 EULAR recommendations on imaging in diagnosis and management of crystal-induced arthropathies in clinical practice. Ann Rheum Dis. 2024;83:752–9. https://doi.org/10.1136/ard-2023-224771.
5. Tan SYW, Stanway J, Ellis S. Crystal arthropathies. Medicine. 2022;50:109–15. https://doi.org/10.1016/j.mpmed.2021.11.008.

6. Scagnellato L, Farah S, Cozzi G, Lorenzin M, Cipolletta E, Raffeiner B, et al. POS0167 Crystal arthropathies in women: a complex presentation and a difficult diagnostic journey. Ann Rheum Dis. 2024;83:310.
7. Vaidya B, Bhochhibhoya M, Nakarmi S. Synovial fluid uric acid level aids diagnosis of gout. Biomed Rep. 2018;9:60–4. https://doi.org/10.3892/br.2018.1097.
8. Cox P, Gupta S, Zhao SS, Hughes DM. The incidence and prevalence of cardiovascular diseases in gout: a systematic review and meta-analysis. Rheumatol Int. 2021;41:1209–19. https://doi.org/10.1007/s00296-021-04876-6.
9. George M, Pullman-Mooar S, Hussain F, Schumacher HR. Evaluating appropriate use of prophylactic colchicine for gout flare prevention. Arthritis Care Res (Hoboken). 2014;66:1258–62. https://doi.org/10.1002/acr.22275.
10. Coburn BW, Mikuls TR. Treatment options for acute gout. Fed Pract. 2016;33:35–40.
11. Voulgari PV, Venetsanopoulou AI, Drosos AA. Recent advances in the therapeutic management of calcium pyrophosphate deposition disease. Front Med (Lausanne). 2024;11:1327715. https://doi.org/10.3389/fmed.2024.1327715.
12. Kravchenko D, Behning C, Bergner R, Schäfer VB. How to differentiate gout, calcium pyrophosphate deposition disease, and osteoarthritis using just four clinical parameters. Diagnostics (Basel). 2021;11:924. https://doi.org/10.3390/diagnostics11060924.
13. Sattui S, Singh JA, Gaffo AL. Comorbidities in patients with crystal diseases and hyperuricemia. Rheum Dis Clin N Am. 2014;40:251–78. https://doi.org/10.1016/j.rdc.2014.01.005.
14. Muiesan ML, Agabiti-Rosei C, Paini A, Salvetti M. Uric and cardiovascular disease: an update. Eur Cardiol. 2016;11:54–9. https://doi.org/10.15420/ecr.2016:4:2.
15. Eun Y, Han K, Lee SW, Kim K, Kang S, Lee S, et al. Increased risk of incident gout in young men with metabolic syndromed: a nationwide population-based cohort study of 3.5 million men. Front Med (Lausanne). 2022;9:1010391. https://doi.org/10.3389/fmed.2022.1010391.
16. Moi JHY, Sriranganathan MK, Edwards CJ, Buchbinder R. Lifestyle interventions for chronic gout. Cochrane Database Syst Rev. 2013;2013:CD010039. https://doi.org/10.1002/14651858.CD010039.pub2.

Pitfalls in Sjögren's Syndrome

14

Abbreviations

CS	Corticosteroids
CsA	Cyclosporine
EMA	European Medicines Agency
FDA	Food and Drug Administration
HCQ	Hydroxychloroquine
ILD	Interstitial lung disease
LFTs	Liver function tests
MALT	Mucosa-associated lymphoid tissue
MSK	Musculoskeletal
MTX	Methotrexate
NHL	Non-Hodgkin's lymphoma
NSAIDs	Non-steroidal anti-inflammatory drugs
PFTs	Pulmonary function tests
pSS	Primary SS
QoL	Quality of life
RA	Rheumatoid arthritis
RMD	Rheumatic disease
RTX	Rituximab
SLE	Systemic lupus erythematosus
SS	Sjögren's syndrome
sSS	Secondary SS

E. Pelechas et al., *Pitfalls in Rheumatology*,
https://doi.org/10.1007/978-3-031-98671-0_14

14.1 Delayed or Missed Diagnosis

SS can be difficult to diagnose due to its often subtle and non-specific symptoms. Dry eyes and mouth are common complaints in the general population, especially in older adults, and can be misattributed to aging, diabetes mellitus or environmental factors. As a result, the disease is often underdiagnosed or diagnosed late, particularly in the primary care setting where symptoms may not be immediately recognised as part of a systemic autoimmune process [1].

Consequences of Delayed Diagnosis (a) *Progressive damage to exocrine glands*: prolonged untreated glandular inflammation can lead to irreversible damage to the salivary and lacrimal glands, worsening dryness and leading to complications like dental caries, oral infections and vision problems [2]; (b) *missed opportunities for early intervention*: delay in diagnosis may result in missed opportunities to manage systemic manifestations early, including potential damage to internal organs, particularly the lungs, kidneys and peripheral nervous system [3]; (c) *patient frustration*: many patients experience frustration and reduced quality of life due to chronic symptoms that are poorly managed in the absence of a clear diagnosis. In Fig. 14.1, eye and oral complications are presented.

Overcoming This Pitfall Clinicians should maintain a high index of suspicion for SS, particularly in patients with chronic dry eyes, dry mouth or unexplained systemic symptoms. Diagnostic tools such as Schirmer's test (for testing tear production), salivary gland imaging and serologic testing (anti-SSA/Ro and anti-SSB/La antibodies) are critical for confirming the diagnosis. Referral to a rheumatologist for further evaluation should be considered when primary care evaluation is inconclusive.

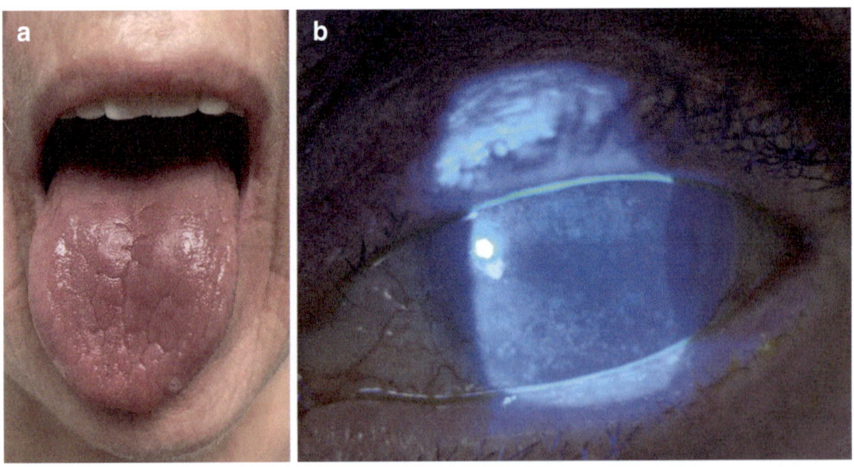

Fig. 14.1 (**a**) Xerostomia or dry mouth in a patient with Sjögren's syndrome. The tongue feels dry and chewing may present difficulties or even pain; (**b**) punctate keratopathy in a patient with Sjögren's syndrome—fluorescein staining—patient under treatment with topical cyclosporine. Severe dry eyes may present significant impact on visual acuity

14.2 Over-Reliance on Serologic Testing

The diagnosis of SS is often delayed or complicated by an over-reliance on serologic testing. Although anti-SSA/Ro and anti-SSB/La antibodies are commonly associated with the disease, not all patients with SS test positive for these markers [4]. Seronegative patients can still have the disease and may be misdiagnosed if their clinical presentation is not fully considered.

Pitfalls in Over-Reliance on Serology (a) *Misdiagnosis of seronegative patients*: relying solely on antibody testing can lead to a missed diagnosis in patients who have clinical symptoms of SS but are seronegative [5]; (b) *incomplete assessment*: a positive serologic test without careful evaluation of symptoms and glandular function can lead to overdiagnosis or misattribution of symptoms of SS when another condition may be responsible.

Overcoming This Pitfall Diagnosis should be based on a combination of clinical symptoms, objective findings (such as reduced tear production, salivary flow rates or abnormal minor salivary gland biopsy) and serology. A multidisciplinary approach involving rheumatologists, ophthalmologists and dentists can help provide a comprehensive evaluation of glandular and systemic involvement. Lip biopsy, which assesses minor salivary glands for lymphocytic infiltration, may be useful in unclear cases [6].

14.3 Overlooking Systemic Manifestations

While SS is primarily known for its effects on exocrine glands, it can involve virtually any organ system. Systemic manifestations, including fatigue, arthralgia, vasculitis, ILD, renal tubular acidosis and neurological complications, are common but often under-recognised, leading to suboptimal management of the disease as a whole [7].

Pitfalls of Focusing Only on Glandular Symptoms (a) *Undertreatment of systemic disease*: by focusing exclusively on dry mouth and dry eyes, clinicians may overlook more serious manifestations like renal dysfunction, peripheral neuropathy or pulmonary involvement, which can have significant morbidity [8]; (b) *failure to address quality of life*: systemic symptoms, such as severe fatigue, chronic pain and cognitive dysfunction (often called "brain fog"), can profoundly impact a patient's QoL, but they may be dismissed or inadequately treated if not directly associated with the glandular disease [9].

Overcoming This Pitfall A thorough and regular assessment of systemic involvement is essential. Routine monitoring for organ involvement, including blood tests (renal and LFTs), urinalysis, PFTs and neurological evaluations, should be incorporated into the management plan. Collaboration with specialists such as nephrologists, pulmonologists and neurologists may be required for comprehensive care [10].

14.4 Inadequate Management of Dryness

The hallmark symptoms of SS (sicca syndrome—dry eyes and dry mouth) are often difficult to manage effectively. Standard treatments, including artificial tears and saliva substitutes, may not provide sufficient relief, and patients may continue to experience significant discomfort and complications from chronic dryness, including corneal damage, dental decay and oral infections.

Pitfalls in Treating Glandular Symptoms (a) *Underutilisation of available therapies*: many patients rely solely on over-the-counter products for symptom relief, but there are prescription options and non-pharmacologic approaches that may be more effective; (b) *neglecting preventive care*: chronic dryness can lead to complications like dental caries, oral candidiasis and corneal ulcers if not properly managed, but preventive care is often overlooked [11, 12].

Overcoming This Pitfall For dry eye, patients should be encouraged to use preservative-free artificial tears frequently, and more advanced treatments like CsA eye drops, Lifitegrast eye solution (not available worldwide), or punctal plugs can be considered for refractory cases. For dry mouth, salivary stimulants like pilocarpine or cevimeline (not available worldwide) may be effective, and patients should be referred to a dentist for regular monitoring and preventive care, including fluoride treatments and the use of sugar-free lozenges to stimulate saliva production [13].

14.5 Insufficient Management of Fatigue and Pain

Fatigue and widespread pain are common in SS and can be debilitating as glandular symptoms. However, these systemic symptoms are often underestimated or attributed to other causes, leading to inadequate treatment and a significant impact on the patient's QoL.

Pitfalls in Addressing Fatigue and Pain (a) *Dismissal of symptoms*: patients with SS often report fatigue, arthralgias and myalgias that are dismissed as unrelated to their autoimmune RMD or are poorly understood, leading to ineffective treatment strategies; (b) *misattribution to depression*: fatigue may be mistakenly attributed to depression or psychosomatic factors, resulting in inappropriate or incomplete management [14].

Overcoming This Pitfall Management of fatigue and pain should include a comprehensive evaluation for other contributing factors, such as anaemia, thyroid dysfunction or fibromyalgia, which may be common in SS patients. Non-pharmacological approaches, including physical therapy, exercise programmes and cognitive–behavioural therapy, can help improve QoL. Pain management strategies should include both pharmacologic (NSAIDs, HCQ or low-dose CS) and non-pharmacologic approaches [15].

14.6 Risk of Lymphoma Development

One of the most serious complications of SS is an increased risk of NHL, particularly MALT lymphoma. Patients with long-standing or severe disease, particularly those with persistent parotid gland swelling, purpura, low complement levels or cryoglobulinaemia, are at heightened risk, yet this complication is often under-recognised. Furthermore, SS presents with symptoms that can overlap with other autoimmune conditions and chronic illnesses, including RA, SLE and even chronic fatigue syndrome. This can complicate the diagnosis [16].

Pitfalls in Identifying Lymphoma Risk (a) *Delayed detection*: the symptoms of lymphoma, such as gland swelling or systemic "B" symptoms (fever, night sweats and weight loss), may be misattributed to SS itself, delaying the diagnosis of this potentially life-threatening complication; (b) *failure to screen high-risk patients*: patients at high risk for lymphoma may not be regularly monitored, leading to delayed recognition of malignancy [17]. In Table 14.1, a list with the bad prognostic factors for lymphoma development is presented.

Overcoming This Pitfall Clinicians should maintain vigilance for signs of lymphoma in patients with SS, particularly those with significant parotid gland enlargement, splenomegaly or systemic symptoms. Regular monitoring of laboratory markers (such as serum complement levels and cryoglobulins) and imaging of the parotid glands may help detect early changes suggestive of lymphoma [18]. Early referral to haematology-oncology for biopsy or further evaluation is essential if lymphoma is suspected.

Table 14.1 Bad prognostic factors for lymphoma development in patients with Sjögren's syndrome

Category	Prognostic factors
Clinical features	Persistent salivary gland enlargement
	Lymphadenopathy
	Recurrent fever—night sweats
Laboratory findings	Low complement levels
	Cryoglobulinaemia
	Monoclonal gammopathy
	High beta-2 microglobulin levels
Histopathological features	Presence of large ectopic germinal centres
	High focus score in minor salivary gland biopsy
Immunological findings	Presence of rheumatoid factor
	Positive anti-Ro/SSA and anti-La/SSB antibodies
	Clonal B-cell expansion detected in salivary glands or peripheral blood

14.7 Limited Treatment Options

Unlike some other autoimmune diseases, there are relatively few FDA/EMA-approved treatments specifically for SS. Many treatments focus on symptom management rather than modifying the disease itself. This lack of targeted therapies can leave patients and clinicians feeling frustrated by the limited efficacy of available treatments, especially for systemic manifestations of the disease [19].

Pitfalls Due to Limited Treatment Choices (a) *Symptomatic treatment only*: current treatments for SS often focus on relieving symptoms (sicca syndrome) without addressing the underlying autoimmune process, leading to persistent disease activity and progression; (b) *lack of disease-modifying agents*: while HCQ and immunosuppressants like MTX or RTX are sometimes used, their efficacy in SS is variable and often modest compared to their use in diseases like RA or SLE.

Overcoming This Pitfall A personalised, multidisciplinary approach is essential in managing SS. While symptom management remains a key focus, clinicians should also consider immunosuppressive or biologic agents in cases with significant systemic involvement. Ongoing clinical trials may offer new therapeutic options in the future, so staying informed about emerging treatments is crucial [20].

14.8 Conclusion

SS presents a complex challenge for both patients and clinicians. The subtlety of its symptoms, the potential for systemic involvement and the limited availability of effective treatments all contribute to the pitfalls encountered in its management. By maintaining a high index of suspicion, employing comprehensive diagnostic and monitoring strategies and addressing both the glandular and systemic components of the disease, healthcare providers can better navigate these challenges and improve patient outcomes.

References

1. Pelechas E, Kaltsonoudis E, Voulgari PV, Drosos AA. Sjögren's syndrome. In: Illustrated handbook of rheumatic and musculo-skeletal diseases. Cham: Springer; 2023. https://doi.org/10.1007/978-3-031-47379-1_6.
2. Mavragani CP, Moutsopoulos HM. Sjögren's syndrome. Annu Rev Pathol. 2014;9:273–85. https://doi.org/10.1146/annurev-pathol-012513-104728.
3. Wang B, Chen S, Zheng Q, Li Y, Zhang X, Xuan J, et al. Early diagnosis and treatment for Sjögren's syndrome: current challenges, redefined disease stages and future prospects. J Autoimmun. 2021;117:102590. https://doi.org/10.1016/j.jaut.2020.102590.
4. Shiboski CH, Chiboski SC, Seror R, Criswell LA, Labetoulle M, Lietman TM, et al. 2016 ACR-EULAR classification criteria for primary Sjögren's syndrome: a consensus and data-driven methodology involving three international patient cohorts. Arthritis Rheumatol. 2016;69:35–45. https://doi.org/10.1002/art.39859.

5. Lee AYS, Rischmueller M. The diagnosis and misdiagnosis of Sjögren disease. Intern Med J. 2024;54:833–5. https://doi.org/10.1111/imj.16395.
6. Fisher BA, Jonsson R, Daniels T, Bombardieri M, Brown RM, Morgan P, et al. Standardisation of labial salivary gland histopathology in clinical trials in primary Sjögrne's syndrome. Ann Rheum Dis. 2017;76:1161–8. https://doi.org/10.1136/annrheumdis-2016-210448.
7. Negrini S, Emmi G, Greco M, Borro M, Sardanelli F, Murdaca G, et al. Sjögren's syndrome: a systemic autoimmune disease. Clin Exp Med. 2021;22:9–25. https://doi.org/10.1007/s10238-021-00728-6.
8. Maleki-Fischbach M, Kastsianok L, Koslow M, Chan ED. Arthritis Res Ther. 2024;26:43. https://doi.org/10.1186/s13075-024-03262-4.
9. Manzo C, Martinez-Suarez E, Kechida M, Isetta M, Serra-Mestres J. Cognitive function in primary Sjögren's syndrome: a systematic review. Brain Sci. 2019;9:85. https://doi.org/10.3390/brainsci9040085.
10. Kokoti M, Zisis V, Andreadis D, Bakopoulou A. Multidisciplinary therapeutic approach of a patient with Sjögren's syndrome: a three-year follow-up study. Cureus. 2024;16:e55148. https://doi.org/10.7759/cureus.55148.
11. Ramos-Casals M, Brito-Zerón P, Bombardieri S, Bootsma H, de Vita S, Dörner T, et al. EULAR recommendations for the management of Sjögren's syndrome with topical and systemic therapies. Ann Rheum Dis. 2020;79:3–18. https://doi.org/10.1136/annrheumdis-2019-216114.
12. Kruszka P, O'Brian RJO. Diagnosis and management of Sjögren syndrome. Am Fam Physician. 2009;79:465–70.
13. Ramos-Casals M, Brito-Zerón P, Sisó-Almirall A, Bosch X, Tzioufas AG. Topical and systemic medications for the treatment of primary Sjögren's syndrome. Nat Rev Rheumatol. 2012;8:399–411. https://doi.org/10.1038/nrrheum.2012.53.
14. Maeland E, Miyamoto ST, Hammenfors D, Valim V, Jonsson MV. Understanding fatigue in Sjögren's syndrome: outcome measures, biomarkers and possible interventions. Front Immunol. 2021;12:703079. https://doi.org/10.3389/fimmu.2021.703079.
15. Hackett KL, Deane KHO, Strassheim V, Deary V, Rapley T, Newton JL, et al. A systematic review of non-pharmacological interventions for primary Sjögren's syndrome. Rheumatology (Oxford). 2015;54:2025–32. https://doi.org/10.1093/rheumatology/kev227.
16. Fragkioudaki S, Mavragani CP, Moutsopoulos HM. Predicting the risk for lymphoma development in Sjögren syndrome. Medicine (Baltimore). 2016;95:e3766. https://doi.org/10.1097/MD0000000000003766.
17. Singh AG, Singh S, Matteson EL. Rate, risk factors and causes of mortality in patients with Sjögren's syndrome: a systematic review and meta-analysis of cohort studies. Rheumatology (Oxford). 2016;55:450–60. https://doi.org/10.1093/rheumatology/kev354.
18. Kapsogeorgou E, Voulgarelis M, Tzioufas AG. Predictive markers of lymphomagenesis in Sjögren's syndrome: From clinical data to molecular stratification. J Autoimmun. 2019;104:102316. https://doi.org/10.1016/j.jaut.2019.102316.
19. Tzioufas AG, Goules AV. Limited efficacy of targeted treatments in Sjögren's syndrome: why? Clin Exp Rheumatol. 2018;36:27–8.
20. Zhao T, Zhang R, Li Z, Qin D, Wang X. Novel and potential future therapeutic options in Sjögren's syndrome. Heliyon. 2024;10:e38803. https://doi.org/10.1016/j.heliyon.2024.e38803.

Pitfalls in Systemic Lupus Erythematosus 15

Abbreviations

ACR	American College of Rheumatology
ANA	Antinuclear antibodies
anti-Sm	Anti-Smith
AZA	Azathioprine
BLM	Belimumab
CNS	Central nervous system
CP	Cyclophosphamide
CRP	c-Reactive protein
CS	Corticosteroids
CVD	Cardiovascular disease
DMARDs	Disease-modifying anti-rheumatic drugs
ESR	Erythrocyte sedimentation rate
ESRD	End-stage renal disease
EULAR	European League Against Rheumatism
HCQ	Hydroxychloroquine
HL	Hodgkin's lymphoma
LN	Lupus nephritis
MMF	Mycophenolate mofetil
MTX	Methotrexate
NHL	Non-Hodgkin's lymphoma
QoL	Quality of life
RA	Rheumatoid arthritis
SLE	Systemic lupus erythematosus
SLEDAI	Systemic lupus erythematosus disease activity index

E. Pelechas et al., *Pitfalls in Rheumatology*,
https://doi.org/10.1007/978-3-031-98671-0_15

15.1 Delayed or Missed Diagnosis

Diagnosing SLE can be notoriously difficult, as tis symptoms often overlap with other conditions and can develop gradually over time. Common initial complaints (fatigue, joint pain and skin rashes) are non-specific and may be mistaken for other disorders, such as RA, fibromyalgia or even viral infections. Furthermore, SLE disproportionately affects women of childbearing age, and symptoms such as fatigue and joint pain can be misattributed to stress, hormonal changes or psychosomatic causes [1]. There are though some signs such as the "butterfly rash", Jaccoud's arthropathy and discoid skin lesions that are more characteristic of the disease and others such as pleuritis that are not so specific. In Fig. 15.1, all the above-mentioned signs are presented.

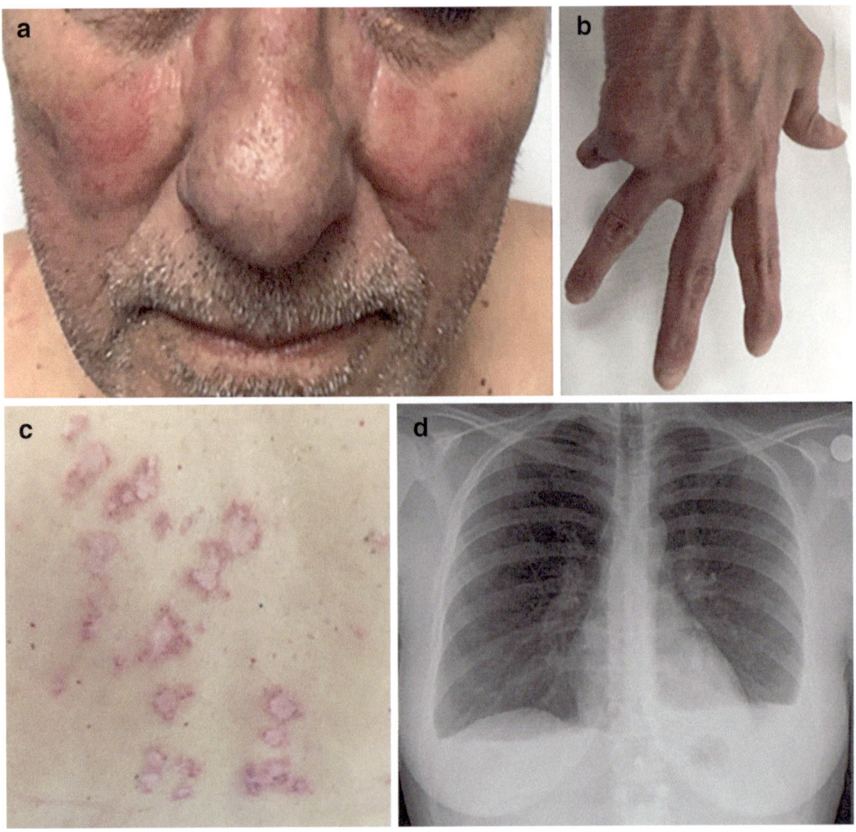

Fig. 15.1 (**a**) The "butterfly or malar rash" is a characteristic finding of the SLE but not pathognomonic; (**b**) Jaccoud's arthropathy is another characteristic sign of SLE, but again not pathognomonic. Jaccoud's arthropathy is a non-erosive reversible joint disorder that can be seen in patients with various autoimmune diseases except SLE; (**c**) discoid skin lesions on the trunk of a patient with SLE. Discoid lesions may present as purplish red, disc-shaped flat or slightly raised and firm areas of skin that may develop scarring or skin atrophy; (**d**) pleuritis in a newly-diagnosed patient with SLE. Serositis is a common finding in SLE patients and one of the causes of raised inflammatory markers

Consequences of Delayed Diagnosis (a) *Increased disease activity*: the longer SLE remains undiagnosed, the more time the immune system has to cause inflammation and damage to organs such as the kidneys, heart and lungs; (b) *organ damage*: delay in diagnosis, particularly in patients with LN or CNS involvement, can lead to irreversible organ damage; (c) *patient frustration and misunderstanding*: a delay in diagnosing SLE often leaves patients feeling frustrated and misunderstood, potentially leading to poor mental health and reduced QoL [2].

Overcoming This Pitfall Clinicians should maintain a high index of suspicion for SLE, particularly in young women presenting with a combination of systemic symptoms such as unexplained fatigue, fever, joint pain, photosensitive rash or kidney abnormalities. Screening for SLE should include a detailed history and physical examination, along with laboratory tests such as ANA testing, anti-dsDNA, anti-Sm antibodies, complement levels, lupus anticoagulant, anti-β2GPI and anti-aCL. Early referral to a rheumatologist can help ensure prompt diagnosis and appropriate treatment [3].

15.2 Over-Reliance on Serologic Testing

While the presence of ANA and other autoantibodies is a key feature of SLE, not all patients with SLE test positive for these antibodies, particularly early in the disease course (this represents a very small percentage of SLE patients). Conversely, a positive ANA test can also be seen in healthy individuals or those with other autoimmune conditions, leading to potential overdiagnosis [4].

Pitfalls of Over-Reliance on Serology (a) *False positives*: a positive ANA test alone (especially in low titer) is not diagnostic of SLE, and over-reliance on this test can lead to the misdiagnosis of SLE in patients who may have other conditions or no autoimmune disease at all [5]; (b) *missed seronegative SLE*: as mentioned before, a small fragment of patients with SLE may test negative for ANA or specific lupus-related antibodies, particularly early in the disease, leading to missed diagnoses if clinicians rely too heavily on serologic testing (although this is a relatively rare scenario) [6].

Overcoming This Pitfall The diagnosis of SLE should be based on a combination of clinical findings and laboratory results, rather than serologic tests alone. The EULAR/ACR classification criteria can be useful tools to guide diagnosis, focusing on a range of clinical and laboratory features. In patients with suggestive clinical symptoms but negative serology, follow-up and re-testing over time may be necessary to capture the evolving disease [7].

15.3 Underappreciation of Organ Involvement

SLE is not confined to the joints and skin. It can involve any organ system, and failure to recognise systemic involvement is a major pitfall. Some of the most serious complications of SLE, such as LN, cardiac involvement and neuropsychiatric lupus, may present with subtle or non-specific symptoms, leading to delayed recognition and treatment [8].

Pitfalls of Failing to Identify Organ Involvement (a) *LN*: kidney involvement can be asymptomatic in its early stages, but if untreated, it can progress to ESRD. Routine monitoring of renal function and urinalysis is essential, even in patients who do not report symptoms [9]; (b) *neuropsychiatric lupus*: neuropsychiatric manifestations of SLE, such as cognitive dysfunction, seizures, psychosis and mood disorders may be mistakenly attributed to other causes such as depression or anxiety, leading to a failure to address the underlying autoimmune process [10]; (c) *CVD*: SLE patients are at increased risk of CVD, including premature atherosclerosis, endocarditis and pericarditis, yet this risk is often underappreciated, leading to a lack of preventive measures [11, 12].

Overcoming This Pitfall A multidisciplinary approach to monitoring organ involvement in SLE is essential. Routine laboratory testing, including urinalysis, renal function tests and complement levels, should be part of regular care to detect early signs of LN. Cardiac monitoring, including echocardiograms and regular blood pressure assessments, can help identify cardiovascular complications early. A detailed neurological assessment should be conducted in patients with neuropsychiatric symptoms to rule out neuropsychiatric lupus [13]. Finally, the modification of coexisting classic risk factors, such as diabetes mellitus, should be addressed promptly, as they contribute to target organ damage.

15.4 Inconsistent Monitoring of Disease Activity

SLE is characterised by periods of flare-ups and remission. Inadequate or inconsistent monitoring of disease activity can result in missed flares of the escalation of treatment without adequate justification. Additionally, the wide variability in symptoms from patient to patient makes standardised monitoring challenging [14].

Consequences of Inconsistent Monitoring (a) *Missed flares*: failure to recognise an impending flare can lead to severe disease activity, causing organ damage, particularly in patients with LN or CNS involvement; (b) *overtreatment or undertreatment*: without regular monitoring, clinicians may overtreat with immunosuppressive medications when disease activity is low or fail to escalate therapy during periods of high disease activity.

Overcoming This Pitfall Disease activity in SLE should be regularly assessed (and should be individualised) using a combination of clinical evaluation, laboratory tests (such as anti-dsDNA antibodies, complement levels and markers of inflammation) and validated disease activity indices such as the SLEDAI. Patients should be educated to recognise early signs of a flare, such as increased fatigue, joint pain or skin rash, and report these symptoms promptly [15, 16].

15.5 Overlooking the Psychological Impact of SLE

The psychological burden of living with SLE is often underestimated. Depression, anxiety and fatigue are common in patients with SLE, and these symptoms can significantly impair the quality of life. However, they are often overlooked in clinical assessments, leading to undertreatment of mental health issues [17].

Pitfalls in Addressing Mental Health (a) *Undiagnosed depression and anxiety*: chronic pain, fatigue and uncertainty about the disease's course can lead to depression and anxiety, but these symptoms may be misattributed solely to the physical aspects of the disease, leading to missed opportunities for mental health interventions; (b) *failure to address QoL*: SLE patients often experience fatigue and reduced physical functioning, which can lead to isolation and impaired social and occupational functioning. These aspects of the disease may not be adequately addressed in routine care.

Overcoming This Pitfall Mental health screenings should be incorporated into routine SLE management. Clinicians should ask about mood, sleep, and fatigue, and consider referrals to mental health professionals or support groups. Treatment of fatigue should include managing both the physical aspects of the disease and addressing psychological contributors. Cognitive–behavioural therapy, regular exercise and social support can all help improve the quality of life [17]. Finally, it is important to distinguish the symptoms of neuropsychiatric SLE from those resulting from the psychological burden of the disease itself, which in some cases may resemble each other and be difficult to differentiate. Nevertheless, this distinction is crucial: if the psychological symptoms are due to active SLE, immunosuppressive treatment is warranted; in contrast, if they are due to anxiety or depression, the condition should be managed with mood-modifying medications.

15.6 Inadequate Treatment or Overtreatment of Mild or Non-Organ-Threatening Disease

In patients with milder forms of SLE or without immediate organ-threatening manifestations, there is a tendency to undertreat the disease, particularly when the symptoms are primarily related to joint pain or fatigue. Inadequate treatment can lead to poor long-term outcomes, including disease progression and organ damage [18]. On the other hand, in cases of non-threatening, mild disease, the administration of heavy immunosuppressive therapy or high doses of CS may result in unnecessary and unjustified immunosuppression, leading to long-term side effects, as described in the following section.

Pitfalls of Undertreatment (a) *Persistent disease activity*: even mild SLE requires appropriate treatment to prevent chronic inflammation and future flares, yet undertreatment may result in ongoing symptoms and cumulative damage; (b) *progression to organ damage*: some patients with seemingly mild disease may later develop more serious organ involvement if the underlying inflammation is not controlled.

Overcoming This Pitfall Treatment of SLE should be tailored to disease severity, but even mild disease requires close monitoring and appropriate management to control symptoms and prevent progression. HCQ is a cornerstone of SLE treatment and should be used in nearly all patients, regardless of disease severity, as it has been shown to reduce flares, improve survival and protect against organ damage. CS and other immunosuppressive agents should be used judiciously, balancing the need to control inflammation with the risk of side effects and following the official guidelines [19].

15.7 Medication Side Effects and Long-Term Toxicity

The medications used to manage SLE, particularly CS and immunosuppressive agents, can cause significant side effects, especially when used long-term. CS, while highly effective at controlling inflammation, can lead to serious complications such as osteoporosis, diabetes, hypertension and infections [20].

Pitfalls Related to Medication Toxicity (a) *Overuse of CS*: high dose or prolonged use of CS can lead to severe side effects, but tapering these drugs can be challenging when the disease is active or flaring; (b) *immunosuppression-related infections*: immunosuppressive medications increase the risk of infections, which can be life-threatening, particularly in patients receiving high-dose CS, CP or biologic DMARDs [21]. Also, medication or rescue therapies may contribute to this direction [22].

Overcoming This Pitfall The goal of SLE management should be to use the lowest effective dose of CS for the shortest possible time. HCQ should be used in all patients to minimise the need of CS. Immunosuppressive agents such as MTX, AZA and MMF can help reduce reliance on CS, and newer biologic agents such as BLM can also be considered for steroid-sparing effects [23]. Particular attention to infections should be given in patients receiving rituximab, and regular screening for malignancy is recommended in patients treated with CP. Regular monitoring for side effects, including bone density testing and screening for infections, is essential in patients on long-term immunosuppression [24].

15.8 SLE and Cancer Development

One of the primary challenges in patients with SLE is differentiating between autoimmune activity and potential malignancy. SLE can mimic the clinical and laboratory features of several cancers, leading to delays or misdiagnosis [25]. For example:

Lymphoma SLE patients often present with lymphadenopathy, splenomegaly and constitutional symptoms such as fever, weight loss and night sweats. These features overlap significantly with NHL and HL, both of which are associated with an increased incidence in SLE [26].

Pleural and Pericardial Effusions In SLE, pleural or pericardial effusions may arise from serositis, an inflammatory condition, whereas similar findings in cancer patients may indicate metastasis or a primary malignancy of the pleura or pericardium.

Laboratory and imaging techniques often fail to make a clear distinction. For instance, anaemia, an elevated ESR or CRP can signal either active SLE or an underlying malignancy. Hence, clinicians must maintain a high index of suspicion when evaluating new symptoms in SLE patients, balancing the investigation of active disease against the potential for malignancy.

Increased Risk of Hematologic Malignancies As mentioned above, SLE patients are at a notably higher risk for NHL and HL, with studies suggesting up to a fourfold increase in risk. Chronic immune activation, B-cell hyperactivity and the prolonged use of immunosuppressive drugs are believed to contribute to this increased risk. SLE-associated NHL tends to present in extranodal sites, complicating its detection and treatment [26].

Decreased Risk of Breast and Endometrial Cancers Interestingly, some epidemiologic studies suggest that SLE patients have a lower risk of breast and endometrial cancers compared to the general population. The reasons for this remain unclear but may involve alterations in hormone metabolism due to chronic inflammation or the immunosuppressive therapies used in SLE management [27].

Lung and Liver Cancers Increased risk of lung and liver cancers have also been observed, particularly among patients with a history of smoking or alcohol use. The complex interaction between environmental risk factors, chronic inflammation and immunosuppressive therapies may drive this increased susceptibility.

Increased Risk of Bladder Cancer The risk of genitourinary malignancy, particularly bladder cancer, is higher following exposure to CP, which is often used in cases of major organ involvement, such as renal disease.

Screening for Cancer In SLE patients presents numerous difficulties. Given their increased risk for certain malignancies, more rigorous screening might seem appropriate, yet several issues make this problematic: (a) *diagnostic confusion*: symptoms such as fatigue, fever and weight loss, which can signal both SLE flares and cancer, may lead to diagnostic delays. Clinicians may mistakenly attribute new symptoms to disease activity rather than considering the possibility of a malignancy; (b) *immunosuppressive therapy interference*: the immunosuppressive treatments used in SLE can suppress tumour markers and alter the immune response, potentially leading to false negatives in cancer screening tests. For example, immunosuppression, and especially CS, may mask the inflammatory response typically seen in malignancies, causing clinicians to overlook early warning signs; (c) *underscreening in the SLE population*: despite an increased risk of certain cancers, SLE patients may not always receive appropriate cancer screening. This may be due to competing priorities in managing the underlying autoimmune disease or a lack of awareness among healthcare providers about the cancer risks specific to SLE [28].

15.9 Conclusion

Managing SLE presents unique challenges due to the complexity of its clinical manifestations, its unpredictable course and the limitations of current treatment options. Early and accurate diagnosis, comprehensive monitoring of disease activity and a personalised approach to treatment that balances disease control with minimising side effects are key to optimising outcomes. Addressing both the physical and psychological aspects of the disease is essential to improve the quality of life for patients living with SLE. Finally, as the relationship between SLE and cancer development is multifaceted, presenting numerous clinical, immunological and psychosocial challenges, patients should be screened appropriately and rheumatologists should have a high index of suspicion, in order to diagnose and treat early different malignancies. In Fig. 15.2, a flowchart shows a proposed way of cancer screening in SLE patients.

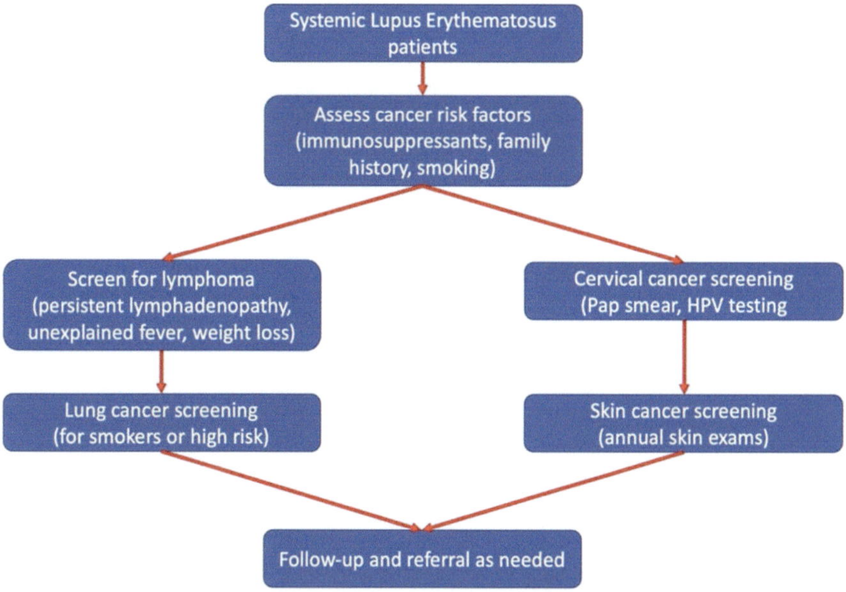

Fig. 15.2 Proposed cancer screening flowchart for systemic lupus erythematosus patients

References

1. Pelechas E, Kaltsonoudis E, Voulgari PV, Drosos AA. Systemic lupus erythematosus. In: Illustrated handbook of rheumatic and musculo-skeletal diseases. Cham: Springer; 2023. https://doi.org/10.1007/978-3-031-47379-1_10.
2. Mitchell JL. Understanding the impact of delayed diagnosis and misdiagnosis of systemic lupus erythematosus (SLE). J Family Med Prim Care. 2024;13:4819–23. https://doi.org/10.4103/jfmpc.jfmpc_1177_24.
3. American College of Rheumatology Ad Hoc Committee on Systemic Lupus Erythematosus Guidelines. Guidelines for referral ANA management of systemic lupus erythematosus in adults. Arthritis Rheum. 1999;42:1785–96.
4. Li QZ, Karp DR, Quan J, Branch VK, Zhou J, Lian Y, et al. Risk factors for ANA positivity in healthy persons. Arthritis Res Ther. 2011;13:R38. https://doi.org/10.1186/ar3271.
5. Grygiel Górniak B, Rogacka N, Puszczewicz M. Antinuclear antibodies in healthy people and non-rheumatic diseases—diagnostic and clinical implications. Reumatologia. 2018;56:243–8. https://doi.org/10.5114/reum.2018.77976.
6. Bakshi N, Munir T, Guma M, Chenitz KB. A rare case of antinuclear antibody (ANA)-negative lupus nephritis. Cureus. 2023;15:e41480. https://doi.org/10.7759/cureus.41480.
7. Aringer M, Costenbader KH, Daikh DI, Brinks R, Mosca M, Ramsey-Goldman R, et al. 2019 EULAR/ACR classification criteria for systemic lupus erythematosus. Arthritis Rheumatol. 2019;71:1400–12. https://doi.org/10.1002/art.40930.
8. Cojocaru M, Cojocaru IM, Silosi I, Vrabie CD. Manifestations of systemic lupus erythematosus. Maedica (Bucur). 2011;6:330–6.

9. Seshan SV, Jennette JC. Renal disease in systemic lupus erythematosus with emphasis on classification of lupus glomerulonephritis: advances and implications. Arch Pathol Lab Med. 2009;133:233–48. https://doi.org/10.5858/133.2.233.
10. Popescu A, Kao AH. Neuropsychiatric Systemic lupus erythematosus. Curr Neuropharmacol. 2011;9:449–57. https://doi.org/10.2174/157015911796557984.
11. Zeller CB, Appenzeller S. Cardiovascular disease in systemic lupus erythematosus: the role of traditional and lupus related risk factors. Curr Cardiol Rev. 2008;4:116–22. https://doi.org/10.2174/157340308784245775.
12. Pieta A, Pelechas E, Gerolymatou N, Voulgari PV, Drosos AA. Calcified constrictive pericarditis resulting in tamponade in a patient with systemic lupus erythematosus. Rheumatol Int. 2021;41:651–70. https://doi.org/10.1007/s00296-020-04747-6.
13. Galoppini G, Marangoni A, Cirilli F, Ruffilli F, Garaffoni C, Govoni M, et al. Optimizing patient care: a systematic review of multidisciplinary approaches for SLE management. J Clin Med. 2023;12:4059. https://doi.org/10.3390/jcm12124059.
14. Mosca M, Tani C, Aringer M, Bombardieri S, Boumpas D, Cervera R, et al. Development of quality indicators to evaluate the monitoring of SLE patients in routine clinical practice. Autoimmun Rev. 2011;10:383–8. https://doi.org/10.1016/j.autrev.2010.12.008.
15. Mathian A, Mouries-Martin S, Dorgham K, Devilliers H, Barnabei L, Salah EB, et al. Monitoring disease activity in systemic lupus erythematosus with single-molecule array digital enzyme-linked immunosorbent assay quantification of serum interferon-α. Arthritis Rheumatol. 2019;71:756–65. https://doi.org/10.1002/art.40792.
16. Bombardier C, Gladman DD, Urowitz MB, Caron D, Chang CH. Derivation of the SLEDAI. A disease activity index fro lupus patients. The committee on prognosis studies in SLE. Arthritis Rheum. 1992;35:630–40. https://doi.org/10.1002/art.1780350606.
17. Figueiredo-Braga M, Cornaby C, Cortez A, Bernardes M, Terroso G, Figueiredo M, et al. Depression and anxiety in systemic lupus erythematosus. Medicine (Baltimore). 2018;97:e11376. https://doi.org/10.1097/MD.0000000000011376.
18. Arnaud L, Tektonidou MG. Long-term outcomes in systemic lupus erythematosus: trends over time and major contributors. Rheumatology (Oxford). 2020;59:v29–38. https://doi.org/10.1093/rheumatology/keaa382.
19. Fanouriakis A, Kostopoulou M, Andersen J, Aringer M, Arnaud L, Bae SC, et al. EULAR recommendations for the management of systemic lupus erythematosus: 2023 update. Ann Rheum Dis. 2024;83:15–29. https://doi.org/10.1136/ard-2023-224762.
20. Popa R, Lautaru LA, Lucretiu R, Ruiu DC, Caragea D, Olteanu M. Therapy side effects in systemic lupus erythematosus. Curr Health Sci J. 2018;44:316–21. https://doi.org/10.12865/CHSJ.44.03.18.
21. Quan XY, Chen HT, Liang SG, Yang C, Yao CW, Xu YZ, et al. Revisited cyclophosphamide in the treatment of lupus nephritis. Biomed Res Int. 2022;2022:8345737. https://doi.org/10.1155/2022/8345737.
22. Pelechas E, Gerolymatou N, Voulgari PV, Drosos AA. Transfusion-related acute lung injury in a patient with systemic lupus erythematosus. Clin Exp Rheumatol. 2017;35:353.
23. Oon S, Huq M, Godfrey T, Nikpour M. Systematic review, and meta-analysis of steroid-sparing effect, of biologic agents in randomized, placebo-controlled phase 3 trials for systemic lupus erythematosus. Semin Arthritis Rheum. 2018;48:221–39. https://doi.org/10.1016/j.semarthrit.2018.01.001.
24. Mejía-Vilet JM, Ayoub I. The use of glucocorticoids in lupus nephritis: new pathways for an old drug. Front Med (Lausanne). 2021;8:622225. https://doi.org/10.3389/fmed.2021.622225.
25. Zhang M, Wang Y, Wang Y, Bai Y, Gu D. Association between systemic lupus erythematosus and cancer morbidity and mortality: findings from cohort studies. Front Oncol. 2022;12:860794.

26. Apor E, O'Brien J, Stephen M, Castillo JJ. Systemic lupus erythematosus is associated with increased incidence of hematologic malignancies: a meta-analysis of prospective cohort studies. Leuk Res. 2014;38:1067–71. https://doi.org/10.1016/j.leukres.2014.06.025.
27. Bernatsky S, Ramsey-Goldman R, Foulkes WD, Gordon C, Clarke AE. Breast, ovarian, and endometrial malignancies in systemic lupus erythematosus: a meta-analysis. Br J Cancer. 2011;104:1478–81. https://doi.org/10.1038/bjc.2011.115.
28. Bernatsky SR, Cooper GS, Mill C, Ramsey-Goldman R, Clarke AE, Pineau CA. Cancer screening in patients with systemic lupus erythematosus. J Rheumatol. 2006;33:45–9.

Pitfalls in Scleroderma

16

Abbreviations

ACA	Anti-centromere antibodies
ANA	Antinuclear antibodies
CP	Cyclophosphamide
CS	Corticosteroids
dcSScl	Diffuse cutaneous systemic sclerosis
GI	Gastrointestinal
GOERD	Gastroesophageal reflux disease
HRCT	High-resolution computed tomography
ILD	Interstitial lung disease
lcSScl	Limited cutaneous systemic sclerosis
MMF	Mycophenolate mofetil
NSIP	Non-specific interstitial pneumonia
NVC	Nailfold videocapillaroscopy
PAH	Pulmonary arterial hypertension
PFTs	Pulmonary function tests
QoL	Quality of life
RA	Rheumatoid arthritis
RMDs	Rheumatic diseases
RP	Raynaud's phenomenon
SLE	Systemic lupus erythematosus
SOB	Shortness of breath
SScl	Systemic sclerosis
UIP	Usual interstitial pneumonia

E. Pelechas et al., *Pitfalls in Rheumatology*,
https://doi.org/10.1007/978-3-031-98671-0_16

16.1 Misinterpreting Early Skin Changes

SScl may present with subtle early signs of skin involvement, such as RP or mild skin tightening, which are easily overlooked or attributed to other less serious conditions like stress or benign skin conditions. The skin changes can initially be limited to the fingers and toes (in the case of lcSScl), and they may be mistaken for non-specific changes related to aging, weather conditions or other inflammatory skin disorders [1]. For example, mouth puckering and telangiectasias sometimes are attributed to age-related changes (Fig. 16.1).

Consequences (a) *Delayed diagnosis*: early skin changes can be mistaken for other common conditions, such as contact dermatitis, eczema or even aging-related skin changes, delaying the recognition of SScl. This can result in significant organ involvement before the diagnosis is made; (b) *missed opportunity for early intervention*: delayed recognition of SScl can result in progression to irreversible organ damage, especially in the lungs and kidneys, where early intervention can improve prognosis [2].

How to Avoid This Pitfall (a) *Vigilant screening*: clinicians should be particularly vigilant in patients presenting with RP, particularly if they also have unexplained joint pain, dysphagia or GOERD. A detailed history of these early symptoms can help identify patients at risk; (b) *systematic skin examination*: pay attention to early signs of skin thickening, which can start insidiously in the fingers, forearms or face. The skin tightening, often referred to as "sclerodactyly", is a distinguishing feature of the disease; (c) *early referral*: if a patient presents with unexplained skin changes, particularly in the presence of RP or other systemic symptoms, early referral to a rheumatologist is crucial for accurate diagnosis and timely intervention [3].

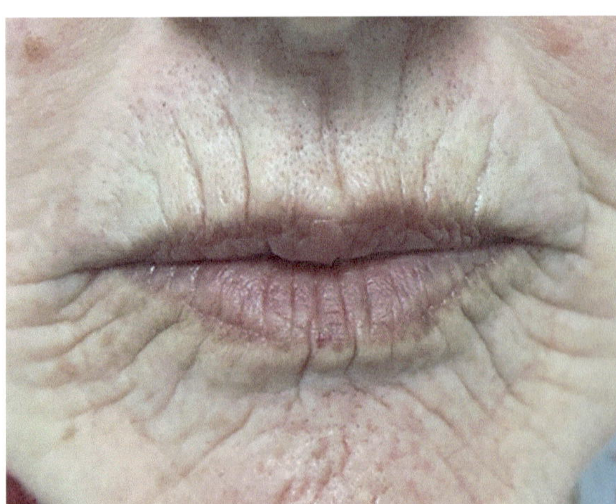

Fig. 16.1 Mouth puckering in a scleroderma patient. Reduced mouth opening occurs due to tightness in the skin on the face around the mouth

16.2 Delayed Diagnosis

SScl often begins with subtle, non-specific symptoms, such as RP, fatigue or mild skin changes, which can be mistaken for other conditions like SLE or RA. The slow onset of more specific signs, such as skin tightening or internal organ involvement, frequently delays diagnosis.

Consequences of Delayed Diagnosis (a) *Irreversible organ damage*: progression of pulmonary fibrosis or renal crisis can occur before SScl is identified [4]; (b) *worsened QoL*: early symptoms like RP or GI dysfunction may escalate without timely intervention; (c) *missed therapeutic window*: early treatment targeting inflammatory pathways that lead to vascular dysfunction or fibrosis may halt progression, but this opportunity is often missed, and it seems that there is also a difference between sexes [5]. In Fig. 16.2, pulmonary fibrosis with honeycombing is seen at both lung bases. In advanced cases, calcinosis cutis, another debilitating complication of SScl, may occur (Fig. 16.3).

Overcoming This Pitfall Clinicians should maintain a high index of suspicion in patients presenting with RP, especially when accompanied by skin thickening, digital ulcers or unexplained organ dysfunction. Routine use of autoantibody panels (ACA and anti-Scl-70) and NVC can aid in early identification [6].

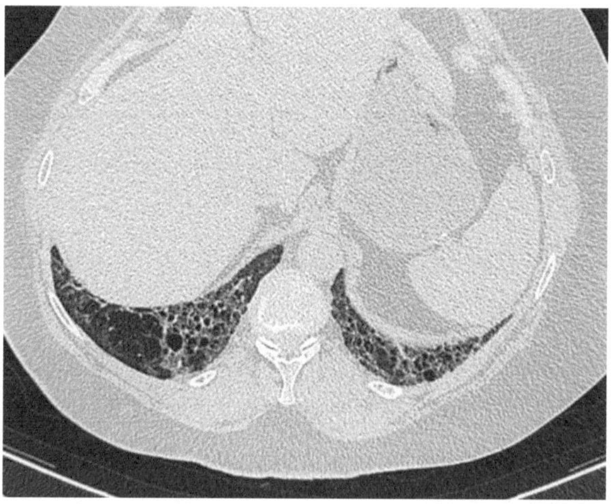

Fig. 16.2 High-resolution CT of a patient with systemic sclerosis. The most common ILD in SScl is NSIP pattern, but this is a UIP pattern which is also prevalent in SScl. The hallmark feature of UIP is honeycombing as you clearly see at both lung bases

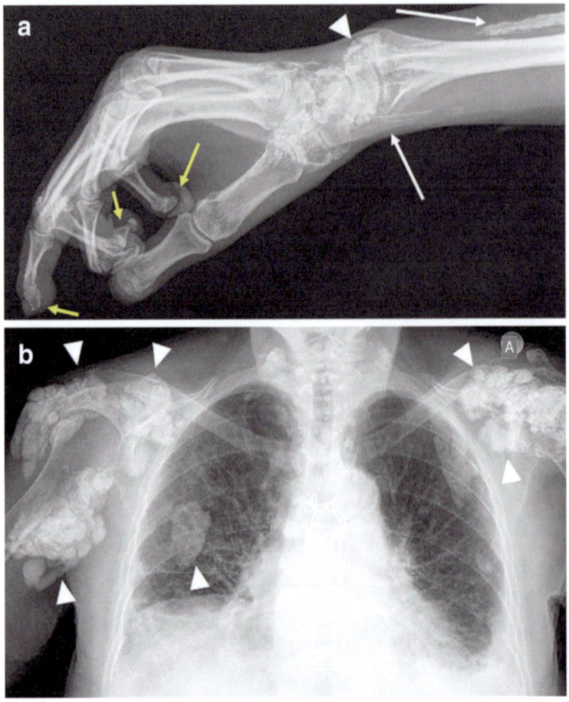

Fig. 16.3 (**a**) Calcinosis cutis is a late onset complication of SScl that can be debilitating. Deposition of insoluble calcium salts occurs in the skin and subcutaneous tissues (white arrowheads). Calcification of tendons can also occur with crepitus and significant pain while moving the affected anatomical region (white arrows). In yellow arrows, bone absorption of the terminal phalanges is also seen due to severe vascular complication of SScl; (**b**) severe accumulation of calcium subcutaneously (white arrowheads)

16.3 Over-Reliance on Serologic Markers

While serologic tests, such as ANA, ACA and anti-topoisomerase I (anti-Scl-70) antibodies, are useful in diagnosing SScl, they should not be relied upon in isolation. These tests are not always definitive and can be positive in other autoimmune condition or even in healthy individuals, particularly ANA. A false-negative result in a patient with early disease can also occur, especially when autoantibodies are not yet detectable [7].

Consequences (a) *False reassurance or misdiagnosis*: negative or inconclusive serologic results may lead clinicians to dismiss SScl as a possible diagnosis, potentially overlooking the early signs of disease. Conversely, a positive ANA or anti-Scl-70 may lead to misdiagnosis in a patient with further clinical evidence of SScl [8]; (b) *missed diagnosis*: given that only 50–70% of SScl patients test positive for specific autoantibodies, a negative test in the setting of suggestive clinical findings may delay diagnosis.

Strategy (a) *Clinical correlation*: always correlate serologic findings with clinical signs and symptoms. For instance, a positive ACA antibody is strongly associated with lcSScl, while anti-Scl-70 antibodies are more common in dcSScl. These markers should be interpreted within the context of the patient's full clinical presentation; (b) *broad differential diagnosis*: use serologic testing to support a clinical suspicion rather than relying on it as the sole diagnostic tool. Many RMDs share ANA positivity, and early forms of SScl may not show detectable autoantibodies at first; (c) *regular monitoring*: serologic tests should be repeated periodically in patients with a suspected diagnosis of SScl, especially if the clinical picture evolves over time.

16.4 Suboptimal Treatment Strategies

Treatment of SScl is not one-size-fits-all and varies based on the subset (lcSScl vs dcSScl) and organ involvement. However, inadequate recognition of disease-specific manifestations can lead to both under- and overtreatment [9].

Pitfalls in Treatment (a) *Undertreatment*: early vascular changes (digital ulcers or RP) may be underestimated, delaying vasodilator therapy. Similarly, systemic complications like pulmonary fibrosis may be overlooked until it gets advanced [10]; (b) *overtreatment*: aggressive immunosuppression in patients with limited disease or stable manifestations may cause more harm than benefit; (c) *failure to personalise therapy*: SScl involves a spectrum of clinical manifestations, requiring individualised care plans [11].

Overcoming This Pitfall Management should involve early initiation of targeted therapies, such as endothelin receptor antagonists for pulmonary hypertension or antifibrotics for lung involvement. A multidisciplinary team, including rheumatologists, pulmonologists and gastroenterologists, is essential for tailored care [12].

16.5 Failure to Recognise Vascular Changes

SScl is known for its vascular involvement, particularly in the form of RP, which causes episodic colour changes in the fingers and toes in response to cold or stress. Although the majority of these episodes are benign, they can often be dismissed as simple as a variant of normal cold intolerance. Additionally, digital ulcers, another hallmark of the disease, may be mistaken for simple mechanical injury or infections [13].

Consequences (a) *Undiagnosed vascular complications*: failure to recognise RP or the early development of digital ulcers can lead to worsening vascular damage leading to more profound ulcers such as the one in Fig. 16.4 and even gangrene, including irreversible loss of blood flow to extremities or other organs, which can be difficult to reverse once established [14]; (b) *delayed diagnosis of internal organ involvement*: vascular complications in SScl can extend beyond the extremities to internal organs, such as the lungs (PAH) or kidneys (SScl renal crisis) [15]. Early recognition of these symptoms allows for better management and prevention of long-term damage.

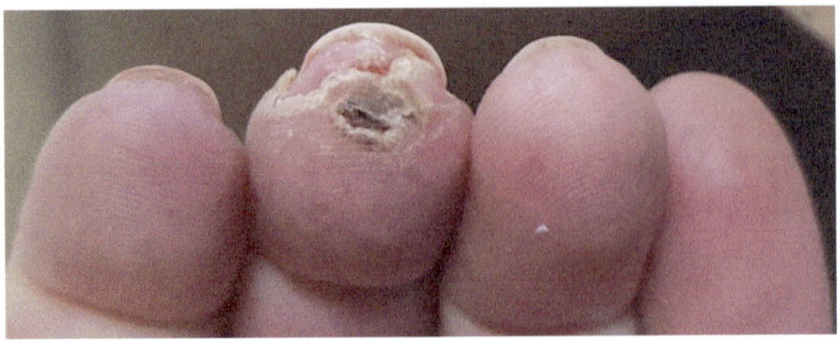

Fig. 16.4 Vascular complication in SScl. Deep ulcer at the tip of the middle finger of a patient with severe secondary Raynaud's phenomenon due to SScl. This kind of skin lesions produce significant pain and disability

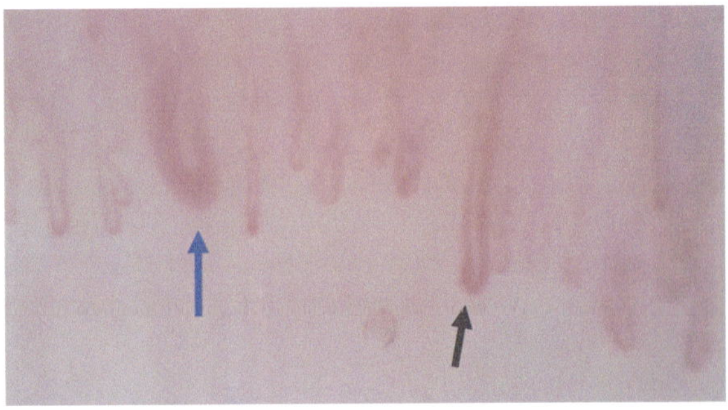

Fig. 16.5 Nailfold videocapillaroscopy showing an early scleroderma pattern. The blue arrow point towards a giant capillary (>50 μm) and the black towards a capillary dilatation

Strategy (a) *Detailed history and physical examination*: always assess for signs of RP and digital ulcers, especially in patients with symptoms like unexplained coldness or colour changes in fingers or toes. Also, note any signs of telangiectasia or RP in the mucosal surfaces or nailfolds; (b) *capillaroscopy*: NVC is a simple, non-invasive test that can be invaluable in detecting microvascular abnormalities characteristic of SScl, with the most characteristic finding being giant capillaries (Fig. 16.5). Even one giant capillary poses significant chances for a positive diagnosis of scleroderma. This test can provide early evidence of disease, especially in patients with vague or early symptoms [16]; (c) *screening for pulmonary and cardiac involvement*: regular screening for pulmonary fibrosis (via chest CT), PAH (via echocardiogram) and kidney function (via blood pressure measurements and serum creatinine) should be part of the initial workup and ongoing monitoring in patients with suspected SScl [17].

16.6 Overlooking Extracutaneous Manifestations

While SScl is most recognised for its skin changes, internal organ involvement significantly impacts morbidity and mortality. Pulmonary, GI, renal and cardiovascular complications are often underdiagnosed or inadequately managed [18], with some of them being life-threatening [19].

Pitfalls of Ignoring Systemic Involvement (a) *Pulmonary complications*: ILD and PAH are the leading causes of mortality in SScl, yet symptoms like mild dyspnoea can be overlooked [20]; (b) *GI dysfunction*: from GOERD to severe malabsorption due to bacterial overgrowth, GI issues are frequently underappreciated. Caution is also required, as in a very small percentage of cases, scleroderma SScl may present without its characteristic skin manifestations, a condition known as systemic sclerosis sine scleroderma [21].

Overcoming This Pitfall Regular screening with HRCT, echocardiography and PFTs is essential. Early referral to appropriate specialists (e.g. pulmonologists or gastroenterologists) ensures comprehensive management [22]. Furthermore, in cases of characteristic imaging or endoscopic patterns suggestive of SScl, immunological testing and/or referral to a rheumatologist should be performed.

16.7 Misdiagnosing Diffuse Cutaneous Scleroderma as Localised Scleroderma

Localised scleroderma (morphoea) and eosinophilic fasciitis can resemble SScl in its initial stages, particularly when the skin is the primary organ involved. However, morphoea is a much less aggressive form of the disease, with no systemic involvement, while dcSScl is more likely to affect internal organs such as the lungs, heart or kidneys. Early misdiagnosis of dcSSc as localised scleroderma can delay the initiation of appropriate systemic treatments [23].

Consequences (a) *Inadequate treatment*: failure to recognise systemic involvement in dcSScl may result in inappropriate treatment, with patients being offered only localised therapies, such as topical CS, rather than more aggressive systemic interventions; (b) *missed organ damage*: delaying the diagnosis of SScl may allow internal organ fibrosis to progress undetected, leading to irreversible damage, particularly in the lungs and kidneys.

Overcoming This Pitfall (a) *Thorough clinical assessment*: a detailed history and physical examination should be performed to assess for any signs of internal organ involvement, such as SOB (suggesting pulmonary fibrosis) or blood pressure changes (suggesting renal involvement); (b) *differentiating morphoea from SScl*: look for signs of systemic disease, such as weight loss, fatigue or internal organ involvement (dysphagia and dyspnoea). SScl is often associated with more widespread skin changes and a history of RP, while morphoea is typically limited to focal skin plaques; (c) *imaging and functional tests*: if internal organ involvement is suspected, consider imaging studies (such as chest X-ray and CT scan) or PFTs to evaluate for early signs of fibrosis and echocardiography or kidney function tests to assess for organ damage [24].

16.8 Medication Side Effects and Monitoring

Medications for SScl, including immunosuppressants (e.g. MMF and CP) and vasodilators, carry significant risks. Side effects may exacerbate patient morbidity if not managed appropriately [25].

Challenges with Medication Toxicity (a) *Inadequate monitoring*: regular follow-ups for organ function (liver, pulmonary and renal) are often overlooked, delaying the detection of adverse effects; (b) *non-adherence*: fear of side effects or lack of understanding about the disease can lead to poor compliance [26].

Overcoming This Pitfall Clinicians should provide detailed patient education about the risks and benefits of therapies. Routine monitoring, including PFTs, liver and kidney function and blood counts, is essential. Prophylactic measures, such as annual influenza and pneumococcal vaccination, can mitigate infection risks.

16.9 Psychosocial and Mental Health Challenges

SScl imposes significant physical and emotional burdens. Patients may experience chronic pain, disfigurement and functional limitations, leading to depression, anxiety and social isolation.

Psychosocial Pitfalls (a) *Under-recognised mental health issues*: depression and anxiety are prevalent but often overlooked in SScl patients; (b) *impact on QoL*: physical limitations, such as difficulty with daily tasks due to skin tightening or fatigue, can lead to reduced independence and social withdrawal [27].

Overcoming This Pitfall Integrating mental health support, including counselling and antidepressant therapy, into SScl care can improve outcomes. Patient support groups and rehabilitation programmes (occupational and physical therapy) can also enhance coping strategies and the quality of life [28].

16.10 Conclusion

SScl management involves navigating numerous pitfalls, from delayed diagnosis to under-recognised systemic complications and psychosocial challenges. Early identification and a holistic, multidisciplinary approach are key to improving outcomes. By addressing these challenges, clinicians can better support patients in managing this complex disease, reducing morbidity and enhancing their QoL.

References

1. Pelechas E, Kaltsonoudis E, Voulgari PV, Drosos AA. Scleroderma. In: Illustrated handbook of rheumatic and musculo-skeletal diseases. Cham: Springer; 2023. https://doi.org/10.1007/978-3-031-47379-1_11.
2. Delisle VC, Hudson M, Baron M, Thombs BD. Sex and time to diagnosis in systemic sclerosis: an updated analysis of 1,129 patients form the Canadian scleroderma research group registry. Clin Exp Rheumatol. 2014;32:S-10–4.
3. Distler O, Allanore Y, Denton CP, Matucci-Cerinic M, Pope JE, Hinzmann B, et al. Factors influencing early referral, early diagnosis and management in patients with diffuse cutaneous systemic sclerosis. Rheumatology (Oxford). 2018;57:813–7. https://doi.org/10.1093/rheumatology/kex504.
4. Herzog EL, Mathur A, Tager AM, Feghali-Bostwick C, Schneider F, Varga J. Interstitial lung disease associated with systemic sclerosis and idiopathic pulmonary fibrosis. Arthritis Rheumatol. 2014;66:1967–78.
5. Koletsos N, Kaltsonoudis E, Trentzidis K, Pelechas E, Gerolymatou N, Memi T, Voulgari PV. Pulmonary involvement in systemic sclerosis: can sex play a role? Rheumatology (Oxford). 2024;25:keae639. https://doi.org/10.1093/rheumatology/keae639.
6. Maciejewska M, Sikora M, Maciejewski C, Alda-Malicka R, Czuwara J, Rudnicka L. Raynaud's phenomenon with focus on systemic sclerosis. J Clin Med. 2022;11:2490. https://doi.org/10.3390/jcm11092490.
7. Mecoli CA, Casciola-Rosen L. An update on autoantibodies in scleroderma. Curr Opin Rheumatol. 2018;30:548–53. https://doi.org/10.1097/BOR.0000000000000550.
8. Salazar GA, Assassi S, Wigley F, Hummers L, Varga J, Hinchcliff M, et al. Antinuclear antibody negative systemic sclerosis. Semin Arthritis Rheum. 2014;44:680–6. https://doi.org/10.1016/j.semarthrit.2014.11.006.
9. Pope JE, Denton CP, Johnson SR, Fernandez-Codina A, Hudson M, Nevskaya T. State-of-the-art evidence in the treatment of systemic sclerosis. Nat Rev Rheumatol. 2023;19:212–26. https://doi.org/10.1038/s41584-023-00909-5.
10. Pattanaik D, Brown M, Postlethwaite A. Vascular involvement in systemic sclerosis (scleroderma). J Inflamm Res. 2011;4:105–25. https://doi.org/10.2147/JIR.S18145.
11. Dobrota R, Jibai C, Distler O. Personalized medicine in systemic sclerosis: facts and promises. Curr Rheumatol Rep. 2014;16:425. https://doi.org/10.1007/s11926-014-0425-8.
12. Farina N, Benanti G, De Luca G, Palmisano A, Peretto G, Tomassetti S, et al. The role of the multidisciplinary health care team in the management of patients with systemic sclerosis. J Multidiscip Healthc. 2022;15:815–24. https://doi.org/10.2147/JMDH.S295478.
13. Guiducci S, Giacomelli R, Matucci-Cerinic M. Vascular complications of scleroderma. Autoimmun Rev. 2007;6:520–3. https://doi.org/10.1016/j.autrev.2006.12.006.
14. Hughes M, Bruni C, Ruaro B, Confalonieri M, Matucci-Cerinic M, Bellando-Randone S. Digital ulcers in systemic sclerosis. Presse Med. 2021;50:104064. https://doi.org/10.1016/j.lpm.2021.104064.
15. Chaisson NF, Hassoun PM. Systemic sclerosis-associated pulmonary arterial hypertension. Chest. 2013;144:1346–56. https://doi.org/10.1378/chest.12.2396.
16. Lambova SN, Müller-Ladner U. Nailfold capillaroscopy in systemic sclerosis—state of the art: the evolving knowledge about capillaroscopic abnormalities in systemic sclerosis. J Scleroderma Relat Disord. 2019;4:200–11. https://doi.org/10.1177/2397198319833486.
17. Guicã A, Mihai C, Jurcut C, Gheorgiu AM, Groseanu L, Dima A, et al. Screening for pulmonary hypertension in systemic sclerosis—a primer for cardio-rheumatology clinics. Diagnostics (Basel). 2021;11:1013. https://doi.org/10.3390/diagnostics11061013.

18. Forbes A, Marie I. Gastrointestinal complications: the most frequent internal complications of systemic sclerosis. Rheumatology (Oxford). 2009;48:iii36–9. https://doi.org/10.1093/rheumatology/ken485.
19. Cossio M, Menon Y, Wilson W, deBiosblanc BP. Life-threatening complications of systemic sclerosis. Crit Care Clin. 2002;18:819–39. https://doi.org/10.1016/s0749-0704(02)00023-4.
20. Mulkoju R, Saka VK, Rajaram M, Kumari R, Negi VS, Mohapatra MM, et al. Pulmonary manifestations in systemic sclerosis: hospital-based descriptive study. Cureus. 2020;12:e8649. https://doi.org/10.7759/cureus.8649.
21. Makris A, Panagiotopoulos A, Distler O, Sfikakis PP. Systemic sclerosis sine scleroderma: a time of reappraisal. J Rheumatol. 2024;51:1060–8. https://doi.org/10.3899/jrheum.2023-1113.
22. Khanna D, Distrler O, Cottin V, Brown KK, Chung L, Goldin JG. Diagnosis and monitoring of systemic sclerosis-associated interstitial lung disease using high-resolution computed tomography. J Scleroderma Relat Disord. 2022;7:168–78. https://doi.org/10.1177/23971983211064463.
23. Dilia G, Michele C, Emanuele C, Amelia S, Federica L, Clodoveo F. From localized scleroderma to systemic sclerosis: coexistence or possible evolution. Dermatol Res Pract. 2018;2018:1284687. https://doi.org/10.1155/2018/1284687.
24. Rutka K, Garkowski A, Karaszewska K, Lebkowska U. Imaging in diagnosis of systemic sclerosis. J Clin Med. 2021;10:248. https://doi.org/10.3390/jcm10020248.
25. Boukhal S, Chouchana L, Saadi M, Casadevall M, Cohen P, Dunogue B, et al. Polypharmacy, drug-drug interactions, and adverse drug reactions among systemic sclerosis patients: a cross-sectional risk factor study. Semin Arthritis Rheum. 2024;67:152469. https://doi.org/10.1016/j.semarthrit.2024;152469.
26. Brijs J, Arat S, Westhovens R, Lenaers JL, De Langhe E. Treatment adherence in systemic sclerosis: a cross-sectional study. Musculoskeletal Care. 2019;17:44–53. https://doi.org/10.1002/msc.1363.
27. Mura G, Krishna MB, Pisano A, Licci G, Carta MG. Psychiatric symptoms and quality of life in systemic sclerosis. Clin Pract Epidemiol Ment Health. 2012;8:30–5. https://doi.org/10.2174/1745017901208010030.
28. Becetti K, Kwakkenbos L, Carrier ME, Gordon JK, Nguyen JT, Mancuso CA, et al. Physical or occupational therapy use in systemic sclerosis: a scleroderma patient-centered intervention network cohort study. J Rheumatol. 2019;46:1605–13. https://doi.org/10.3899/jrheum.181130.

Pitfalls in Inflammatory Myopathies

17

Abbreviations

ALS	Amyotrophic lateral sclerosis
AZA	Azathioprine
CK	Creatinine kinase
CS	Corticosteroids
CTDs	Connective tissue diseases
DM	Dermatomyositis
DMARDs	Disease-modifying anti-rheumatic drugs
EMG	Electromyography
IBM	Inclusion body myositis
ILD	Interstitial lung disease
IM	Inflammatory myopathies
IVIG	Intravenous immunoglobulin
MSAs	Myositis-specific autoantibodies
MTX	Methotrexate
NAM	Necrotising autoimmune myopathy
PM	Polymyositis
QoL	Quality of life
RA	Rheumatoid arthritis
RMDs	Rheumatic diseases
RTX	Rituximab
SLE	Systemic lupus erythematosus
SRP	Signal recognition particle

E. Pelechas et al., *Pitfalls in Rheumatology*,
https://doi.org/10.1007/978-3-031-98671-0_17

17.1 Understanding Inflammatory Myopathies: Overview

IM are chronic, autoimmune-mediated muscle diseases marked by inflammation of muscle tissue. These disorders affect skeletal muscle and, in some cases, the skin and other organs. The most common clinical feature is muscle weakness, primarily affecting the proximal muscles (shoulders, hips and thighs), which can severely impact a patient's mobility and QoL. While MSAs have improved diagnostic capabilities, the variability in disease presentation, testing limitations and overlap with other conditions make diagnosis challenging. The four major subtypes of IM include: (a) *PM*: affects muscles symmetrically, primarily those closest to the body's core; (b) *DM*: involves muscle weakness with a characteristic skin rash; (c) *IBM*: progressive muscle weakness with both proximal and distal muscle involvement, primarily affecting older adults; (d) *NAM*: features severe muscle weakness and rapid muscle tissue destruction, often associated with statin use or malignancy [1]. There are also subcategories of the inflammatory myopathies such as the "DM sine myositis" or amyopathic myositis [2, 3].

17.2 Misdiagnosis Due to Overlapping Symptoms

The first and perhaps most common pitfall in diagnosing IMs arises from the nonspecific symptoms of muscle weakness and fatigue, which overlap with many other neuromuscular and systemic conditions. The result is frequent misdiagnosis, particularly in the early stages of the disease [3].

Overlap with Other Neuromuscular Disorders Muscle weakness, the hallmark of IMs, can be seen in a wide range of neuromuscular conditions, including muscular dystrophies, motor neuron disease such as ALS and metabolic myopathies. Many of these conditions can mimic the clinical presentation of IMs, especially in the absence of clear skin findings or unique features of IBM. IBM, for instance, often presents with slowly progressive muscle weakness in older adults, mimicking conditions like motor neuron disease or age-related muscle loss (sarcopenia). Its involvement of both proximal and distal muscles, particularly the quadriceps and finger flexors, can be misattributed to normal aging or other neuromuscular diseases [4].

Overlap with Rheumatic Diseases IMs can also be mistaken for systemic RMDs, such as PMR, RA or SLE, due to shared features like fatigue, joint pain and muscle pain. Moreover, some patients with autoimmune CTDs can develop secondary myositis, further complicating the diagnosis. DM, which involves skin rashes, may be misdiagnosed as SLE or psoriasis due to its cutaneous manifestations. The classic heliotrope rash around the eyes or Gottron's papules (rash over the knuckles) can resemble other dermatologic conditions, leading to diagnostic delay if not carefully evaluated [5].

17.3 Limitations of Diagnostic Testing

Diagnostic testing is critical for confirming IMs, but it is not without its limitations. A thorough clinical evaluation must be combined with laboratory tests, imaging, EMG and muscle biopsy. However, these tests are not always definitive, and their results can be misleading, leading to diagnostic confusion. In Table 17.1, a summary of the types of IMs, including their clinical characteristics, CK levels and histopathological features, is presented.

Serum Creatinine Kinase and Myositis-Specific Antibodies CK is often elevated in patients with IMs, reflecting muscle damage. However, CK levels can be normal or mildly elevated in some patients, particularly those with IBM or in the later stages of disease, leading to false reassurance or missed diagnosis. MSAs, such as anti-Jo-1, anti-Mi-2 and anti-SRP, can aid in the diagnosis of certain myositis subtypes. However, these antibodies are not universally present, and their absence does not exclude the diagnosis of IM. Furthermore, MSAs are not highly specific to individual disease subtypes, and some patients may test positive for MSAs without having clinically significant myositis [6].

Muscle Biopsy Interpretation Muscle biopsy remains the gold standard for diagnosing IM, particularly in cases where other diagnostic modalities are inconclusive. However, interpreting muscle biopsy findings requires considerable expertise, and biopsies can sometimes yield non-specific results, especially in milder cases. Inflammatory changes may be patchy, and a biopsy of an uninvolved muscle can yield false-negative results. Additionally, certain features of muscle biopsy, such as perifascicular atrophy, seen in DM, or inclusion bodies, seen in IBM, can be missed or misinterpreted by less experienced pathologists. This can lead to inappropriate diagnoses, delayed treatment or incorrect prognostication [6].

Table 17.1 Summary of the types of inflammatory myopathies and their characteristics

Type of IM	Clinical characteristics	CK levels	Histopathology
DM	Proximal muscle weakness, heliotrope rash, Gottron's papules, photosensitive rash on face and neck	Elevated (moderate to high)	Perifascicular atrophy, perivascular and perimysial inflammation, capillary dropout, membrane attack complex deposition
PM	Proximal muscle weakness, no skin findings, associated with ILD	Elevated (moderate to high)	Endomysial inflammation, predominantly CD8+ T-cells, myofiber necrosis without perifascicular atrophy
IBM	Distal and proximal muscle weakness, finger flexor and quadriceps involvement, poor response to treatment	Normal to mildly elevated	Endomysial inflammation, rimmed vacuoles, myofiber atrophy, intracellular amyloid deposits
NAM	Severe proximal weakness, associated with statin use or anti-SRP/anti-HMGCR antibodies	Elevated (very high)	Myofibre necrosis, minimal or absent inflammation, macrophage infiltration, no rimmed vacuoles

17.4 Delayed Recognition of Inclusion Body Myositis

IBM is often under-recognised, leading to significant diagnostic delays. This form of myositis has a slower progression compared to PM or DM and predominantly affects individuals over the age of 50. IBM is unique in its involvement of both proximal and distal muscles, and patients may present with weakness in the quadriceps, leading to frequent falls, or weakness in the finger flexors, causing difficulty with fine motor tasks like gripping objects [7].

Confusion with Other Diseases of Aging Because IBM develops slowly and affects older adults, it is often mistaken for age-related muscle loss (sarcopenia) or neurological conditions such as motor neuron disease. Additionally, IBM is typically resistant to CS therapy, further complicating its differentiation from PM or DM, which often responds to immunosuppressive treatment [8].

The misdiagnosis of IBM as PM can result in patients being placed on long-term immunosuppressive therapy, which is ineffective in IBM and exposes patients to unnecessary side effects, such as osteoporosis, infections and metabolic disturbances.

Lack of Early Biomarkers There are no highly specific biomarkers for IBM, which further contributes to delayed recognition. While certain biopsy findings, such as rimmed vacuoles, are characteristic of IBM, these features may be subtle or missed altogether, particularly in the early stages of the disease [9].

17.5 Misinterpretation of Response to Treatment

The treatment response in IM can provide important diagnostic clues, but interpreting this response also presents pitfalls. The standard treatment for most inflammatory myopathies is high-dose CS, often in combination with other immunosuppressive agents such as MTX or AZA. However, not all patients respond uniformly to treatment [10]. On the other hand, other mimicking conditions such as PMR may significantly benefit from, or even enter remission with, the aforementioned pharmacological treatment.

Lack of Response in IBM As noted earlier, IBM is generally resistant to CS therapy. Patients with IBM who are misdiagnosed as having PM may be subjected to prolonged courses of ineffective therapy, leading to a delay in more appropriate care, such as physical therapy and assistive devices.

Incomplete or Delayed Responses Some patients with PM or DM may experience an incomplete or delayed response to treatment, which can be misinterpreted as treatment failure. In these cases, clinicians should consider the possibility of an incorrect diagnosis or the need for alternative treatments, such as IVIG, RTX or other DMARDs. Additionally, some patients with NAM, particularly those associated with statin use, may require discontinuation of statins and aggressive immunosuppression, including IVIG or RTX, if standard therapies fail. Recognising these treatment-resistant forms of myopathy is crucial to avoid prolonged disease activity and irreversible muscle damage [11].

17.6 Overlooking Extramuscular Manifestations

While muscle weakness is the primary manifestation of IMs, these diseases can affect multiple organ systems, including the skin, lungs and heart. Overlooking these extramuscular manifestations can lead to incomplete diagnoses and suboptimal management [12], with a higher risk of being overlooked in patients who lack the typical muscular presentation—that is, myositis sine myositis.

ILD A significant proportion of patients with myositis, particularly those with antisynthetase syndrome, develop ILD, which can cause dyspnoea and cough. Failure to recognise ILD early can result in irreversible lung damage. In some cases, ILD may be the presenting feature, preceding the onset of muscle weakness, which can lead to misdiagnosis as a primary pulmonary condition rather than an IM [13].

Cardiac Involvement Though less common, it can occur in patients with IMs, manifesting as myocarditis, arrhythmias or heart failure. Routine cardiac monitoring is essential in these patients, as cardiac complications may be silent or misattributed to other causes, particularly in older patients [14].

Skin and Subcutaneous Tissue Calcifications in DM are a hallmark of dystrophic calcification where calcium deposits form in damaged or inflamed tissues. The can occur in skin, subcutaneous tissues, muscles and fascia, and they may be palpable. These calcifications are usually visible as soft tissue calcifications on X-rays. They cause discomfort or even pain, especially if they are large or near joints. One of the most significant clinical impacts of those calcifications are infections. Secondary bacterial infections may occur in ulcerated areas, in patients that are already on immunosuppressant treatment, and sometimes a combination of immunosuppressants. In Fig. 17.1, two different cases of DM with dystrophic calcifications are presented.

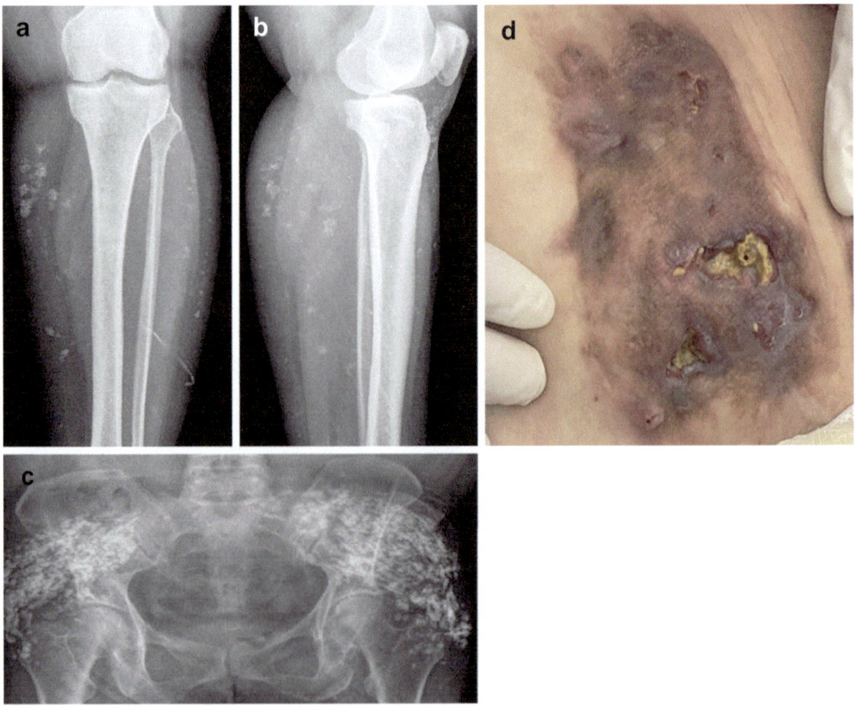

Fig. 17.1 Dystrophic calcifications in dermatomyositis. In (**a**) and (**b**) small calcifications scattered in the subcutaneous tissue of the calves; (**c**) pelvis X-ray of a female patient with severe dystrophic calcifications of the gluteal regions; (**d**) the same patient as in figure (c) with secondary bacterial infection. Note also the chalky material under the skin

17.7 Conclusion

The diagnosis and management of IMs require a high index of suspicion, detailed clinical assessment and judicious use of diagnostic tests. The overlap with other neuromuscular diseases, limitations of diagnostic testing, misinterpretation of treatment response and the potential for missed extramuscular manifestations all contribute to the complexity of managing these conditions. Clinicians must remain vigilant to these pitfalls, ensuring that patients with IMs receive timely and accurate diagnoses, appropriate treatment and comprehensive care that addresses both muscle and extramuscular disease.

References

1. Pelechas E, Kaltsonoudis E, Voulgari PV, Drosos AA. Inflammatory myopathies. In: Illustrated handbook of rheumatic and musculo-skeletal diseases. Cham: Springer; 2023. https://doi.org/10.1007/978-3-031-47379-1_12.
2. Kaltsonoudis E, Pelechas E, Drosos AA. Dermatomyositis sine myositis—case presentation. Mediterr J Rheumatol. 2017;28:57–8. https://doi.org/10.31138/mjr.28.1.57.
3. Oldroyd A, Lilleker J, Chinoy H. Idiopathic inflammatory myopathies—a guide to subtypes, diagnostic approach and treatment. Clin Med (Lond). 2017;17:322–8. https://doi.org/10.7861/clinmedicine.17-4-322.
4. Mathis S, Magy L, Corcia P, Ghorab K, Richard L, Ciron J, Duchesne M, et al. Simultaneous combined myositis, inflammatory polyneuropathy, and overlap myasthenic syndrome. Case Rep Neurol Med. 2016;2016:6108234. https://doi.org/10.1155/2016/6108234.
5. Lepreux S, Hainfellner JA, Vital A. Idiopathic inflammatory myopathies overlapping with systemic diseases. Clin Neuropathol. 2017;37:6–15. https://doi.org/10.5414/NP301077.
6. Tsamis KI, Boutsoras C, Kaltsonoudis E, Pelechas E, Nikas IP, Simos YV, et al. Clinical features and diagnostic tools in idiopathic inflammatory myopathies. Crit Rev Clin Lab Sci. 2022;59:219–40. https://doi.org/10.1080/10408363.2021.2000584.
7. Namsrai T, Parkinson A, Chalmers A, Lowe C, Cook M, Phillips C, et al. Diagnostic delay of myositis: an integrated systematic review. Orphanet J Rare Dis. 2022;17:420. https://doi.org/10.1186/s13023-022-02570-9.
8. Acosta I, Hofer M, Hilton-Jones D, Squier W, Brady S. Treatment resistance in inclusion body myositis: the role of mast cells. Neuromuscul Disord. 2024;41:20–3. https://doi.org/10.1016/j.nmd.2024.05.001.
9. Tebo AE. Autoantibody evaluation in idiopathic inflammatory myopathies. Adv Clin Chem. 2024;120:45–67. https://doi.org/10.1016/bs.acc.2024.04.001.
10. Joffe MM, Love LA, Leff RL, Frases DD, Targoff IN, Hicks JE, et al. Drug therapy of the idiopathic inflammatory myopathies: predictors of response to prednisone, azathioprine, and methotrexate and a comparison of their efficacy. Am J Med. 1993;94:379–87. https://doi.org/10.1016/0002-9343(93)90148-i.
11. Oldroyd AGS, Lilleker JB, Amin T, Aragon O, Bechman K, Cuthbert V, et al. British Society of Rheumatology guideline on management of paediatric, adolescent and adult patients with idiopathic inflammatory myopathy. Rheumatology (Oxford). 2022;61:1760–8. https://doi.org/10.1093/rheumatology/keac115.
12. Spiera R, Kagen L. Extramuscular manifestations in idiopathic inflammatory myopathies. Curr Opin Rheumatol. 1998;10:556–61. https://doi.org/10.1097/00002281-199811000-00008.
13. Hervier B, Uzunhan Y. Inflammatory myopathy-related interstitial lung disease: from pathophysiology to treatment. Front Med (Lausanne). 2020;6:326. https://doi.org/10.3389/fmed.2019.00326.
14. Shah M, Shinjo SK, Day J, Gupta L. Cardiovascular manifestations in idiopathic inflammatory myopathies. Clin Rheumatol. 2023;42:2557–75. https://doi.org/10.1007/s10067-023-06599-4.

18 Pitfalls in Vasculitides in Rheumatology

Abbreviations

AAV	ANCA-associated vasculitis
ACR	American College of Rheumatology
ANCA	Anti-neutrophil cytoplasmic antibodies
Anti-GBM	Anti-glomerular basement membrane
AZA	Azathioprine
cANCA	Cytoplasmic ANCA
CHCC	Chapel Hill Consensus Conference
CP	Cyclophosphamide
CS	Corticosteroids
CT	Computed tomography
CTA	CT angiography
DMARDs	Disease-modifying anti-rheumatic drugs
GCA	Giant cell arteritis
GN	Glomerulonephritis
GPA	Granulomatosis with polyangiitis
LN	Lupus nephritis
LVV	Large-vessel vasculitis
MPA	Microscopic polyangiitis
MRA	MRI angiography
MRI	Magnetic resonance imaging
MSK	Musculoskeletal
MTX	Methotrexate
MVV	Medium-vessel vasculitis
pANCA	Perinuclear ANCA
PET-CT	Positron-emission tomography—computed tomography
PMR	Polymyalgia rheumatica

E. Pelechas et al., *Pitfalls in Rheumatology*,
https://doi.org/10.1007/978-3-031-98671-0_18

RPGN	Rapidly progressive glomerulonephritis
RTX	Rituximab
SLE	Systemic lupus erythematosus
SScl	Systemic sclerosis
SVV	Small-vessel vasculitis
TA	Takayasu arteritis
US	Ultrasound

18.1 Overlooking Vasculitis as a Differential Diagnosis

One of the most common pitfalls in diagnosing vasculitides is failing to consider them in the differential diagnosis, particularly when the initial presentation mimics more common conditions. Given the wide range of manifestations, from constitutional symptoms to organ-specific signs, vasculitis can be mistaken for infections, malignancies or other autoimmune disorders [1].

In Order to Avoid This Pitfall

Maintain a high index of suspicion: consider vasculitis in patients with systemic symptoms such as fever, weight loss and fatigue, combined with multisystem involvement, such as skin rash, peripheral neuropathy or renal dysfunction. This is especially important in younger patients who present with unexplained systemic symptoms or organ failure [2].

Look for red flags: certain symptoms should trigger suspicion of vasculitis including: (a) *mononeuritis multiplex*: this is often seen in MVV such as polyarteritis nodosa (Fig. 18.1) and cryoglobulinaemic vasculitis and is an important clue [3]; (b) *palpable purpura*: this skin manifestation is a hallmark of SVV [4]; (c) *unexplained haematuria or proteinuria and dyspnoea*: these can be signs of renal or pulmonary involvement, particularly in AAV [5]; (d) *sudden vision loss*: GCA should be considered in patients >50 with acute visual disturbances, especially if they have a history of headache or jaw claudication [6].

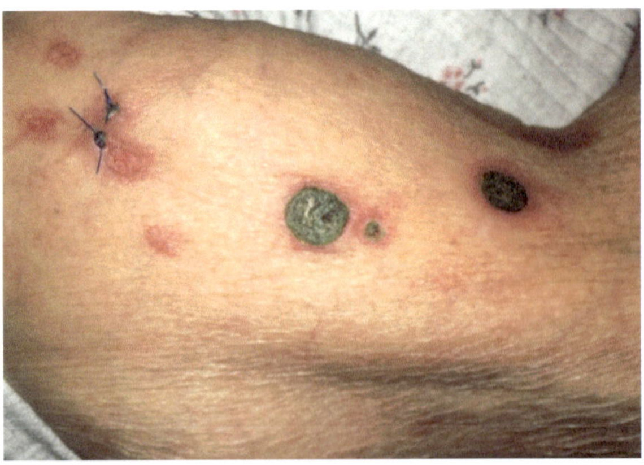

Fig. 18.1 Skin lesions of polyarteritis nodosa. Skin manifestations appear in 40% and can be from erythematous nodules and petechiae, to painful subcutaneous nodules and skin ulceration and necrosis such as the lesions in this figure

18.2 Misdiagnosis Based on Overlapping Symptoms

Vasculitides share clinical features with other systemic diseases, such as SLE, SScl, infections or malignancies. This can lead to misdiagnosis or delayed diagnosis, especially in cases with atypical presentations.

In Order to Avoid This Pitfall

Use diagnostic criteria and classification: familiarise yourself with the diagnostic criteria for various vasculitides, such as the CHCC definitions and the ACR criteria. These tools can help differentiate vasculitis from other systemic diseases [7–9]. In Fig. 18.2, the distribution of vessel involvement is presented.

Exclude infections and malignancy: many forms of vasculitis, particularly AAV, can mimic infections. For example, endocarditis can present with fever, anaemia and embolic phenomena similar to vasculitis. Always rule out (latent) infection and malignancy, as initiating immunosuppressive therapy in an undiagnosed infection can worsen patient outcomes [10].

Use biopsy and imaging: when clinical features overlap with other diseases, tissue biopsy and advanced imaging (PET-CT for LVV) can provide definitive diagnostic information. For example, renal biopsy can differentiate between LN and pauci-immune GN seen in AAV [11].

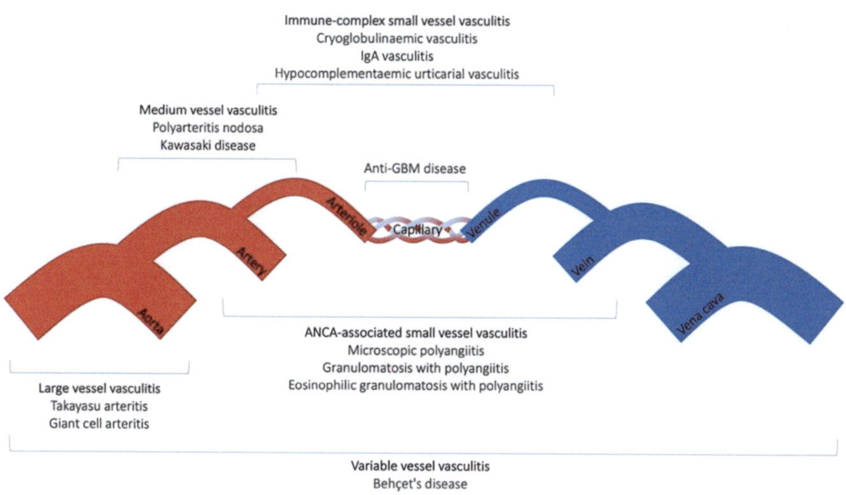

Fig. 18.2 Distribution of vessel involvement by large-vessel, medium-vessel, and small-vessel vasculitis

18.3 Over-Reliance on Autoantibodies

Autoantibody testing, particularly ANCA, plays an important role in diagnosing vasculitis. However, over-reliance on autoantibodies can lead to diagnostic errors. Not all patients with vasculitis have detectable antibodies, and false-positive results can occur, particularly in the setting of infections, malignancies or other autoimmune diseases. On the other hand, the presence of low-titre positive autoantibodies without any symptoms may be found in non-vasculitic conditions.

In Order to Avoid This Pitfall

Use autoantibodies as part of a broader diagnostic workup: positive ANCA tests (cANCA for GPA, and pANCA for MPA) should be interpreted in the context of clinical presentation and other diagnostic findings. A positive ANCA alone does not confirm vasculitis, nor does a negative ANCA exclude it, as ANCA-negative forms or vasculitis exist [12].

Avoid over testing: testing for ANCA should be reserved for patients with clinical features suggestive of vasculitis, such as RPGN, pulmonary–renal syndrome or unexplained multisystem disease. Avoid indiscriminate testing, as it may lead to false-positives and unnecessary treatment.

Consider other diagnostic tools: tissue biopsy (skin, renal or temporal artery) and imaging modalities (US, CT and MRI) often provide more definitive evidence of vasculitis than serologic testing alone [13].

18.4 Delayed or Missed Diagnosis of Large-Vessel Vasculitis

LVV, including GCA and TA, often presents with non-specific symptoms such as fever, malaise or MSK pain, leading to diagnostic delays. The consequences of delayed diagnosis can be severe, particularly in GCA, where untreated disease can lead to irreversible vision loss. Furthermore, anatomical disfigurements may occur, such as the saddle nose deformity in GPA (Fig. 18.3).

In Order to Avoid This Pitfall

Consider GCA in patients >50 with new-onset headache: GCA should be suspected in older adults presenting with new-onset headache, scalp tenderness or jaw claudication. Visual symptoms or PMR-like features increase the likelihood of GCA [14].

Early use of temporal artery biopsy or imaging: temporal artery biopsy remains the gold standard for diagnosing GCA, but imaging techniques such as Doppler US or PET-CT can provide valuable information when biopsy is not feasible or non-diagnostic. In TA, cross-sectional imaging such as CTA or MRA can reveal vessel wall thickening or stenosis [15].

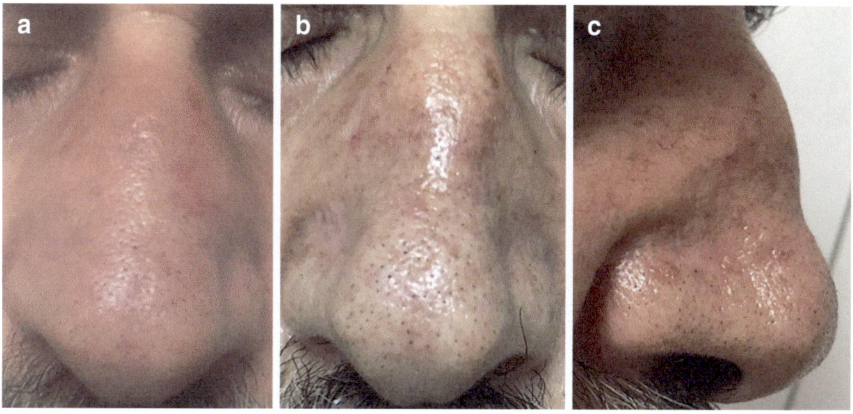

Fig. 18.3 Saddle nose deformity in a patient diagnosed with granulomatosis with polyangiitis. A saddle nose deformity refers to a marked depression or collapse along the mid portion of the nasal bridge. In (**a**) at the time of diagnosis; (**b**, **c**) 6 months after diagnostic delay

Start CS promptly: if GCA is strongly suspected, initiate high-dose CS immediately to prevent complications such as vision loss, even before confirmatory biopsy or imaging results are available.

18.5 Mismanagement of Corticosteroid Therapy

CSs are the cornerstone of treatment for most vasculitides, but their long-term use is associated with significant adverse effects, including osteoporosis, diabetes, hypertension and increased infection risk. Managing the balance between controlling disease activity and minimising CS toxicity is a common challenge.

How to Avoid This Pitfall

Taper CS appropriately: the goal should be to taper CS to the lowest effective dose or discontinue them as soon as possible while maintaining disease control. Too rapid a taper may lead to disease flares, while prolonged high-dose use increases the risk of side effects. Individualise the tapering schedule based on disease activity, biomarkers and the patient's response to treatment.

Use steroid-sparing agents: immunosuppressive or DMARD therapies (MTX, AZA, RTX or CP) can be used to control disease and reduce the need for prolonged high-dose CS. In cases of relapsing disease, steroid-sparing agents are essential to minimise CS toxicity [16].

Monitor and manage side effects: regularly assess for CS side effects and implement preventive measures, such as bone protection (calcium, vitamin D and bisphosphonates) and glucose control.

18.6 Inadequate Monitoring for Disease Relapse

Vasculitides often follow a relapsing–remitting course. Failure to recognise early signs of relapse can lead to delayed treatment and increased organ damage. Conversely, mistaking non-specific symptoms for relapse can lead to overtreatment and unnecessary side effects.

How to Avoid This Pitfall

Regular follow-up and use of biomarkers: patients with vasculitis should be monitored regularly with clinical assessments and laboratory tests, including inflammatory markers. Biomarkers like ANCA can be useful in some cases but should not be relied upon exclusively, as clinical symptoms may precede changes in serologic markers [17]. Furthermore, in a patient with specific findings such as uveitis, clinical monitoring and patient education are also important. In Fig. 18.4, a GPA patient with recurrent anterior uveitis is presented.

Differentiate relapse from damage of side effects: patients with vasculitis often have residual organ damage or side effects from treatment such as fatigue, muscle weakness and joint pain. Carefully assess symptoms to distinguish between true disease relapse and chronic damage or drug-related side effects.

Imaging for disease monitoring: in LVV, serial imaging such as US or CTA can help detect subclinical relapse or progression of vascular lesions, even in the absence of systemic symptoms [18].

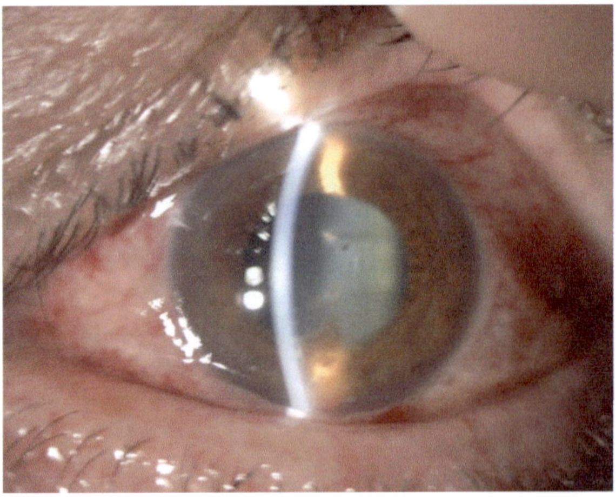

Fig. 18.4 Anterior uveitis with cell aggregates that are visible in the anterior chamber during examination in a GPA patient

18.7 Failure to Recognise and Manage Organ-Specific Involvement

Vasculitis can affect virtually an organ system, leading to complications such as GN, pulmonary haemorrhage or peripheral neuropathy. Failure to recognise organ-specific involvement early can result in irreversible damage.

How to Avoid This Pitfall

Comprehensive evaluation at diagnosis: at the time of diagnosis, conduct a thorough evaluation to assess for organ involvement, including renal function tests, chest imaging and neurological assessments. Early identification of organ-specific involvement allows for timely intervention and prevents long-term damage [19].

Multidisciplinary care: management of vasculitis often requires input from multiple specialists. In complex cases, a multidisciplinary approach ensures that all aspects of the disease are addressed.

Prompt and aggressive treatment of severe organ involvement: organ-threatening vasculitis, such as RPGN or alveolar haemorrhage, requires prompt initiation of aggressive immunosuppressive therapy, often including pulses of CS and agents like CP or RTX [20, 21].

18.8 Conclusion

The diagnosis and management of vasculitides in rheumatology are fraught with challenges due to the heterogeneity of clinical presentations, overlapping symptoms with other conditions and the potential for severe organ damage if treatment is delayed. A high index of suspicion, careful clinical assessment, appropriate use of diagnostic tools and aggressive or judicious use of immunosuppressive therapy are critical to optimising outcomes. By recognising and avoiding these common pitfalls, clinicians can improve the accuracy of diagnosis, prevent disease-related complications and minimise treatment-related toxicity.

References

1. Pelechas E, Kaltsonoudis E, Voulgari PV, Drosos AA. Vasculitides. In: Illustrated handbook of rheumatic and musculo-skeletal diseases. Cham: Springer; 2023. https://doi.org/10.1007/978-3-031-47379-1_13.
2. Saadoun D, Vautier M, Cacoub P. Medium-and-large-vessel vasculitis. Circulation. 2021;143:267–82. https://doi.org/10.1161/circulationaha.120.046657.

3. Chae HJ, Kim JW, Lee YL, Park JH, Lee SY. Mononeuropathy multiplex associated with systemic vasculitis: a case report. World J Clin Cases. 2021;9:1741–7. https://doi.org/10.12998/wjcc.v9.i7.1741.
4. Lotti T, Ghersetich I, Comacchi C, Jorizzo JL. Cutaneous small-vessel vasculitis. J Am Acad Dermatol. 1998;39:667–87. https://doi.org/10.1016/s0190-9622(98)70039-8.
5. Benichou N, Charles P, Terrier B, Jones RB, Hiemstra T, Mouthon L, et al. Proteinuria and hematuria after remission induction are associated with outome in ANCA-associated vasculitis. Kidney Int. 2023;103:1144–55. https://doi.org/10.1016/j.kint.2023.02.0239.
6. Héron E, Sedira N, Dahia O, Jamart C. Ocular complications of giant cell arteritis: an acute therapeutic emergency. J Clin Med. 2022;11:1997. https://doi.org/10.3390/jcm11071997.
7. Pyo JY, Lee LE, Park YB, Lee SW. Comparison of the 2022 ACR/EULAR classification criteria for antineutrophil cytoplasmic antibody-associated vasculitis with previous criteria. Yonsei Med J. 2023;64:11–7. https://doi.org/10.3349/ymj.2022.0435.
8. Jannette JC. Overview of the 2012 revised international Chapel Hill consensus conference nomenclature of vasculitides. Clin Exp Nephrol. 2013; https://doi.org/10.1007/s10157-013-0869-6.
9. Karassa FB, Pelechas E, Zouzos G. The immunogenetics of vasculitis. Adv Exp Med Biol. 2022;1367:299–334. https://doi.org/10.1007/978-3-030-92616-8_11.
10. Greer JM, Longley S, Edwards NL, Elfenbein GJ, Panush RS. Vasculitis associated with malignancy. Experience with 13 patients and literature review. Medicine (Baltimore). 1099;67:220–30. https://doi.org/10.1097/00005792-1988070000-00003.
11. Chapman GB, Farrah TE, Chapman FA, Pugh D, Bellamy COC, Lahiri R, et al. Utility of interval kidney biopsy in ANCA-associated vasculitis. Rheumatology (Oxford). 2022;61:1966–74.
12. Fijołek J, Wiatr E. Antineutrophil cytoplasmic antibodies (ANCA)—their role in pathogenesis, diagnosis, and treatment monitoring of ANCA-associated vasculitis. Cent Eur J Immunol. 2020;45:218–27. https://doi.org/10.5114/ceji.2019.92494.
13. Dejaco C, Ramiro S, Bond M, Bosch P, Ponte C, Mackie SL, Bley TA. EULAR recommendations for the use of imaging in large vessel vasculitis in clinical practice: 2023 update. Ann Rheum Dis. 2024;83:741–51.
14. Ponte C, Grayson PC, Robson JC, Suppiah R, Gribbons KB, Judge A, et al. 2022 American College of Rheumatology/EULAR classification criteria for giant cell arteritis. Arthritis Rheumatol. 2022;74:1881–9. https://doi.org/10.1002/art.42325.
15. Kaltsonoudis E, Pelechas E, Papoudou-Bai A, Markatseli TE, Elisaf M, Voulgari PV, et al. The impact of temporal artery biopsy for the diagnosis of giant cell arteritis in clinical practice in a tertiary university hospital. PLoS One. 2019;14:e0210845. https://doi.org/10.1371/journal.pone.0210845.
16. Chung SA, Langford CA, Maz M, Abril A, Gorelik M, Guyatt G, et al. 2021 American College of Rheumatology/Vasculitis foundation guideline for the management of antineutrophil cytoplasmic antibody-associated vasculitis. Arthritis Rheumatol. 2021;73:1366–83. https://doi.org/10.1002/art.41773.
17. Scurt FG, Hirschfeld V, Schubert L, Mertens P, Chatzikyrkou C. Monitoring disease activity in antineutrophil antibody-associated vasculitis. Scand J Immunol. 2023;98:e13284. https://doi.org/10.1111/sji.13284.
18. Allam MN, Ali NB, Mahmoud AK, Scalia IG, Farina JM, Abbas MT, et al. Multi-modality imaging in vasculitis. Diagnostics (Basel). 2024;14:838.
19. Suresh E. Diagnostic approach to patients with suspected vasculitis. Postgrad Med J. 2006;82:483–8. https://doi.org/10.1136/pgmj.2005.042648.
20. Singh A, Everest S, Nguyen L, Kasari M. ANCA-Associated vasculitis in a patient presenting with rapid progressive glomerulonephritis. Cureus. 2021;13:e20227. https://doi.org/10.7759/cureus.20227.
21. Krause ML, Cartin-Ceba R, Specks U, Peikert T. Update on diffuse alveolar hemorrhage and pulmonary vasculitis. Immunol Allergy Clin N Am. 2012;32:587–600. https://doi.org/10.1016/j.iac.2012.08.001.

Pitfalls in Sarcoidosis

19

Abbreviations

ACE	Angiotensin-converting enzyme
ACPA	Anti-citrullinated protein antibodies
AZA	Azathioprine
bDMARDs	Biologic disease-modifying anti-rheumatic drugs
CS	Corticosteroids
ECG	Electrocardiogram
HRCT	High-resolution computed tomography
MRI	Magnetic resonance imaging
MTX	Methotrexate
PFTs	Pulmonary function tests
pSS	Primary SS
RA	Rheumatoid arthritis
RF	Rheumatoid factor
RMDs	Rheumatic diseases
SLE	Systemic lupus erythematosus
SS	Sjögren's syndrome
TB	Tuberculosis
TNFi	Tumour necrosis factor alpha inhibitor

19.1 Clinical Mimicry: Confusion with Other Autoimmune Diseases

Sarcoidosis may be diagnosed incidentally by a simple chest X-ray (Fig. 19.1), but one of the most significant challenges in sarcoidosis, in some cases, is its ability to mimic other autoimmune and inflammatory diseases. Given its systemic nature,

E. Pelechas et al., *Pitfalls in Rheumatology*,
https://doi.org/10.1007/978-3-031-98671-0_19

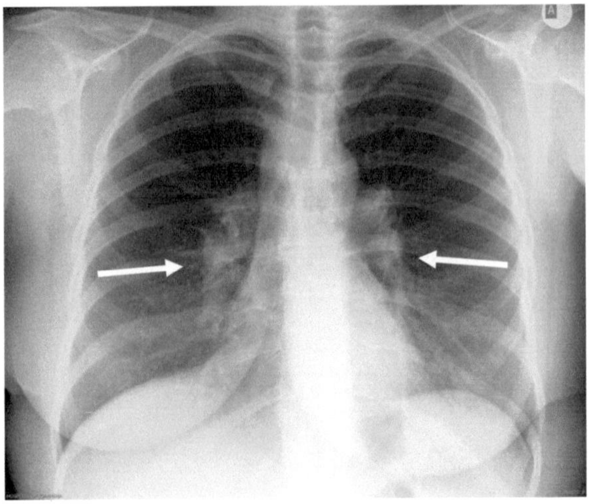

Fig. 19.1 Pulmonary sarcoidosis stage 1 after Scadding classification system. Note the bilateral hilar lymph node enlargement (arrows)

sarcoidosis can present with joint pain, arthritis, myalgia, more often skin lesions and ocular symptoms (Fig. 19.2), which are all hallmarks of RMDs such as SLE, RA or SS.

RA: symmetric polyarthritis, particularly involving the hands, can be confused with RA. However, the absence of RF and ACPA, the presence of hilar lymphadenopathy on chest imaging and distinct structural lesions on hand radiographs (e.g. moth-eaten bone appearance) should prompt consideration of sarcoidosis.

SS: dry eyes and dry mouth (sicca syndrome) in sarcoidosis can be mistaken for pSS. A lack of anti-SSA/SSB antibodies and characteristic salivary gland biopsy findings (granulomas rather than lymphocytic infiltration) can help differentiate the two conditions. Acute bilateral painless parotid swelling, with or without associated submandibular and sublingual gland involvement and oral dryness, may sometimes be part of Heerfordt's syndrome when accompanied by uveitis, fever and facial nerve paralysis.

SLE: skin rashes, arthralgias and organ involvement (most commonly kidneys and lungs) in sarcoidosis may closely resemble SLE. The absence of ANA or anti-dsDNA antibodies, normal complement levels, absence of leucopenia or other suggestive laboratory findings and the presence of granulomas (accumulation of CD4 lymphocytes and activated macrophages in the affected organs) on tissue biopsy should suggest sarcoidosis.

How to Avoid These Pitfalls (a) *Comprehensive evaluation*: a detailed history, thorough physical examination and targeted laboratory investigations (e.g. ACE levels, calcium levels and autoantibody panels) are essential; (b) *biopsy*: when appropriate, tissue biopsy demonstrating non-caseating granulomas remains the gold standard for sarcoidosis diagnosis [1].

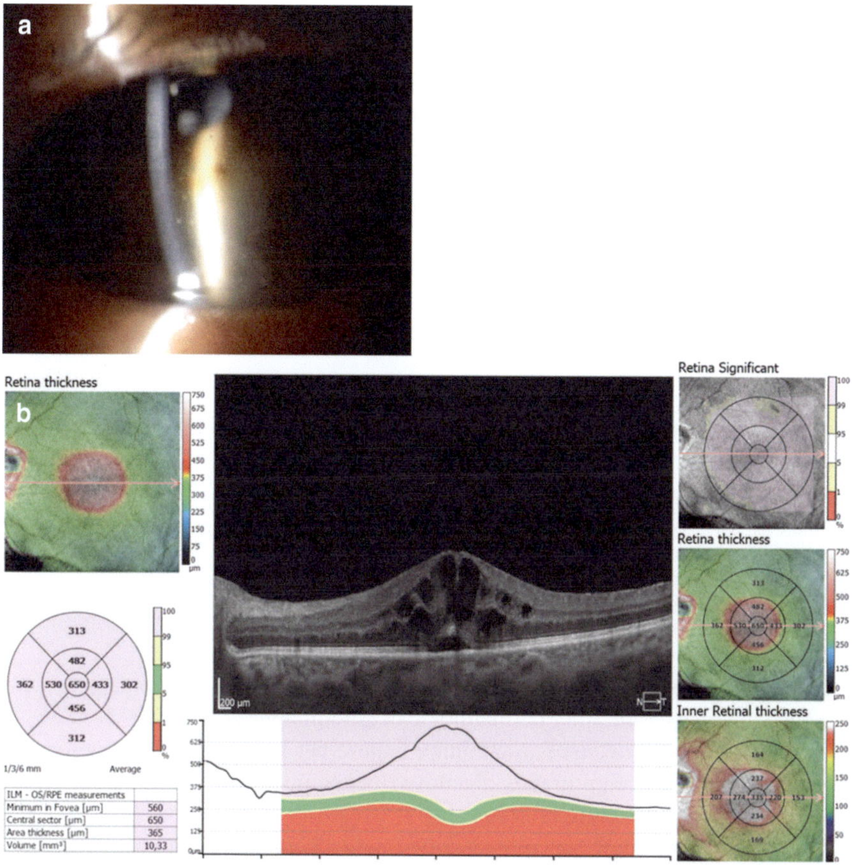

Fig. 19.2 (**a**) Uveitis and mutton fat keratic precipitates in a patient with sarcoidosis; (**b**) cystoid macular oedema and anterior/posterior uveitis in a patient with sarcoidosis

19.2 Over-Reliance on Serum Angiotensin-Converting Enzyme Levels

ACE levels are often elevated in sarcoidosis and are sometimes used as a diagnostic marker. However, reliance on ACE levels can be misleading for several reasons:

Non-specificity: elevated ACE levels are not exclusive to sarcoidosis and can be seen in other granulomatous conditions such as TB, berylliosis, and even some malignancies.

False-negatives: not all patients with sarcoidosis have elevated ACE levels, particularly in chronic or inactive disease states.

Non-diagnostic nature: ACE levels alone cannot confirm sarcoidosis. And while several biomarkers have been proposed for the diagnosis and prognosis of sarcoidosis, none is ideal for diagnostic purposes. Other investigations, such as imaging and biopsy, are necessary to establish a diagnosis.

Pitfall Avoidance Use ACE levels as a supportive test rather than a diagnostic tool. Always correlate ACE levels with clinical findings, imaging studies and histopathological evidence [2, 3].

19.3 Failure to Recognise Extrapulmonary Sarcoidosis

Sarcoidosis is most well-known for its pulmonary involvement, yet rheumatologists must remain vigilant for its extrapulmonary manifestations, which can be subtle or atypical. Sarcoidosis can be diagnosed based on both pulmonary and extrapulmonary manifestations. In many cases, these may or may not be obvious, typical, easily accessible for biopsy or severe. Potentially, it can affect any organ or system.

Musculoskeletal involvement: sarcoidosis can cause arthritis, tenosynovitis and muscle involvement, often leading to misdiagnosis as a primary rheumatologic disorder [4].

Cutaneous sarcoidosis: skin manifestations (lupus pernio and erythema nodosum) may be mistaken for other dermatologic or autoimmune conditions [5].

Ocular sarcoidosis: uveitis is a common feature but is not always recognised as sarcoid-related. If not promptly diagnosed, ocular involvement can lead to severe complications, including blindness [6].

Cardiac and neurologic sarcoidosis: often underdiagnosed due to their insidious onset, these manifestations can be life-threatening. Cardiac involvement can present as arrhythmias or heart failure, while neurological sarcoidosis can cause seizures, cranial nerve palsies or peripheral neuropathy [7].

How to Avoid These Pitfalls (a) *Multidisciplinary approach*: close collaboration with pulmonologists, dermatologists, ophthalmologists and cardiologists is crucial for the comprehensive care of patients with multisystem sarcoidosis; (b) *high index of suspicion*: maintain awareness of atypical presentations and always consider sarcoidosis in cases of unexplained systemic inflammation or organ dysfunction.

19.4 Inadequate Screening for Organ Involvement

Sarcoidosis has the potential to involve nearly any organ system, and underestimating the extent of disease can result in inadequate treatment or missed complications. For instance, a patient may present with isolated skin or joint symptoms, but a thorough evaluation may reveal occult pulmonary, cardiac or neurologic involvement.

Table 19.1 Scadding staging system for radiographic sarcoidosis

Stage	Radiographic findings	Clinical implications
Stage 0	Normal chest radiograph	No radiographic evidence of lung involvement
Stage I	Bilateral hilar lymphadenopathy	Often asymptomatic or with mild systemic symptoms. Good prognosis
Stage II	Bilateral hilar lymphadenopathy and parenchymal infiltrates	Involves lung parenchyma. Symptoms may include cough or dyspnoea
Stage III	Parenchymal infiltrates without hilar lymphadenopathy	Progressive lung disease with significant respiratory symptoms
Stage IV	Pulmonary fibrosis	Advanced, irreversible lung damage, often with respiratory failure

For pulmonary involvement, the Scadding staging system is used, and it is presented in Table 19.1 along with the clinical implications.

How to Avoid These Pitfalls Perform a baseline screening for organ involvement in all newly diagnosed sarcoidosis patients including: (a) *pulmonary involvement*: PFTs and HRCT; (b) *ophthalmic involvement*: a thorough ophthalmologic exam; (c) *cardiac involvement*: ECG and, if indicated, cardiac MRI; (d) *renal involvement*: serum calcium and kidney function tests for hypercalcaemia [4–7].

19.5 Mismanagement of Steroid Therapy

More than 50% of patients do not require treatment at the time of diagnosis. Many of them will never need any therapy during follow-up, while some will require delayed treatment once disease progression meets the criteria for initiating therapy. CS remain the cornerstone of treatment for sarcoidosis, but their use requires caution. Many pitfalls in treatment arise from inappropriate dosing or duration of CS therapy:

Overtreatment: some patients may have asymptomatic or self-limiting sarcoidosis, particularly with isolated pulmonary or cutaneous disease. In such cases, aggressive CS therapy can lead to unnecessary side effects without improving outcomes.

Undertreatment: conversely, underestimating the severity of extrapulmonary sarcoidosis (especially for cardiac or neurological involvement) can result in irreversible damage if CS are not initiated early and aggressively.

Long-term complications: prolonged CS use leads to well-known side effects such as osteoporosis, diabetes, hypertension and increased infection risk, which can be particularly problematic in patients with chronic or recurrent disease [8, 9].

How to Avoid These Pitfalls (a) *Individualised treatment plans*: tailor the CS dose and duration to the severity of organ involvement and patient-specific factors. The decision to withhold treatment is based on the absence of "at-risk target organ involvement". For mild disease, consider NSAID options or a steroid-sparing approach. For example, local therapies may be recommended for the skin and eyes in cases of limited involvement; (b) *steroid-sparing agents*: immunosuppressive agents like MTX, AZA or bDMARDs (such as TNFi) may be needed to reduce CS exposure in chronic or severe sarcoidosis; (c) *monitor for side effects*: ensure close follow-up to assess for both disease activity and complications of therapy [10, 11].

19.6 Conclusion

Sarcoidosis poses a diagnostic and therapeutic challenge for clinicians due to its ability to mimic other autoimmune diseases, its variable and often subtle manifestations and the complex management of systemic involvement. Awareness of the common pitfalls in diagnosing and treating sarcoidosis can help clinicians avoid misdiagnosis, inappropriate treatments and missed complications. A multidisciplinary approach and a high index of suspicion are vital to optimise outcomes for patients with this multifaceted disease.

References

1. Pelechas E, Kaltsonoudis E, Voulgari PV, Drosos AA. Sarcoidosis. In: Illustrated handbook of rheumatic and musculo-skeletal diseases. Cham: Springer; 2023. https://doi.org/10.1007/978-3-031-47379-1_17.
2. Kahkoucc S, Samadi K, Alai A, Abedini A, Rezaiian L. Serum ACE level in sarcoidosis patients with typical and atypical HRCT manifestations. Pol J Radiol. 2016;81:458–61. https://doi.org/10.12659/PJR.897708.
3. Zheng SY, Du X, Dong JZ. Re-evaluating serum antiotensin-converting enzyme in sarcoidosis. Front Immunol. 2023;14:950095. https://doi.org/10.3389/fimmu.2023.950095.
4. Nessrine A, Zahra AF, Taoufik H. Musculoskeletal involvement in sarcoidosis. J Bras Pneumol. 2014;40:175–82. https://doi.org/10.1590/S1806-37132014000200012.
5. Reddy RR, Kumar BMS, Harish MR. Indian J Dermatol. 2011;56:568–72. https://doi.org/10.4103/0019-5154.87158.
6. Yang S, Salek S, Rosenbaum JT. Ocular sarcoidosis: new diagnostic modalities and treatment. Curr Opin Pulm Med. 2017;23:458–67. https://doi.org/10.1097/MCP.0000000000000409.
7. Gilandehi SN, Wong KH, Francis T, Wright MA, Lord J, Stehlik J, et al. Cardiac involvement in neurosarcoidosis: a single-center investigation. Neurol Neuroimmunol Neuroinflamm. 2024;11:e200196.
8. Grutters JC, van den Bosch JMM. Corticosteroid treatment in sarcoidosis. Eur Respir J. 2006;28:627–36. https://doi.org/10.1183/09031936.06.00105805.
9. Khan NA, Donatelli CV, Tonelli AR, Wiesen J, Neto MLR, Sahoo D, et al. Toxicity risk from glucocorticoids in sarcoidosis patients. Respir Med. 2017;132:9–14. https://doi.org/10.1016/j.rmed.2017.09.003.
10. Vorselaars ADM, Wuyts WA, Vorselaars VMM, Zanen P, Deneer VHM, Veltkamp M, et al. Methotrexate vs azathioprine in second-line therapy of sarcoidosis. Chest. 2013;144:805–12.
11. Adler BL, Wang CJ, Bui TL, Schilperoort HM, Armstrong AW. Semin Arthritis Rheum. 2019;48:1093–104. https://doi.org/10.1016/j.semarthrit.2018.10.005.

Pitfalls in Primary Immunodeficiencies 20

Abbreviations

AHA	Autoimmune haemolytic anaemia
ALPS	Autoimmune lymphoproliferative syndrome
A-T	Ataxia–telangiectasia
bDMARDs	Biologic disease-modifying anti-rheumatic drugs
CGD	Chronic granulomatous disease
CS	Corticosteroids
CVID	Common variable immunodeficiency
FBC	Full blood count
GI	Gastrointestinal
i.v.	Intravenous
IBD	Inflammatory bowel disease
IRT	Immunoglobulin replacement therapy
ITP	Immune thrombocytopaenic purpura
LAD	Leucocyte adhesion deficiency
MTX	Methotrexate
NGS	Next-generation sequencing
PFTs	Pulmonary function tests
PIDs	Primary immunodeficiencies
QoL	Quality of life
RMDs	Rheumatic diseases
s.c.	Subcutaneous
SCID	Severe combined immunodeficiency
SLE	Systemic lupus erythematosus
WAS	Wiskott–Aldrich syndrome
WES	Whole exome sequencing
WGS	Whole genome sequencing
XLA	X-linked agammaglobulinaemia

E. Pelechas et al., *Pitfalls in Rheumatology*,
https://doi.org/10.1007/978-3-031-98671-0_20

20.1 Delayed or Missed Diagnosis

One of the most frequent pitfalls in PIDs is the failure to recognise the condition early. Given the variability in presentations and overlap with other diseases, PIDs often go undiagnosed with environmental exposure, allergies or isolated incidents, missing the underlying immunodeficiency. This can result in cumulative damage from infections, complications from RMDs or even death due to untreated disease [1]. Some of the major categories of PIDs are presented in Table 20.1, even if they consist of >200 known conditions.

How to Avoid This Pitfall A high index of suspicion is necessary, particularly in patients presenting with: (a) *recurrent, severe or unusual infections*: multiple episodes of pneumonia, sinusitis, otitis media or abscesses, particularly when caused by unusual organisms or requiring prolonged antibiotic courses; (b) *infections with opportunistic pathogens*: fungi, viruses and atypical mycobacteria should raise concern; (c) *chronic or severe autoimmune manifestations*: many PIDs present with autoimmune conditions like ITP, AHA or SLE; (d) *failure to thrive or chronic diarrhoea*: especially in paediatric patients, failure to thrive, malabsorption or chronic

Table 20.1 Major categories of primary immunodeficiencies

Category	Conditions	Defect	Key clinical features
Humoral immunodeficiencies	X-linked agammaglobulinaemia, common variable immunodeficiency, selective IgA deficiency	Impaired B-cell development or antibody production	Recurrent bacterial infections mainly of the respiratory and gastrointestinal tract
Cellular immunodeficiencies	DiGeorge syndrome, chronic mucocutaneous candidiasis	T-cell defects (e.g. thymic aplasia in DiGeorge syndrome)	Viral, fungal, and opportunistic infections
Combined immunodeficiencies	Severe combined immunodeficiency, hyper-IgM syndrome	Impairment in both T- and B-cell functions	Severe infections, failure to thrive, early-onset infections
Complement deficiencies	C1q, C2, C4 deficiencies and terminal pathway defects (C5–C9)	Defects in complement cascade	Recurrent *Neisseria* infections, autoimmune diseases
Defects in immune regulation	Autoimmune lymphoproliferative syndrome, IPEX syndrome	Dysregulated immune tolerance	Autoimmune diseases, lymphadenopathy, chronic diarrhoea
Syndromic immunodeficiencies	Wiskott–Aldrich syndrome, Ataxia–telangiectasia syndrome, hyper-IgE syndrome	Multi-system syndromic effects	Eczema, thrombocytopenia, gain abnormalities, skin infections
Phagocytic defects	Chronic granulomatous disease, leucocyte adhesion deficiency	Impaired phagocyte function or migration	Recurrent abscesses, granuloma formation, poor wound healing

GI symptoms can be a sign of an underlying immunodeficiency; (e) *family history of PIDs*: genetic inheritance plays a key role in many immunodeficiencies.

If PID is suspected, early referral to an immunologist and targeted immune function testing should be performed, including quantitative immunoglobulins, lymphocyte subsets and neutrophil function tests [2].

20.2 Inadequate Screening Tests

A common pitfall in diagnosing PIDs is the over-reliance on basic laboratory tests such as FBC and serum immunoglobulin levels. While these tests are valuable initial screening tools, they may miss subtler immunodeficiencies, such as functional antibody T-cell defects, where quantitative measures are normal but functional deficits exist. Similarly, relying solely on genetic tests can result in missed diagnoses since not all genetic variants are well understood.

How to Avoid This Pitfall When initial tests are normal but clinical suspicion for PID remains high, further specialised testing should be conducted. This can include: (a) *functional antibody testing*: assessing the patient's ability to mount an appropriate response to vaccines; (b) *flow cytometry*: to evaluate T-cell, B-cell and NK-cell function; (c) *neutrophil oxidative burst tests*: to assess for chronic granulomatous disease; (d) *complement assays*: to evaluate for complement deficiencies; (e) *genetic testing*: NGS panels for known PIDs can identify mutations associated with these disorders. WES or WGS can help diagnose patients with atypical or unclear presentations.

Referral to a specialised centre with expertise in PIDs is often necessary to perform and interpret these advanced tests [3].

20.3 Overlooking Non-infectious Manifestations

Many clinicians focus on recurrent infections as the hallmark of PIDs, but non-infectious manifestations such as RMDs, autoinflammatory conditions or malignancies are also common. Autoimmune cytopenias, IBD, vasculitis or unexplained organ inflammation may all be signs of underlying PID. Failing to recognise these symptoms as part of a PID can result in ineffective treatments or worsening disease [4].

How to Avoid This Pitfall PIDs should be considered in patients with: (a) *recurrent or treatment-refractory RMDs*: especially when multiple autoimmune conditions coexist; (b) *unexplained inflammatory syndromes*: such as granulomatous disease, vasculitis or sarcoid-like presentations [5]; (c) *early-onset cancers*: particularly lymphomas or other haematologic malignancies, which are more common in certain PIDs.

In such cases, collaboration with an immunologist for further diagnostic workup is essential to identify the underlying immunodeficiency.

20.4 Inappropriate Use of Immunosuppressive Therapies

In some PIDs, autoimmune or inflammatory symptoms may dominate the clinical picture, leading to treatment with immunosuppressive drugs such as CS, MTX or bDMARDs. However, excessive or prolonged immunosuppression in patients with undiagnosed PIDs can worsen infections and lead to life-threatening complications. Mismanagement of immunosuppression is a major pitfall in these patients [6].

Hot to Avoid This Pitfall Before initiating long-term immunosuppressive therapy, clinicians should consider an underlying PID, especially in patients with a history of severe or recurrent infections. When treating autoimmunity in the context of known PID, collaboration with an immunologist is crucial to balance immune modulation without oversuppressing the immune system. In certain PIDs, such as CVID, selective use of immunomodulatory therapies may be necessary but should be done cautiously with ongoing monitoring for infections.

20.5 Failure to Initiate Immunoglobulin Replacement Therapy

For patients with antibody deficiencies, such as CVID or XLA, IRT can result in severe infections, chronic lung disease (such as bronchiectasis) or other complications. In some cases, even when PID is diagnosed, clinicians may be hesitant to initiate IRT due to concerns about cost, access or patient compliance [7].

How to Avoid This Pitfall IRT should be considered in any patient with a significant antibody deficiency, even in the absence of frequent infections, to prevent long-term complications. There are multiple routes of administration (i.v. or s.c.), and regimens can be tailored to the patient's needs and preferences. Early initiation of IRT has been shown to reduce infection rates, prevent organ damage and improve QoL. Patients and their families should be educated about the importance of ongoing IRT, and regular monitoring of immunoglobulin levels and clinical response should be performed [8].

20.6 Neglecting Long-Term Monitoring and Follow-Up

PIDs are lifelong conditions, and even with appropriate treatment, patients remain at risk for infections, RMDs, malignancies and organ damage. Neglecting long-term monitoring is a common pitfall that can lead to significant morbidity and mortality (Table 20.2). Patients may experience complications such as bronchiectasis, liver disease or cancer if not closely followed [9].

Hot to Avoid This Pitfall Patients with PIDs require regular follow-up with an immunologist to monitor for complications, optimise therapies and adjust treatment

Table 20.2 Long-term complications of primary immunodeficiencies

Category	Complications	Associated primary immunodeficiency	Clinical features
Infections	Chronic/recurrent infections, bronchiectasis	CVID, XLA and in general humoral immunodeficiencies	Persistent respiratory infections, chronic sinusitis, otitis media
Autoimmune diseases	Autoimmune cytopenias such as ITP and haemolytic anaemia, autoimmune thyroiditis	CVID, ALPS, IPEX	Fatigue, pallor, petechiae, thyroid dysfunction
Chronic lung disease	Bronchiectasis, pulmonary fibrosis	SCID, CVID	Chronic cough, sputum production, dyspnoea
Malignancies	Lymphoma, gastric carcinoma, skin cancer	CVID, Wiskott-Aldrich syndrome	Lymphadenopathy, abdominal pain, skin lesions
Gastrointestinal	Inflammatory bowel disease-like symptoms, malabsorption	CVID, SCID	Chronic diarrhoea, abdominal pain, weight loss
	Liver dysfunction	CVID, XLA	Elevated liver enzymes, hepatomegaly, proteinuria
Chronic inflammation	Granuloma formation, lymphoproliferative disorders	CVID, CGD	Non-caseating granulomas, lymphadenopathy, splenomegaly
Musculoskeletal	Osteoporosis, septic arthritis	CVID, hyper-IgE syndrome	Fractures, joint pain, reduced mobility
Skin	Eczema, recurrent abscesses, poor wound healing	Hyper-IgE syndrome, CGD	Chronic rash, skin infections, delayed healing
Cardiovascular	Pulmonary hypertension, vasculitis	CVID, SCID	Dyspnoea, fatigue, digital ulcers, Raynaud's phenomenon
Psychosocial impact	Anxiety, depression, social isolation	All PIDs	Poor QoL, emotional distress, reduced social engagement

as needed. Long-term monitoring should include: (a) *PFTs and imaging*: to assess for bronchiectasis or other chronic lung diseases; (b) *liver function and abdominal imaging*: to screen for liver disease or GI involvement; (c) *routine cancer surveillance*: particularly for lymphomas or other haematologic malignancies; (d) *monitoring of immunoglobulin levels*: in patients receiving IRT, regular assessments ensure adequate dosing and clinical efficacy [10].

Patients should also be counselled on the importance of preventive measures, including vaccinations and early intervention for infections.

20.7 Conclusion

PIDs present unique challenges due to their diverse presentations and complexities in diagnosis and management. By recognising and addressing common pitfalls, such as delayed diagnoses, inappropriate use of immunosuppressive therapies and failure to initiate IRT, clinicians can improve patient outcomes. A multidisciplinary approach involving immunologists and other specialists is essential for the optimal care of patients with PIDs. Through early detection, personalised treatment and regular follow-up, it is possible to prevent complications and improve the QoL for these patients.

References

1. McCusker C, Upton J, Warrington R. Primary immunodeficiency. Allergy Asthma Clin Immunol. 2018;14:61. https://doi.org/10.1186/s13223-018-0290-5.
2. Yarmohammadi H, Estrella L, Doucette J, Cunningham-Rundles C. Recognizing primary immune deficiency in clinical practice. Clin Vaccine Immunol. 2006;13:329–32. https://doi.org/10.1128/CVI.13.3.329-332.2006.
3. Oliveira JB, Fleisher TA. Laboratory evaluation of primary immunodeficiencies. J Allergy Clin Immunol. 2009;125:S297–305. https://doi.org/10.1016/j.jaci.2009.08.043.
4. Berger M, Geng B, Cameron DW, Murphy LM, Schulman ES. Primary immune deficiency diseases as unrecognized causes of chronic respiratory disease. Respir Med. 2017;132:181–8. https://doi.org/10.1016/j.rmed.2017.10.016.
5. Verbsky JW, Routes JM. Sarcoidosis and common variable immunodeficiency: similarities and differences. Semin Respir Crit Care Med. 2014;35:330–5. https://doi.org/10.1055/s-0034-1376862.
6. Chapel H, Prevot J, Gaspar HB, Español T, Bonilla FA, Solís L, et al. Primary immune deficiencies—principles of care. Front Immunol. 2014;5:627. https://doi.org/10.3389/fimmu.2014.00627.
7. Sriaroon P, Ballow M. Immunoglobulin replacement therapy for primary immunodeficiency. Immunol Allergy Clin N Am. 2015;35:713–30. https://doi.org/10.1016/j.iac.2015.07.006.
8. Peter JG, Chapel H. Immunoglobulin replacement therapy for primary immunodeficiencies. Immunotherapy. 2014;6:853–69. https://doi.org/10.2217/imt.14.54.
9. Caldirola MS, Martínez MP, Bezrodnik L, Zwirner NW, Gaillard MI. Immune monitoring of patients with primary immune regulation disorders unravels higher frequencies of follicular T cells with different profiles that associate with alterations in B cell subsets. Front Immunol. 2020;11:576724. https://doi.org/10.3389/fimmu.2020.576724.
10. Haberstroh H, Hirsch A, Goldacker S, Zessack N, Warnatz K, Grimbacher B, et al. A toolkit for monitoring immunoglobulin G levels from dried blood sport of patients with primary immunodeficiencies. J Clin Immunol. 2023;43:1185–92. https://doi.org/10.1007/s10875-023-01464-0.

Pitfalls in IgG4-Related Disease

21

Abbreviations

AIP	Autoimmune pancreatitis
AZA	Azathioprine
CS	Corticosteroids
CT	Computed tomography
HPF	High-power field
IgG4-RD	Immunoglobulin G4-related disease
MMF	Mycophenolate mofetil
MRI	Magnetic resonance imaging
RMDs	Rheumatic diseases
RTX	Rituximab
TB	Tuberculosis

21.1 Overlapping Features with Other Diseases

One of the major pitfalls in diagnosing IgG4-RD is its clinical and histopathological overlap with other diseases. IgG4-RD can mimic malignancies, infections or RMDs, leading to delays or misdiagnoses [1]. Common examples include:

Malignancies IgG4-RD often presents as mass-forming lesions that can be mistaken for cancers such as pancreatic cancer, lymphoma or salivary gland tumours. For instance, AIP, a form of IgG4-RD, can present with a mass in the pancreas, mimicking pancreatic adenocarcinoma. Misdiagnosis can lead to unnecessary surgeries or treatments [2].

E. Pelechas et al., *Pitfalls in Rheumatology*,
https://doi.org/10.1007/978-3-031-98671-0_21

Sarcoidosis Both diseases can involve multiple organs and present with granulomatous inflammation. Without proper immunostaining and IgG4 testing, these two diseases are often indistinguishable on histology alone [3].

Infectious or Inflammatory Disorders TB and other granulomatous diseases can have similar imaging and histological findings as IgG4-RD, leading to diagnostic confusion [4].

How to Avoid This Pitfall A thorough history, careful organ-specific imaging and attention to serological and immunohistochemical findings are critical. When in doubt, IgG4 immunostaining and serum IgG4 levels should be obtained. However, an elevated serum IgG4 is neither necessary nor sufficient for diagnosis and should not be the sole criterion. Multidisciplinary teams involving radiologists, pathologists and specialists in rheumatology, gastroenterology and other fields can help differentiate between these conditions. Due to the significant overlapping of the disease and the difficulty in diagnosis, in Table 21.1, key features that may help in the diagnosis of IgG4-RD are presented.

Table 21.1 Key features that may help in the diagnosis of IgG4-related disease

Category	Criteria	Key features
Clinical features	Characteristic organ involvement or mass-forming lesions	Commonly affected organs: Pancreas, salivary glands, lacrimal glands, lymph nodes, kidneys, lungs
Serological findings	Elevated serum IgG4 levels	Elevated IgG4 levels are suggestive but not diagnostic on its own
Histopathological findings	Dense lymphoplasmacytic infiltration, storiform fibrosis, obliterative phlebitis	Histological hallmark features such as storiform fibrosis required for definitive diagnosis
Immunohistochemical findings	Increased IgG4 plasma cells (>40% of total IgG plasma cells), IgG4 plasma cells >10 per high-power field	Confirms IgG4 predominance in tissue
Radiological features	Enlargement or masses in affected organs, "hypoattenuating lesions" on imaging	Findings consistent with organ-specific involvement but not diagnostic
Response to steroids	Rapid response to CS treatment	A hallmark of IgG4-RD but not always the case as other mimickers may respond well to CS treatment as well

Definite diagnosis: requires characteristic histopathological and immunohistochemical findings along with typical clinical, serological or radiological features; **probable diagnosis:** meets clinical, serological and radiological criteria but lacks histopathological confirmation; **possible diagnosis:** when suggestive clinical features with supportive serology or imaging but insufficient data for a firm diagnosis

21.2 False Reliance on Serum IgG4 Levels

Serum IgG4 elevation is frequently used as a marker for diagnosing IgG4-RD (but also as a prognostic factor). However, this reliance can be misleading. Up to 30% of patients with IgG4-RD may have normal serum IgG4 levels, while non-IgG4-RD can also exhibit elevated IgG4 levels. This may occur in atopic conditions, parasitic infections and some malignancies. Therefore, although higher IgG4 serum levels strengthen the suspicion of the syndrome, these levels alone are not diagnostic, as other diagnostic criteria must also be met. Consequently, they cannot serve as a standalone prognostic marker.

How to Avoid This Pitfall The diagnosis of IgG4-RD requires a combination of clinical, radiological and histopathological findings. Serum IgG4 levels are helpful but should not be over-relied upon. A tissue biopsy is often necessary for a definitive diagnosis. When biopsy results show storiform fibrosis, obliterative phlebitis and dense lymphoplasmacytic infiltration with IgG4-positive plasma cells, the diagnosis is more secure. Plasma cells should typically be >10 per HPF [5].

21.3 Misinterpretation of Histopathology

Pathological analysis is essential for diagnosing IgG4-RD, but interpreting the histology can be tricky. Some clinicians and pathologists may overlook the characteristic features of IgG4-RD or may misinterpret non-specific findings as suggestive of the disease. Moreover, the distribution of IgG4-positive plasma cells can be patchy, and the disease may not be uniformly present in all parts of the biopsy sample [6].

How to Avoid This Pitfall When IgG4-RD is suspected, clinicians should request a biopsy from a representative lesion or organ, and pathologists should be familiar with the histological hallmarks, including: (a) *lymphoplasmacytic infiltration:* especially with IgG4-positive plasma cells; (b) *storiform fibrosis:* a whorled pattern of fibrosis is often a key feature; (c) *obliterative phlebitis:* involvement of veins with inflammatory cells, leading to occlusion.

Immunostaining for IgG4 and calculation of the IgG4-to-IgG ratio in tissue should be performed. A ratio >40% supports the diagnosis, although it is not exclusive to IgG4-RD. If uncertainty persists, obtaining a second pathology opinion from centres with expertise in IgG4-RD can be helpful [7, 8].

21.4 Failure to Recognise Systemic Involvement

IgG4-RD can affect virtually any organ system. Focusing on only one organ may cause clinicians to miss systemic involvement, resulting in suboptimal treatment. For example, a patient presenting with orbital pseudotumour may have undiagnosed pancreatic or renal involvement, which may only be identified if additional tests are ordered [9].

How to Avoid This Pitfall Systemic involvement should always be suspected, even in patients presenting with what seems to be an isolated organ involvement. Comprehensive imaging such as CT or MRI and screening for involvement of other organs, such as the pancreas, kidneys and salivary glands, should be considered in patients with confirmed or suspected IgG4-RD [10]. Furthermore, collaboration between specialists across disciplines is crucial in managing the systemic nature of this disease.

21.5 Underappreciation of Relapsing Disease

IgG4-RD is a chronic condition, and relapses are common. Some clinicians may overlook the possibility of relapse, especially if the patient had initially responded well to treatment. Relapses of the disease occur when maintenance therapy is stopped prematurely or the disease is not adequately suppressed.

How to Avoid This Pitfall Regular follow-up and monitoring are critical to managing IgG4-RD. Patients should be educated about the potential for relapse, and clinicians should remain vigilant for new symptoms or signs of recurrence. Serum IgG4 levels may help in monitoring disease activity, but imaging and repeat biopsies may be required in some cases to confirm a relapse [11].

21.6 Suboptimal Use of Corticosteroids and Immunosuppressants

CS are the first-line treatment for IgG4-RD, but inappropriate dosing or tapering schedules can lead to inadequate disease control or unnecessary side effects. Long-term use of CS without steroid-sparing agents such as RTX, AZA and MMF may also lead to significant adverse effects, such as osteoporosis, diabetes and hypertension [12].

How to Avoid This Pitfall While CS are effective in the acute phase, long-term management should focus on minimising steroid exposure. Tapering schedules should be individualised, and steroid-sparing immunosuppressive agents should be considered early in the treatment course. RTX has shown particular efficacy in treating refractory or relapsing disease and in patients who cannot tolerate CS [13].

21.7 Inadequate Monitoring for Complications

Chronic IgG4-RD can lead to irreversible organ damage if not adequately managed. Untreated or poorly controlled disease can cause fibrosis, resulting in loss of organ function, such as chronic renal failure or permanent visual loss.

How to Avoid This Pitfall Early diagnosis, appropriate treatment and regular follow-up are essential to prevent irreversible damage. In patients with progressive fibrosis, aggressive treatment with CS and immunosuppressants may not reverse the damage, making early intervention crucial [14].

21.8 Conclusion

IgG4-RD is a challenging condition to diagnose and manage due to its protean manifestations, histopathological complexities and overlap or even coexistence with other conditions. Avoiding common pitfalls such as over-reliance on serum IgG4 levels, misinterpretation of histopathology, undertreatment and underappreciation of systemic involvement is critical for timely diagnosis and effective management. By maintaining a high index of suspicion and employing a multidisciplinary approach, clinicians can improve outcomes for patients with this complex disease.

References

1. Pelechas E, Kaltsonoudis E, Voulgari PV, Drosos AA. Miscellaneous conditions. In: Illustrated handbook of rheumatic and musculo-skeletal diseases. Cham: Springer; 2023. https://doi.org/10.1007/978-3-031-47379-1_18.
2. Wallace ZS, Wallace CJ, Lu N, Choi HK, Stone JH. Association of IgG4-related disease with history of malignancy. Arthritis Rheumatol. 2016;68:2283–9. https://doi.org/10.1002/art.39773.
3. Cler SJ, Ogden MA, Farrell NF, Roland LT, Diffie CE, Schneider JS. When inflammation is not just inflammation – a review of systemic diseases of the nose and sinuses part 1: IgG4-related disease and sarcoidosis. Am J Otolaryngol. 2024;45:104213. https://doi.org/10.1016/j.amjoto.2023.104213.
4. Fenderson J, Berenberg J, Tom L, Gress F. IgG4-related disease: imitating a great imitator. Hawaii J Med Public Health. 2015;74:22–6.
5. Abraham M, Khosroshahi A. Diagnostic and treatment workup for IgG4-related disease. Expert Rev Clin Immunol. 2017;13:867–75. https://doi.org/10.1080/1744666X.2017.1354698.
6. Umehara H, Okazaki K, Kawa S, Takahashi H, Goto H, Matsui S, et al. The 2020 revised comprehensive diagnostic (RCD) criteria for IgG4-RD. Mod Rheumatol. 2021;31:529–33. https://doi.org/10.1080/14397595.2020.1859710.
7. Deshpande V, Zen Y, Chan JK, Yi EE, Sato Y, Yoshino T, et al. Consensus statement on the pathology of IgG4-related disease. Mod Pathol. 2012;25:1181–92. https://doi.org/10.1038/modpathol.2012.72.
8. Avincsal MO, Zen Y. The histopathology of IgG4-related disease. Curr Top Microbiol Immunol. 2017;401:45–60. https://doi.org/10.1007/82_2016_38.
9. Hamano H, Tanaka E, Ishizaka N, Kawa S. IgG4-related disease – a systemic disease that deserves attention regardless of one's subspecialty. Intern Med. 2017;57:1201–7. https://doi.org/10.2169/internalmedicine.9533-17.
10. Ichikawa S, Onishi H. Imaging findings of immunoglobulin G4-related disease: from the head to the pelvis. Singapore Med J. 2021;62:574–81. https://doi.org/10.11622/smedj.2021226.
11. Zongrei J, Lingli C, Ying S, Lingying M, Lijuan Z, Dongmei L, et al. Clinical and pathological predictors of relapse in IgG4-related disease. Arthritis Res Ther. 2022;24:106. https://doi.org/10.1186/s13075-022-02792-z.

12. Kamisawa T, Okazaki K. Diagnosis and treatment of IgG4-related disease. Curr Top Microbiol Immunol. 2017;401:19–33. https://doi.org/10.1007/82_2016-36.
13. Yoshifuji H, Umehara H. Glucocorticoids in the treatment of IgG4-related disease-prospects for new international treatment guidelines. Mod Rheumatol. 2023;33:252–7. https://doi.org/10.1093/mr/roac097.
14. Wallace ZS, Katz G, Hernandez-Barco Y, Baker MC. Current and future advances in practice: IgG4-related disease. Rheumatol Adv Pract. 2024;8:rkae020. https://doi.org/10.1093/rap/rkae020.

Pitfalls in Osteoarthritis

22

Abbreviations

ACL	Anterior cruciate ligament
CS	Corticosteroids
GI	Gastrointestinal
MRI	Magnetic resonance imaging
NSAIDs	Non-steroidal anti-inflammatory drugs
OA	Osteoarthritis
PCL	Posterior cruciate ligament
QoL	Quality of life
SNRI	Serotonin–norepinephrine reuptake inhibitor

22.1 Underdiagnosis and Delayed Diagnosis

Despite its high prevalence, OA can often be underdiagnosed, particularly in younger patients or those with atypical joint involvement. OA is traditionally viewed as a disease of aging, which can lead to a delay in diagnosis in younger individuals and in patients with metabolic causes such as diabetes mellitus who present with joint pain. Similarly, non-weight-bearing joints like the hands or shoulders are often overlooked in early stages, as OA is frequently associated with weight-bearing joints like the knees and hips [1].

E. Pelechas et al., *Pitfalls in Rheumatology*,
https://doi.org/10.1007/978-3-031-98671-0_22

How to Avoid These Pitfalls (a) *Recognise atypical presentations*: OA can affect individuals in their 30s and 40s, particularly those with a history of joint injury, obesity or genetic predisposition. Younger patients presenting with persistent joint pain should be evaluated for early OA [2]; (b) *use appropriate imaging*: radiographic signs of OA, such as joint space narrowing and osteophytes, may not always correlate with the severity of symptoms. Early disease may not be obvious on X-rays, so consider advanced imaging (MRI) if clinical suspicion is high despite normal X-rays [3]; (c) *comprehensive joint assessment*: OA can affect multiple joints, not just weight-bearing ones. Hand, shoulder and spine involvement should be considered in patients with pain in these regions, regardless of age in cases of secondary causes, such as trauma to the affected area.

22.2 Over-Reliance of Radiographic Findings

One of the most common pitfalls in diagnosing OA is an over-reliance on radiographic findings. There is often a poor correlation between the extent of radiographic changes and clinical symptoms. Some patients with severe radiographic OA may have minimal symptoms, while others with early-stage disease or few radiographic signs may have significant pain and functional limitations.

How to Avoid This Pitfall (a) *Clinical diagnosis remains key*: diagnosis of OA is primarily clinical, based on history and physical examination findings, such as joint pain that worsens with activity, morning stiffness lasting <30 min and crepitus on joint movement [4] and absence of inflammatory signs such as warmth or redness; (b) *tailor management to symptoms*: treatment decisions should be based on the severity of symptoms and the impact on the patient's QoL, rather than the degree or radiographic damage [5]. Typical joints that can be affected are presented in Fig. 22.1 such as the first metacarpophalangeal, the first metatarsophalangeal, knees and hips.

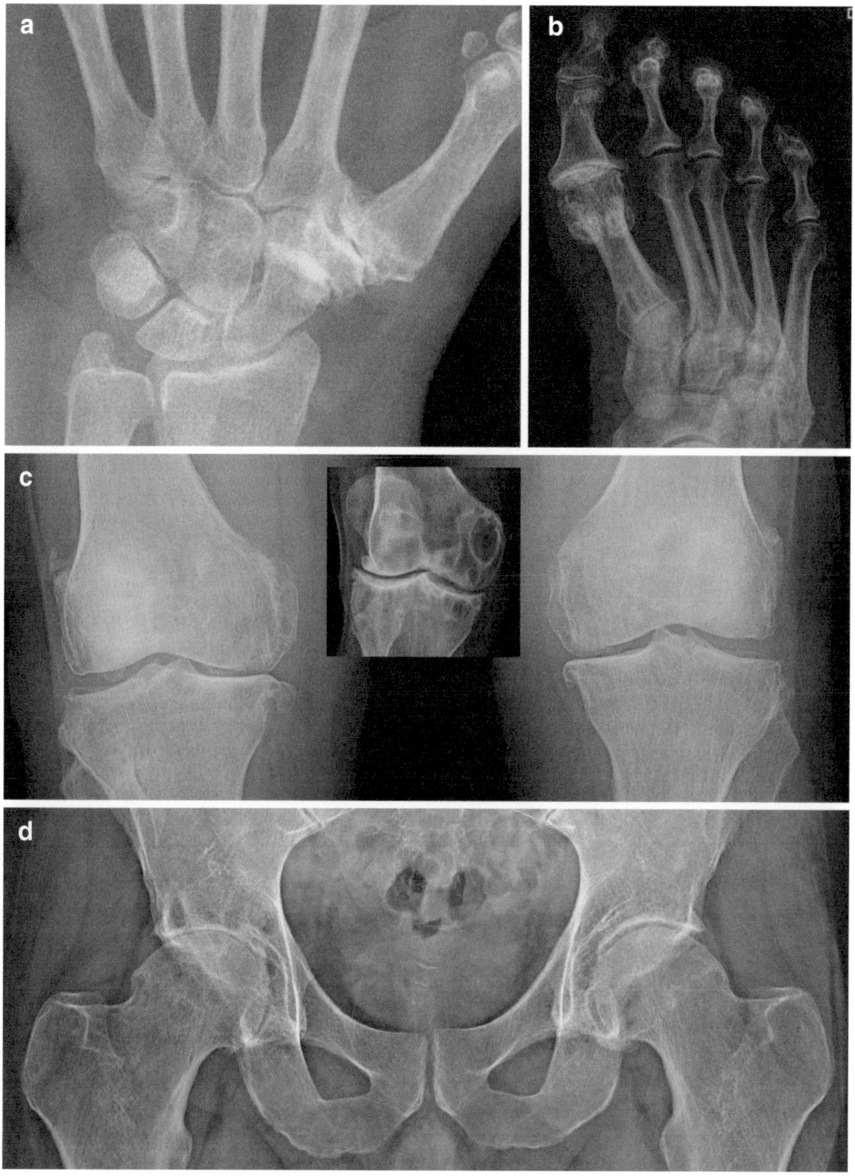

Fig. 22.1 Osteoarthritis; (**a**, **b**) degenerative changes of the first MCP and first MTP respectively consistent with OA; (**c**) knee osteoarthritis Kellgren-Lawrence grade 3–4 (insert figure shows also large cysts named "geode"); (**d**) hip osteoarthritis R > L. Osteoarthritis due to its wear and tear mechanical nature, usually presents the first symptoms in one of these joints

22.3 Failure to Address Modifiable Risk Factors

While OA is often considered a degenerative condition associated with aging and genetic factors, several modifiable risk factors play a significant role in its progression. These include obesity, several metabolic causes, joint injury, muscle weakness and mechanical malalignment. Failure to address these factors can lead to the worsening of symptoms and accelerated joint degeneration.

How to Avoid This Pitfall (a) *Weight management*: obesity is one of the most significant risk factors for knee and hip OA, and even modest weight loss can significantly reduce pain and improve function. Encouraging patients to adopt sustainable weight loss strategies should be a cornerstone of OA management [6]; (b) *joint protection and injury prevention*: previous joint injuries, especially in younger individuals such as ACL/PCL tears or meniscal injuries, can predispose patients to early OA. Rehabilitation and joint protection strategies, including bracing and avoiding high-impact activities, can help reduce the risk of further joint damage [7]; (c) *strengthening and conditioning*: muscle weakness, particularly of the quadriceps in knee OA, is a modifiable risk factor too. Physical therapy and regular exercise programmes that emphasize strengthening, stretching and low-impact aerobic activities can significantly improve pain and function [8]. In addition, use a knee brace, cane or other supportive devices to protect the joints.

22.4 Inadequate Use on Non-Pharmacological Therapies

Non-pharmacological therapies are the cornerstone of OA management. However, they are often underutilised, with clinicians and patients focusing primarily on pharmacological or surgical interventions. Physical therapy, exercise, weight management and education are essential components of OA care but are sometimes overlooked.

How to Avoid This Pitfall (a) *Exercise as medicine*: exercise therapy, particularly low-impact aerobic activities such as swimming, cycling and walking, has been shown to improve pain and joint function in OA. Strengthening exercises targeting the muscles surrounding affected joints are particularly beneficial. Encouraging patient adherence to an exercise programme is crucial [9]; (b) *physical therapy*: physical therapists can play an essential role in providing targeted interventions, including manual therapy, strength training and joint protection techniques. Referral to a physical therapist should be considered early in the management of OA [10]; (c) *patient education*: educating patients about the chronic nature of OA, the importance of lifestyle modifications and the realistic outcomes of treatment can empower them to take an active role in managing their condition. Shared decision-making improves treatment adherence and satisfaction [11].

22.5 Overuse of Pharmacological Treatments

Pharmacological treatments, particularly NSAIDs, are commonly prescribed to manage OA pain. However, over-reliance on these medications can lead to several problems, including side effects like GI ulcers, renal dysfunctions and cardiovascular risks. Additionally, CS injections are sometimes overused, leading to potential joint damage when used too frequently.

How to Avoid This Pitfall (a) *Use pharmacologic therapy as an adjunctive, not primary, treatment*: pharmacological treatments should complement non-pharmacological therapies and be tailored to the individual patient's needs and comorbidities. For mild-to-moderate OA, topical NSAIDs or acetaminophen may be sufficient to control pain, reducing the need for systemic treatments [12]; (b) *limit CS injections*: while CS injections can provide significant pain relief in acute flares, frequent injections may contribute to cartilage damage and further joint degeneration. Limit injections to a few per year, and only in patients with significant pain that impairs function [13]; (c) *consider other pharmacological options*: in patients who cannot tolerate NSAIDs, consider alternative therapies such as duloxetine (SNRI), which has been shown to modify and reduce OA pain [14]. On the other hand, caution is required when prescribing opioids and other narcotic substances for pain control due to the high risk of addiction and dependence.

22.6 Failure to Consider Surgical Referral at the Right Time

Surgical interventions, such as joint replacement, are often viewed as a last resort in OA management. However, delaying surgical referral too long can result in prolonged suffering, decreased QoL and worsening functional impairment. On the other hand, referring patients too early may expose them to unnecessary risks.

How to Avoid This Pitfall (a) *Recognise surgical indications*: patients with severe pain, functional limitation and radiographic evidence of advanced joint damage that is unresponsive to conservative treatments should be considered for surgical referral. Hip and knee replacements, when performed at the appropriate time, can be highly effective in relieving pain and improving function [15]; (b) *collaborative decision-making*: engage in a shared decision-making process with patients regarding the timing of surgery, considering both clinical indications and the patient's goals and preferences. Early referral to an orthopaedic surgeon may be beneficial for patients with rapidly progressing disease.

22.7 Neglecting the Psychosocial Impact of Osteoarthritis

OA is not just a physical condition. It has a significant psychological and social impact. Chronic pain and functional limitations can lead to depression, anxiety, social isolation and reduced QoL. Failure to address these psychosocial aspects can lead to suboptimal outcomes, even when physical symptoms are managed.

How to Avoid This Pitfall (a) *Screen for mental health issues*: regularly assess patients with OA for signs of depression, anxiety or other psychological stressors. Referral to a mental health professional may be necessary for patients struggling with the emotional toll of chronic pain [16]; (b) *pain management strategies*: incorporating pain management strategies, such as cognitive–behavioural therapy and mindfulness techniques, can help patients cope with the chronic nature of OA and its impact on their daily life [17]; (c) *support networks*: encourage patients to engage in support groups, community programmes or online forums where they can share their experiences and coping strategies with others dealing with OA [18].

22.8 Conclusion

OA is a multifaceted disease with significant clinical and therapeutic challenges. The common pitfalls in diagnosing and managing OA include underdiagnosis, overreliance on imaging, failure to address modifiable risk factors and overuse of pharmacologic treatments. A comprehensive, patient-centred approach that emphasizes early diagnosis, lifestyle modifications, appropriate use of pharmacological and non-pharmacological therapies and timely surgical referral can greatly enhance patient outcomes.

References

1. Pelechas E, Kaltsonoudis E, Voulgari PV, Drosos AA. Osteoarthritis. In: Illustrated handbook of rheumatic and musculo-skeletal diseases. Cham: Springer; 2023. https://doi.org/10.1007/978-3-031-37379-1_14.
2. Wilfong JM, Badley EM, Perruccio A. Old before their age? The impact of osteoarthritis on younger adults. Arthritis Care Res (Hoboken). 2024;76:1400–8. https://doi.org/10.1002/acr.25374.
3. Roemer FW, Guermazi A, Demehri S, Wirth W, Kijowski R. Imaging in osteoarthritis. Osteoarthr Cartil. 2022;30:913–34. https://doi.org/10.1016/j.joca.2021.018.
4. Ahbishek A, Doherty M. Diagnosis and clinical presentation of osteoarthritis. Rheum Dis Clin N Am. 2013;39:45–66. https://doi.org/10.1016/j.rdc.2012.10.007.
5. Johnson CB. A personalized shared decision-making tool for osteoarthritis management of the knee. Orthop Nurs. 2020;40:64–70. https://doi.org/10.1097/NOR.0000000000000739.
6. Bliddal H, Leeds AR, Christensen R. Osteoarthritis, obesity and weight loss: evidence, hypotheses and horizons – a scoping review. Obes Rev. 2014;15:578–86. https://doi.org/10.1111/obr.12173.

7. Ratzlaff CR, Liang MH. New developments in osteoarthritis. Prevention of injury-related knee osteoarthritis: opportunities of the primary and secondary prevention of knee osteoarthritis. Arthritis Res Ther. 2010;12:215. https://doi.org/10.1186/ar3113.
8. Shorter E, Sannicandro AJ, Poulet B, Goljanek-Whysall K. Skeletal muscle wasting and its relationship with osteoarthritis: a mini-review of mechanisms and current interventions. Curr Rheumatol Rep. 2019;21:40. https://doi.org/10.1007/s11926-019-0839-4.
9. Semanik P, Chang RW, Dunlop DD. Aerobic activity in prevention & symptom control of osteoarthritis. PM R. 2012;4:S37–44. https://doi.org/10.1016/j.pmrj.2012.02.015.
10. Wang W, Niu Y, Jia Q. Physical therapy as a promising treatment for osteoarthritis: a narrative review. Front Physiol. 2022;13:1011407. https://doi.org/10.3389/fphys.2022.1011407.
11. Sinatti P, Romero EAS, Martínez-Pozas O, Villafañe JH. Effects of patient education on pain and function and its impact on conservative treatment in elderly patients with pain related to hip and knee osteoarthritis: a systematic review. Int J Environ Res Public Health. 2022;19:6194. https://doi.org/10.3390/ijerph19106194.
12. Hochbert MC, Altman RD, Brandt KD, Clark BM, Diepe PA, Griffin MR, et al. Guidelines for the medical management of osteoarthritis. Part II. Osteoarthritis of the knee. American College of Rheumatology. Arthritis Rheum. 1995;38:1541–6. https://doi.org/10.1002/art.1780381104.
13. Guermazi A, Hunter DJ, Kloppenburg M. Debate: intra-articular steroid injections for osteoarthritis – harmful or helpful? Osteoarthr Imaging. 2023;3:100163. https://doi.org/10.1016/j.ostima.2023.100163.
14. Osani MC, Bunnuru RR. Efficacy and safety of duloxetine in osteoarthritis: a systematic review and meta-analysis. Korean J Intern Med. 2019;34:966–73. https://doi.org/10.3904/kjim.2018.460.
15. Srivastava AK. American academy of orthopaedic surgeons clinical practice guideline summary of surgical management of osteoarthritis of the knee. J Am Acad Orthop Surg. 2023;31:1211–20. https://doi.org/10.5435/JAAOS-D-23-00338.
16. Wang ST, Ni GX. Depression in osteoarthritis: current understanding. Neuropsychiatr Dis Treat. 2022;18:375–89. https://doi.org/10.2147/NDT.S346183.
17. Farinelli L, Riccio M, Gigante A, De Francesco F. Pain management strategies in osteoarthritis. Biomedicines. 2024;12:805. https://doi.org/10.3390/biomedicines12040805.
18. Ali SA, Kokorelias KM, MacDermid JC, Kloseck M. Education and social support as key factors in osteoarthritis management programs: a scoping review. Arthritis. 2018;2018:2496190. https://doi.org/10.1155/2018/2496190.

Pitfalls in Osteoporosis

23

Abbreviations

BMD	Bone mineral density
BP	Bisphosphonates
CKD	Chronic kidney disease
CS	Corticosteroid
DEXA	Dual-energy X-ray absorptiometry
FRAX	Fracture risk assessment tool
GI	Gastrointestinal
IA	Inflammatory arthritis
IBD	Inflammatory bowel disease
MSK	Musculoskeletal
ONJ	Osteonecrosis of the jaw
OP	Osteoporosis
PTH	Parathormone
QoL	Quality of life
RA	Rheumatoid arthritis
RANKL	Receptor activator of nuclear factor kappa beta ligand
SERMs	Selective oestrogen receptor modulators
VTE	Venous thromboembolism

23.1 Underdiagnosis and Lack of Screening

OP is often underdiagnosed, particularly because it is asymptomatic until a fracture occurs (Fig. 23.1). Many patients at risk for OP do not receive adequate screening, either due to lack of awareness or misperceptions about who should be tested [1] and treated.

E. Pelechas et al., *Pitfalls in Rheumatology*,
https://doi.org/10.1007/978-3-031-98671-0_23

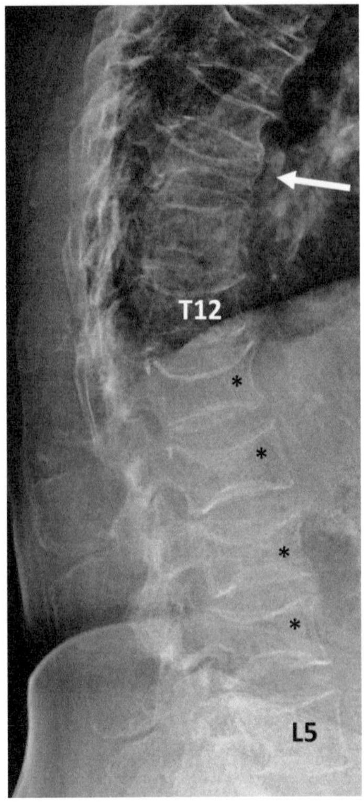

Fig. 23.1 Multiple vertebral fracture of the spine. L1-L4 fractures of the lumbar spine (asterisks), T12 and T10 of the thoracic spine. The white arrow points out the T10 vertebral fracture which is called "vertebra plana" because of the full thickness fracture of *the vertebra*

How to Avoid This Pitfall (a) *Adhere to screening guidelines*: bone density screening using DEXA should be performed in women aged >65 and men >70, postmenopausal women, men aged 50–69 with clinical risk factors (family history of OP, previous fractures, smoking and low body weight) and anyone over age 50 who has had a fragility fracture; (b) *consider secondary OP*: be vigilant for secondary causes of OP, such as CS use, hyperthyroidism or CKD, which may require earlier screening or more aggressive or even prophylactic treatment [2].

23.2 Misinterpretation of Bone Mineral Density Results

While DEXA scans are the gold standard for diagnosing OP, misinterpretation of BMD results is common. T-scores, which compare a patient's BMD to that of a healthy young adult, are often used to diagnose OP. However, BMD is just one factor in fracture risk, and over-reliance on T-scores can lead to missed opportunities for intervention.

How to Avoid This Pitfall (a) *Consider absolute fracture risk*: tools like the FRAX score estimate the 10-year risk of major OP and hip fractures by integrating BMD with clinical risk factors (age, gender, history of fractures, smoking, alcohol use, etc.). This can help identify patients who may benefit from treatment, even if their T-score does not meet the threshold for OP; (b) *monitor for progression*: patients with osteopenia (T-scores between −1.0 and −2.5) should be monitored regularly as they are at risk for progressing to OP. Implementing early preventive strategies in these patients can help prevent fractures [3]. Furthermore, application of the Z-score in younger individuals and premenopausal women is indicated.

23.3 Failure to Recognise and Treat Osteoporosis After a Fragility Fracture

One of the biggest missed opportunities in OP care is the failure to initiate treatment after a fragility fracture. Patients who suffer a fragility fracture are at high risk for future fractures, yet many do not receive appropriate evaluation or treatment to reduce this risk.

How to Avoid This Pitfall (a) *Post-fracture evaluation*: any patient over 50 who experiences a fragility fracture should be evaluated for OP. This includes a thorough history, physical examination, DEXA scan and evaluation for secondary causes of bone loss [4]; (b) *timely initiation of treatment*: if OP is confirmed or strongly suspected, initiate treatment to reduce the risk of subsequent fractures. This is especially important for hip and vertebral fractures, which carry significant morbidity and mortality [5]; (c) *fracture liaison services*: implementing a fracture liaison service or a similar model of care can help ensure that patients who suffer fragility fractures receive appropriate evaluation and treatment for OP [6].

23.4 Over-Reliance on Calcium and Vitamin D Supplementation Alone

While calcium and vitamin D play a crucial role in bone health, relying solely on supplementation for the treatment or prevention of OP is insufficient. In many cases, this leads to undertreatment of the underlying disease and fails to address the increased fracture risk.

How to Avoid This Pitfall (a) *Calcium and vitamin D are foundational but not curative*: ensure patients receive adequate calcium (1000–1200 mg/day) and vitamin D (800–1000 IU/day) through diet or supplements. However, supplementation alone is not enough to treat OP. Pharmacologic therapies are often necessary for patients at high fracture risk [7]; (b) *pharmacotherapy for high-risk individuals*: use anti-resorptive agents such as BP and denosumab or anabolic agents such as teriparatide and romosozumab to reduce fracture risk in patients diagnosed with OP, particularly those with a history of fragility fractures or high FRAX scores [8].

23.5 Mismanagement of Pharmacological Treatment

Pharmacological treatment of OP is effective at reducing fracture risk, but several pitfalls exist, particularly regarding the choice of therapy, duration of treatment and patient adherence.

How to Avoid These Pitfalls (a) *Tailor treatment to individual needs*: BP such as alendronate and risedronate are first-line therapies, but patients with severe OP or multiple fractures may benefit from anabolic therapies, such as teriparatide and romosozumab. Denosumab is another effective option but requires long-term adherence, as discontinuation can lead to rapid bone loss; (b) *monitor treatment duration*: BP are typically given for 3–5 years, after which a "drug holiday" may be considered to reduce the risk of rare but serious side effects such as atypical femoral fractures, osteomalacia or ONJ. However, high-risk patients may need continued therapy or switching to another agent [9]; (c) *ensure adherence*: poor adherence to OP medications is common due to the asymptomatic nature of the disease. Side effects like GI symptoms from oral BP can reduce compliance. Consider less frequent dosing regimens (e.g. annual zoledronic acid infusion) or switching to a different class of medication if adherence is an issue [10]. In Table 23.1, a summary of all available medications with their mechanism of action and side effects is presented.

Table 23.1 Summary of medications for the treatment of osteoporosis

Drug class	Drugs	MOA	Special considerations	Side effects
BP	Alendronate, risedronate, ibandronate, zoledronic acid	Inhibit osteoclast-mediated bone resorption, increasing bone density	Take on an empty stomach with water; remain upright for at least 30 min to prevent oesophageal irritation	GI irritation, oesophageal ulcers, MSK pain, rare ONJ, atypical femoral fractures
RANKL inhibitor	Denosumab	Monoclonal antibody that inhibits RANKL, reducing osteoclast formation and activity	Administered subcutaneously every 6 months; monitor for hypocalcaemia; reversible upon discontinuation	Hypocalcaemia, infections, MSK pain, rash, rare ONJ, atypical femoral fractures, injection site reactions
SERMs	Raloxifene	Mimics oestrogen's protective effects on bone without affecting breast or uterine tissue	May reduce risk of breast cancer; may increase risk of VTE	Hot flashes, leg cramps, increased risk of VTE and stroke

(continued)

Table 23.1 (continued)

Drug class	Drugs	MOA	Special considerations	Side effects
PTH analogues	Teriparatide, abaloparatide	Stimulate new bone formation by activating osteoblasts	Limited to 2 years of use due to potential risk of osteosarcoma in animal studies; follow with antiresorptive therapy	Nausea, dizziness, leg cramps, hypercalcaemia, injection site reactions
Tissue-selective oestrogen complex	Bazedoxifene with conjugated oestrogens	Combines SERM and oestrogen effects for bone protection and menopausal symptom management	Approved for postmenopausal women with a uterus; not first-line treatment for OP	Hot flashes, leg cramps, VTE, nausea
Sclerostin inhibitor	Romosozumab	Monoclonal antibody that increases bone formation and decreases resorption by inhibiting sclerostin	Monthly injections; may increase cardiovascular risk; limit to 1 year of use	Arthralgias, headache, injection site reactions, and rare cardiovascular events
Calcium and Vitamin D	Calcium carbonate, calcium citrate, Cholecalciferol (D3), ergocalciferol (D2)	Essential for bone health; supports other osteoporosis therapies	Adequate intake necessary for efficacy of all treatments	Constipation, bloating, hypercalcaemia, and kidney stones

23.6 Inadequate Attention to Fall Prevention

Fracture risk in OP is not just a matter of bone strength but also the likelihood of falls. Focusing solely on improving bone density while neglecting fall prevention can leave patients vulnerable to fractures.

How to Avoid This Pitfall (a) *Implement fall prevention strategies*: advise patients on fall prevention measures such as home safety modifications (removing rugs and installing handrails), vision correction and balance training. Refer patients for physical therapy if needed [11]; (b) *encourage exercise*: weight-bearing exercises like walking and resistance training can improve bone density, while balance exercises such as tai chi can reduce fall risk. Encourage regular exercise as part of OP management [12]; (c) *address medications that increase fall risk*: review medications that may contribute to dizziness or balance problems, such as sedatives, antihypertensives or antidepressants. Adjust doses or switch medications where possible to reduce fall risk.

23.7 Failure to Address Secondary Causes of Osteoporosis

OP can be primary (age-related or postmenopausal) or secondary, arising from underlying medical conditions or medications. Failure to recognise and treat secondary OP can lead to suboptimal management [13]. In Table 23.2, an extensive list of possible secondary causes of osteoporosis is presented.

Table 23.2 Secondary causes of osteoporosis

Category	Conditions/risk factors	Notes
Endocrine disorders	Hyperthyroidism	Excess thyroid hormone increases bone resorption
	Hyperparathyroidism	Increased PTH leads to calcium loss from bones
	Cushing's syndrome	Excess cortisol decreases bone formation and increases resorption
	Diabetes mellitus	Alters bone metabolism; more pronounced in Type 1
	Hypogonadism	Decreased sex hormones reduce bone density
	Hyperprolactinaemia	Suppresses gonadal function, reducing bone density
	Acromegaly	Abnormal bone turnover due to growth hormone excess
Gastrointestinal disorders	Malabsorption syndromes (coeliac disease, IBD)	Reduced calcium, vitamin D, and nutrient absorption
	Chronic liver disease	Impaired vitamin D metabolism
	Gastrectomy	Reduced calcium and vitamin D absorption
	Chronic pancreatitis	Reduced absorption of fat-soluble vitamins, including vitamin D
Rheumatologic disorders	RA (and practically any long-standing IA)	Inflammation and corticosteroid use contribute to bone loss
	Ankylosing spondylitis	Chronic inflammation impacts bone turnover
Haematologic disorders	Multiple myeloma	Increased osteoclast activity leads to bone loss
	Leukaemia/lymphoma	Bone marrow infiltration impacts bone health
	Sickle cell anaemia	Bone infarctions and marrow changes contribute to osteoporosis
Renal disorders	Chronic kidney disease	Disturbs calcium-phosphate balance and vitamin D metabolism

(continued)

Table 23.2 (continued)

Category	Conditions/risk factors	Notes
Medications	Corticosteroids	Directly impair bone formation and increase resorption
	Anticonvulsants	Induce vitamin D metabolism leading to deficiency
	Proton pump inhibitors	Long-term use may reduce calcium absorption
	Aromatase inhibitors	Decrease oestrogen levels, leading to bone loss
	GnRH agonists/antagonists	Suppress gonadal hormones, reducing bone density
	Heparin	Impairs bone formation
	Chemotherapy	Impacts bone marrow and metabolism
Lifestyle factors	Chronic alcohol use	Directly toxic to osteoblasts
	Smoking	Decreases calcium absorption and sex hormone production
	Excessive caffeine intake	May reduce calcium absorption if excessive
Nutritional deficiencies	Vitamin D deficiency	Impairs calcium absorption
	Calcium deficiency	Limits bone mineralisation
	Protein-energy malnutrition	Reduces bone turnover and density
Miscellaneous	Immobility/bed-bound patients	Mechanical unloading reduces bone strength

How to Avoid This Pitfall A thorough evaluation for secondary causes must be carried out regarding: *CS use* (chronic use of CS is a major cause of secondary OP), *endocrine disorders* (hyperthyroidism, hyperparathyroidism and Cushing's disease can all lead to bone loss), *GI diseases* (conditions like coeliac disease, IBD or gastric bypass surgery can impair calcium absorption) and *CKD* (renal osteodystrophy should be considered in patients with kidney disease and low bone density). In the aforementioned cases, a tailored treatment should be applied. Treat the underlying condition when possible. For example, in patients on long-term CS, use bone-protective agents like BP or teriparatide early in treatment [13], and in cases of metabolic causes, therapeutically address the underlying metabolic condition.

23.8 Inadequate Follow-Up and Monitoring

OP is a chronic condition requiring ongoing management. Inadequate follow-up or failure to monitor treatment response can lead to missed opportunities to adjust therapy, assess fracture risk or intervene early in disease progression.

How to Avoid This Pitfall (a) *Regular follow-up*: reassess patients every 1–2 years with repeat DEXA scans to monitor changes in BMD and adjust treatment as needed. More frequent follow-up may be needed in high-risk patients; (b) *monitor* *for medication side effects*: long-term use of some OP treatments, such as BP or denosumab, can lead to rare complications. Regular follow-up allows for the monitoring of adverse effects and the potential need for drug holidays or therapy changes [14].

23.9 Conclusion

OP management presents unique challenges, from early identification and screening to individualised treatment and long-term follow-up. The common pitfalls in diagnosis and management, including underdiagnosis, misinterpretation of BMD results and inadequate pharmacologic therapy, can significantly impact patient outcomes. A proactive approach, integrating fracture risk assessment, appropriate pharmacotherapy, fall prevention and regular monitoring, is crucial to preventing fractures and improving QoL for patients with OP.

References

1. Pelechas E, Kaltsonoudis E, Voulgari PV, Drosos AA. Osteoporosis. In: Illustrated handbook of rheumatic and musculo-skeletal diseases. Cham: Springer; 2023. https://doi.org/10.1007/978-3-031-47379-1_16.
2. Camacho PM, Petak SM, Binkley N, Diab DL, Eldeiry LS, Farooki A, et al. American Association of Clinical Endocrinologists/American College of Endocrinology clinical practice guidelines for the diagnosis and treatment of postmenopausal osteoporosis – 2020 update executive summary. Endocr Pract. 2020;26:564–70. https://doi.org/10.4158/GL-2020-0524.
3. Rehman O, Sharif M, Khan MS, Tahir S, Zammurad S, Shabbır K, et al. FRAX calculation with and without bone mineral density for assessment of osteoporotic fracture risk in patients of rheumatic disease: a cross-sectional study. Ann Med Surg (Lond). 2023;85:1743–9. https://doi.org/10.1097/MS9.0000000000000656.
4. Weaver J, Sajjan S, Lewiecki EM, Harris ST. Diagnosis and treatment of osteoporosis before and after fracture: a side-by-side analysis of commercially insured and medicare advantage osteoporosis patients. J Manag Care Spec Pharm. 2017;23:735–44. https://doi.org/10.18553/jmcp.2017.23.7.735.
5. Wang CY, Fu SH, Yang RS, Chen LK, Shen LJ, Hsiao FY. Timing of anti-osteoporosis medications initiation after a hip fracture affects the risk of subsequent fracture: a nationwide cohort study. Bone. 2020;138:115452. https://doi.org/10.1016/j.bone.2020.115452.
6. Bonanni S, Sorensen AA, Dubin J, Drees B. The role of the fracture liaison service in osteoporosis care. Mo Med. 2017;114:295–8.
7. Reid IR, Bolland MJ. Calcium and/or vitamin D supplementation for the prevention of fragility fractures: who needs it? Nutrients. 2020;12:1011. https://doi.org/10.3390/nu12041011.
8. Curtis EM, Reginster JY, Al-Daghri N, Biver E, Brandi ML, Cavalier E, et al. Management of patients at very high risk of osteoporotic fractures through sequential treatments. Aging Clin Exp Res. 2022;34:695–714. https://doi.org/10.1007/s40520-022-02100-4.
9. Hayes KN, Winter EM, Cadarette SM, Burden AM. Duration of bisphosphonate drug holidays in osteoporosis patients: a narrative review of the evidence and considerations for decision-making. J Clin Med. 2021;10:1140. https://doi.org/10.3390/jcm10051140.
10. Papaioannou A, Kennedy CC, Dolovich L, Lau E, Adachi JD. Patient adherence to osteoporosis medications: problems, consequences and management strategies. Drugs Aging. 2007;24:37–55. https://doi.org/10.2165/00002512-200724010-00003.

11. Karlsson MK, Magnusson H, von Schewelov T, Rosengren BE. Prevention of falls in the elderly – a review. Osteoporos Int. 2013;24:747–62. https://doi.org/10.1007/s00198-012-2256-7.
12. Benedetti MG, Furlini G, Zati A, Mauro GL. The effectiveness of physical exercise on bone density in osteoporotic patients. Biomed Res Int. 2018;2018:4840531. https://doi.org/10.1155/2018/4840531.
13. Fitzpatrick LA. Secondary causes of osteoporosis. Mayo Clin Proc. 2002;77:453–68. https://doi.org/10.4065/77.5.453.
14. Tu KN, Lie JD, Wan CKV, Cameron M, Austel AG, Nguyen JK, Van K, Hyun D. Osteoporosis: a review of treatment options. P T. 2018;43:92–104.

Pitfalls in Paget's Disease 24

Abbreviations

ALP	Alkaline phosphatase
MRI	Magnetic resonance imaging
NSAIDs	Non-steroidal anti-inflammatory drugs
PD	Paget's disease
QoL	Quality of life

24.1 Delayed Diagnosis and Misinterpretation of Symptoms

PD can be insidious in onset, with many patients remaining asymptomatic for years. When symptoms do occur, they may be mistakenly attributed to other conditions, such as arthritis or normal age-related changes in bone.

Consequences of Delayed Diagnosis (a) *Worsening bone deformities*: prolonged undiagnosed disease can lead to significant bone deformities, increasing the risk of fractures and impairing mobility [1]; (b) *chronic pain*: patients may experience persistent pain that is inadequately addressed if the underlying cause is not recognised [2]; (c) *inappropriate treatment*: symptoms such as bone pain may lead to unnecessary treatment for conditions such as arthritis, delaying the appropriate management of PD [3].

Overcoming This Pitfall Clinicians should maintain a high index of suspicion for PD in older adults presenting with unexplained bone pain, deformities or fractures. A thorough clinical history, including family history and assessment of previous imaging studies, is essential. Laboratory tests, including serum ALP levels, and imaging studies such as X-rays, scintigraphy (Fig. 24.1) or MRI can aid in establishing the diagnosis.

E. Pelechas et al., *Pitfalls in Rheumatology*,
https://doi.org/10.1007/978-3-031-98671-0_24

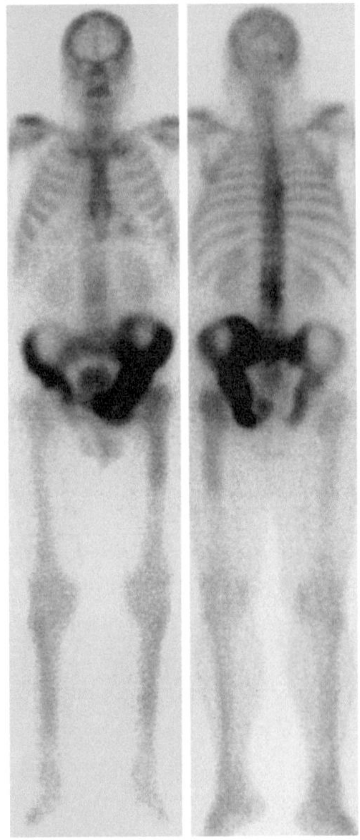

Fig. 24.1 Scintigraphy of a patient diagnosed with Paget's disease. Note the increased uptake of the radiotracer in almost the entire extent of the bones of the left pelvis

24.2 Inadequate Recognition of Asymptomatic Cases

PD is often discovered incidentally on radiographs performed for other reasons, such as routine screening or evaluation of fractures. Asymptomatic patients may not require treatment, but the failure to recognise these cases can lead to unnecessary interventions.

Pitfalls of Mismanaging Asymptomatic Patients (a) *Unnecessary treatment*: in cases where PD is discovered incidentally and patients are asymptomatic, unnecessary bisphosphonate therapy may be initiated without proper consideration of the patient's overall health and comorbidities [4]; (b) *inadequate monitoring*: asymptomatic patients may be overlooked in terms of regular monitoring, potentially leading to disease progression without intervention.

Overcoming This Pitfall In asymptomatic patients with radiographic evidence of PD, a conservative approach may be warranted. Regular monitoring of serum ALP levels and periodic imaging can help assess disease progression and the need for treatment. Clinicians should educate patients about the nature of the disease, emphasizing the importance of monitoring over immediate treatment [5].

24.3 Underestimation of Disease Severity

The severity of PD can vary widely among patients, with some exhibiting significant bone deformities and others showing minimal changes. Clinicians may underestimate the impact of the disease on bone health and overall QoL, particularly in those with mild manifestations.

Consequences of Underestimation (a) *Failure to provide appropriate management*: patients with significant bone involvement may require more aggressive management, including pharmacotherapy, orthopaedic interventions or pain management strategies. Underestimating the disease can lead to inadequate treatment, fractures and poorer outcomes [6]; (b) *increased risk of complications*: severe cases of PD can lead to complication such as osteosarcoma and heart failure. Failure to recognise the potential severity can increase the risk of adverse outcomes [7].

Overcoming This Pitfall Clinicians should assess disease severity through a combination of clinical evaluation, imaging studies and laboratory tests. Comprehensive evaluations should include assessments of bone pain, the rate of progression, mobility and functional status. Referrals to specialists, such as orthopaedic surgeons or pain management specialists, may be necessary for patients with significant disease burden and of younger age.

24.4 Failure to Recognise Extraskeletal Complications

While PD primarily affects the skeleton, it can also be associated with various extraskeletal complications, including osteosarcoma, hearing loss and cardiovascular issues. These complications may be overlooked, particularly in patients with long-standing disease. In Table 24.1, all potential extraskeletal complications are presented in more detail.

Pitfalls of Overlooking Extraskeletal Manifestations (a) *Delayed diagnosis of osteosarcoma*: patients with PD are at increased risk of developing osteosarcoma, particularly in areas of previously affected bone. Misinterpretation of new bone pain as a recurrence of PD or attributing the pain to other causes can delay the diagnosis of malignancy [8]; (b) *unaddressed hearing loss*: bone remodelling in the skull can lead to conductive hearing loss, which may be attributed to age-related changes rather than being recognised as a complication of PD [9].

Overcoming This Pitfall Clinicians should conduct thorough assessments of patients with PD, looking for signs of extraskeletal complications. Regular monitoring for new or worsening symptoms, particularly persistent pain or changes in hearing, is essential. Early referral to specialists for further evaluation and management of complication can improve outcomes.

Table 24.1 Extraskeletal complications of Paget's disease

Complication	Details	Mechanism/association
Hearing loss	Conductive or sensorineural hearing	Bone involvement in the skull (mainly when in temporal bone) affecting the auditory ossicles of cochlea
Neurological compression	Cranial nerve palsies, spinal cord compression, or radiculopathy	Bone overgrowth leading to narrowing of foramina and compression of nerves or spinal cord
Cardiovascular complications	High-output cardiac failure due to increased blood flow to the bones	Increased vascularity of pagetic bone creates a significant arteriovenous shunt burden on the heart
	Cardiac arrhythmias secondary to high-output cardiac failure or hypercalcaemia	Changes in calcium homeostasis and cardiac stress from increased circulatory demands
Hypercalcaemia	Elevated calcium levels (rare)	Increased bone turnover releases calcium into the bloodstream, worsened by immobilisation
Kidney stones	Renal calculi related to hypercalcaemia (rare)	Increased calcium excretion through the kidneys due to excessive bone resorption
Osteosarcoma	Secondary bone cancer	Rare transformation of pagetic bone into malignant osteosarcoma (rare)
Psychological effects	Depression, anxiety, or reduced QoL	Chronic pain, deformities and functional limitations may impact mental health

24.5 Inadequate Treatment for Bone Pain

Bone pain is a common symptom in PD, yet it is often inadequately managed. Clinicians may focus on bisphosphonate therapy without addressing pain control, leading to patient dissatisfaction and reduced QoL.

Pitfalls in Pain Management (a) *Over-reliance on bisphosphonates*: while bisphosphonates can reduce osteoclastic activity and stabilise the disease, they do not always provide sufficient relief for bone pain. Some patients may require additional analgesic strategies [10]; (b) *failure to address comorbid pain syndromes*: many patients with PD are older adults with comorbidities that may contribute to pain, including arthritis or neuropathic pain. These conditions may be overlooked, leading to inadequate pain management.

Overcoming This Pitfall A comprehensive approach to pain management is essential. Clinicians should assess pain intensity, quality and impact on daily activities and consider a multimodal approach, including NSAIDs, analgesics, physical therapy and interventions such as nerve blocks if necessary. Collaboration with pain management specialists may be beneficial for complex cases.

24.6 Neglecting the Role of Lifestyle Modifications

While pharmacotherapy is a cornerstone of PD management, lifestyle modifications are equally important and often neglected. Patients may not receive adequate guidance on dietary changes, exercise and fall prevention strategies.

Consequences of Neglecting Lifestyle Changes (a) *Increased risk of fractures*: patients with PD are at higher risk of fractures, particularly if they have significant bone deformities. Lack of attention to fall prevention strategies can lead to complications [11]; (b) *worsening QoL*: poor nutrition, inactivity and lack of support can negatively impact patients' overall well-being, leading to increased pain and functional limitations [12].

Overcoming This Pitfall Clinicians should emphasize the importance of lifestyle modifications in managing PD. Recommendation should include maintaining a balanced diet rich in calcium and vitamin D, engaging in regular low-impact exercise to improve bone health and mobility and implementing fall prevention strategies to minimise fracture risk. Referrals to dietitians or physical therapists may enhance patient adherence to lifestyle changes.

24.7 Underutilisation of Surgical Interventions

In cases where PD leads to significant bone deformities, fractures or joint instability, surgical intervention may be necessary. However, surgical options are often underutilised due to misconceptions about the disease or concerns about surgical risks.

Pitfalls of Underutilisation (a) *Delayed orthopaedic referral*: clinicians may hesitate to refer patients for orthopaedic evaluation, believing that bisphosphonate therapy alone is sufficient to manage complications. This can lead to worsening deformities and functional impairment [13]; (b) *inadequate surgical planning*: surgical management may be complicated by the presence of PD, requiring careful planning and multidisciplinary collaboration [14].

Overcoming This Pitfall Clinicians should maintain an open dialogue with orthopaedic surgeons regarding the management of patients with severe PD. Patients exhibiting significant symptoms related to deformities or complications should be promptly referred for surgical evaluation. Early intervention can improve functional outcomes and QoL.

24.8 Conclusion

PD presents unique challenges in diagnosis and management due to its varied clinical manifestations and potential complications. Clinicians must be vigilant in recognising the disease and its associated pitfalls to optimise patient outcomes. A thorough understanding of the disease process, along with an individualised approach to treatment and lifestyle modifications, can enhance care for patients with PD. Early diagnosis, appropriate management of symptoms and complications and proactive lifestyle interventions are essential for improving the quality of life and overall health outcomes in affected individuals.

References

1. Pelechas E, Kaltsonoudis E, Voulgari PV, Drosos AA. Miscellaneous conditions. In: Illustrated handbook of rheumatic and musculo-skeletal diseases. Cham: Springer; 2023. https://doi.org/10.1007/978-3-031-47379-1_18.
2. Berg K, Dockrell D, Colvin L, Fraser WD, Tang JC, Aspray T, et al. Causes of musculoskeletal pain in Paget's disease of bone. Calcif Tissue Int. 2024;115:533–41. https://doi.org/10.1007/s00223-024-01279-0.
3. Reid IR. Recent advances in understanding and managing Paget's disease. F1000Res. 2019;8:F1000 Faculty Rev-1485. https://doi.org/10.12688/f1000research.19676.1.
4. Singer FR, Bone HG 3rd, Hosking DJ, Lyles KW, Murad MH, Reid IR, et al. Paget's disease of bone: an endocrine society clinical practice guideline. J Clin Endocrinol Metab. 2014;99:4408–22. https://doi.org/10.1210/jc.2014-2910.
5. Ralston SH, Corral-Gudino L, Cooper C, Francis RM, Fraser WD, Gennari L, et al. Diagnosis and management of Paget's disease of bone in adults: a clinical guideline. J Bone Miner Res. 2019;34:579–604. https://doi.org/10.1002/jbmr.3657.
6. Siris ES. Paget's disease of bone. J Bone Miner Res. 1998;13:1061–5. https://doi.org/10.1359/jbmr.1998.13.7.1061.
7. Tiegs RD. Paget's disease of bone: indications for treatment and goals of therapy. Clin Ther. 1997;19:1309–29. Discussion 1523–4. https://doi.org/10.1016/s0149-2918(97)800007-0.
8. Hansen MF, Seton M, Merchant A. Osteosarcoma in Paget's disease of bone. J Bone Miner Res. 2006;21(Suppl 2):P58–63. https://doi.org/10.1359/jbmr.06s211.
9. Monsell EM. The mechanism of hearing loss in Paget's disease of bone. Laryngoscope. 2009;114:598–606. https://doi.org/10.1097/00005537-200404000-00002.
10. Corral-Gudino L, Tan AJH, Pino-Montes J, Ralston SH. Bisphosphonates for Paget's disease of bone in adults. Cochrane Database Syst Rev. 2017;12:CD004956. https://doi.org/10.1002/14651858.CD004956.pub3.
11. Melton LJ 3rd, Tiegs RD, Atkinson EJ, O'Fallon WM. Fracture risk among patients with Paget's disease: a population-based cohort study. J Bone Miner Res. 2000;15:2123–8. https://doi.org/10.1359/jbmr.2000.15.11.2123.
12. Gold DT, Boisture J, Ship KM, Pieper CF, Lyles KW. Paget's disease of bone and quality of life. J Bone Miner Res. 1996;11:1897–904. https://doi.org/10.1002/jbmr.5650111210.
13. Kaplan FS. Severe orthopaedic complications of Paget's disease. Bone. 1999;24:43S–6S. https://doi.org/10.1016/s8756-3282(99)00048-4.
14. Parvizi J, Klein GR, Sim FH. Surgical management of Paget's disease of bone. J Bone Miner Res. 2006;21(Suppl 2):P75–82. https://doi.org/10.1359/jbmr.06s214.

Pitfalls in Autoinflammatory Diseases 25

Abbreviations

AIDs	Autoinflammatory diseases
ANA	Antinuclear antibodies
bDMARDs	Biologic disease-modifying anti-rheumatic drugs
CAPS	Cryopyrin-associated periodic syndromes
CRP	C-reactive protein
CS	Corticosteroids
ESR	Erythrocyte sedimentation rate
FMF	Familial Mediterranean fever
HIDS	Hyperimmunoglobulin D syndrome
IBD	Inflammatory bowel disease
IL	Interleukin
IMs	Inflammatory markers
JIA	Juvenile idiopathic arthritis
MEFV	Mediterranean fever gene
MTX	Methotrexate
MVK	Mevalonate kinase
NGS	Next-generation sequencing
NLRP3	Nucleotide-binding domain, leucine-rich-containing family, pyrin domain-containing-3 inflammasome
PFAPA	Periodic fever, aphthous stomatitis, pharyngitis, adenitis
QoL	Quality of life
RA	Rheumatoid arthritis
RF	Rheumatoid factor
SAA	Serum amyloid A
SLE	Systemic lupus erythematosus
TCZ	Tocilizumab

E. Pelechas et al., *Pitfalls in Rheumatology*,
https://doi.org/10.1007/978-3-031-98671-0_25

TNFi	Tumour necrosis factor α inhibitors
TNFRSF1A	Tumour necrosis factor receptor superfamily member 1A
TRAPS	Tumour necrosis factor receptor-associated periodic syndrome
VUS	Variants of uncertain significance

25.1 Misdiagnosis as Autoimmune Diseases

A frequent pitfall is the misdiagnosis of AIDs as autoimmune disorders. While autoimmune diseases, such as SLE and RA, are driven by adaptive immune responses involving autoantibodies B- and T-cells, AIDs are primarily mediated by dysregulated innate immune responses. Since both types of diseases may present with systemic inflammation, fevers and elevated acute-phase reactants, distinguishing between them can be challenging, particularly when ANA or RF are tested before considering the possibility of an autoinflammatory disorder.

How to Avoid This Pitfall Clinicians should consider AIDs in patients with recurrent fevers, systemic inflammation and the absence of autoantibodies or T-cell-mediated features. Important clinical clues include [1]: (a) *episodic fevers*: fevers occurring in a cyclical periodic manner without evidence of infection; (b) *non-specific inflammatory symptoms*: such as rash, serositis (pleuritis or pericarditis) or arthritis, which may come and go spontaneously; (c) *absence of typical autoimmune markers*: negative ANA or RF can point towards an autoinflammatory process, particularly in patients with recurrent symptoms and elevated IMs such as CRP or ESR. In Table 25.1, the most prevalent autoinflammatory diseases along with their clinical features and treatment are presented.

Table 25.1 Summary of the most prevalent autoinflammatory diseases

Autoinflammatory disease	Clinical features	Genetic basis	Treatment
FMF	Recurrent fevers, abdominal pain, arthritis, erysipelas-like skin lesions	MEFV gene mutation (pyrin protein)	Colchicine as first-line treatment. IL-1 inhibitors such as anakinra and canakinumab, and IL-6 inhibitors for colchicine-resistant cases
CAPS and Muckle–Wells syndrome (a type of CAPS)	Fever, urticaria-like rash, joint pain, sensorineural hearing loss, amyloidosis	NLRP3 gene mutation (cryopyrin protein)	IL-1 inhibitors and CS for acute symptoms
TRAPS	Recurrent fevers, rash, periorbital oedema, abdominal pain, myalgia	TNFRSF1A gene mutation (TNF receptor)	IL-1 inhibitors, TNF inhibitors, CS for symptom control

(continued)

Table 25.1 (continued)

Autoinflammatory disease	Clinical features	Genetic basis	Treatment
HIDS	Fever, lymphadenopathy, abdominal pain, diarrhoea, rash, arthralgia	MVK gene mutation (mevalonate kinase)	IL-1 inhibitors, CS for acute episodes and supportive care for symptom relief
PFAPA	Recurrent fevers, aphthous ulcers, sore throat, cervical lymphadenopathy	Idiopathic	CS, sometimes tonsillectomy in refractory cases may help resolve the symptoms

Genetic testing for mutations in genes such as MEFV for FMF, NLRP3 for CAPS, MVK for HIDS and TNFRSF1A for TRAPS should be considered when clinical suspicion is high, as this can definitively establish the diagnosis [2–4].

25.2 Overlooking Genetic Testing

Many AIDs are caused by specific gene mutations that affect the innate immune system. However, the importance of genetic testing is sometimes overlooked, leading to delayed or missed diagnoses. This is especially problematic in paediatric patients who present with symptoms early in life, as timely diagnosis is crucial for preventing long-term complications such as amyloidosis.

How to Avoid This Pitfall Clinicians should have a low threshold for ordering genetic testing in patients with recurrent fevers and systemic inflammation of unknown aetiology. Key points include: (a) *early testing in childhood-onset disease*: many autoinflammatory diseases present in childhood and early genetic testing can lead to prompt diagnosis and treatment [5]; (b) *broad genetic panels*: for patients with non-specific symptoms or where the clinical picture does now match a single syndrome, NGS panels for AIDs can help identify less common mutations [6]; (c) *interpretation of VUS*: in cases where a VUS is identified, collaboration with geneticists and immunologists is important for interpreting these findings in the clinical context.

25.3 Failure to Recognise Atypical Presentations

AIDs can present with a broad and sometimes atypical spectrum of symptoms, making diagnosis difficult. Symptoms such as unexplained fevers, arthritis and abdominal pain can be mistaken for more common conditions like infections, IBD or JIA. Additionally, some patients may not have all the "classic" features of a specific AID, leading to diagnostic uncertainty.

How to Avoid This Pitfall Clinicians should consider the possibility of an AID when evaluating patients with unexplained, recurrent systemic inflammation, especially when there are periodic symptoms. A careful history of: (a) *fever patterns*: the timing and regularity of fever episodes can be diagnostic. For example, FMF typically presents with fevers lasting 1–3 days [7]; (b) *family history*: many AIDs are inherited in an autosomal recessive or autosomal dominant pattern, so family history of similar symptoms should raise suspicion; (c) *unusual organ involvement*: chronic serositis, peritonitis or amyloidosis in a young patient may suggest an underlying AID [8].

Collaboration with specialists familiar with AIDs, such as immunologists or rheumatologists, is essential when evaluating patients with atypical presentations.

25.4 Inappropriate Use of Immunosuppressive Drugs

Given the inflammatory nature of AIDs, patients are often mistakenly treated with broad immunosuppressive drugs such as CS, MTX or even bDMARDs such as TNFi. While these drugs may control symptoms in some cases, they are often not the most effective treatment for AIDs and may lead to complications such as infections. Moreover, inappropriate use of these therapies can delay more targeted treatments, such as IL-1 or IL-6 inhibitors.

How to Avoid This Pitfall The treatment of AIDs should focus on targeted therapies that address the underlying molecular defect: (a) *IL-1 inhibitors*: medications like anakinra and canakinumab are effective in many AIDs, including CAPS and FMF, as they target the overproduction of IL-1, a key cytokine in many autoinflammatory pathways [9]; (b) *IL-6 inhibitors*: for conditions such as systemic JIA or Still's disease, TCZ may be effective; (c) *CS*: while sometimes necessary for acute symptom control, CS should be minimised due to long-term side effects and their failure to prevent complications like amyloidosis.

For patients requiring immunomodulatory therapy, the treatment should be individualised based on the specific genetic defect and molecular pathway involved. Consultation with an immunologist or rheumatologist is advised to guide therapy [10].

25.5 Delayed Treatment of Amyloidosis

Amyloidosis, particularly AA amyloidosis, is a severe complication of several AIDs, including FMF, TRAPS and CAPS. In patients with long-standing uncontrolled inflammation, the continuous overproduction of SAA protein can lead to the deposition of amyloid in various organs, particularly the kidneys. Unfortunately, once amyloidosis develops, it is often irreversible, making prevention through early treatment critical.

How to Avoid This Pitfall Early and aggressive control of inflammation is key to preventing amyloidosis in patients with AIDs. Strategies include: (a) *regular monitoring of SAA levels*: in patients with autoinflammatory diseases, SAA levels should be monitored regularly. Persistently elevated levels, even in the absence of clinical symptoms, indicate ongoing subclinical inflammation that requires treatment [11]; (b) *use of colchicine*: in FMF, colchicine has been shown to prevent amyloidosis and should be started as soon as the diagnosis is confirmed; (c) *switching to bDMARD therapy if needed*: for patients who do not respond adequately to first-line treatments, bDMARDs such as IL-1 inhibitors should be initiated early to control inflammation and prevent amyloidosis [12].

25.6 Inadequate Recognition of Environmental and Lifestyle Triggers

Certain environmental and lifestyle factors, such as stress, infections and physical exertion, can exacerbate autoinflammatory symptoms. Failure to recognise and manage these triggers may lead to more frequent or severe flare-ups. For example, patients with FMF may experience attacks triggered by cold exposure, and physical trauma can exacerbate symptoms in patients with TRAPS.

How to Avoid This Pitfall Educating patients about potential triggers is crucial in minimising flare-ups. Clinicians should discuss: (a) *trigger avoidance*: patients should be made aware of known triggers such as infection, cold exposure or stress and take steps to minimise them [13]; (b) *lifestyle modifications*: regular, moderate physical activity, stress management techniques and prompt treatment of infections can reduce the frequency of disease flares; (c) *infection prevention*: immunisation and appropriate prophylactic measures, such as vaccinations against pneumococcus or meningococcus, are important, particularly in patients on bDMARD therapies that may increase the risk of infections [14].

25.7 Conclusion

AIDs are rare and often under-recognised conditions that present significant challenges in diagnosis and management. By recognising common pitfalls, such as misdiagnosis as AIDs, failure to perform genetic testing, inappropriate treatment with broad immunosuppressives and delayed prevention and management of amyloidosis, clinicians can significantly improve outcomes for patients with these conditions. A multidisciplinary approach involving immunologists, rheumatologists and geneticists is essential for the accurate diagnosis and management of AIDs. Through early identifications, targeted therapy and patient education, it is possible to reduce complications and improve the QoL for individuals living with AIDs.

References

1. Krainer J, Siebenhandl S, Weinhäusel A. Systemic autoinflammatory diseases. J Autoimmun. 2020;109:102421. https://doi.org/10.1016/j.jaut.2020.102421.
2. Tezcan ME, Avci M, Mercan R, Aliustaoglu M, Sargin M. MEFV gene testing may guide physicians for early diagnosis of familial Mediterranean fever. Int J Rheum Dis. 2018;21:1452–7. https://doi.org/10.1111/1756-185X.13258.
3. Moltrasio C, Romagnuolo M, Marzano AV. NLRP3 inflammasome and NLRP3-related autoinflammatory diseases: from cryopyrin function to targeted therapies. Front Immunol. 2022;13:1007705. https://doi.org/10.3389/fimmu.2022.1007705.
4. Aksentijevich I, Galon J, Soares M, Mansfield E, Hull K, Oh HH, et al. The tumor-necrosis-factor receptor-associated periodic syndrome: new mutations in TNFRSF1A, ancestral origins, genotype-phenotype studies, and evidence for further genetic heterogeneity of periodic fevers. Am J Hum Genet. 2001;69:301–14. https://doi.org/10.1086/321976.
5. Yildiz M, Haslak F, Adrovic A, Barut K, Kasapçopur. Autoinflammatory diseases in childhood. Balkan Med J. 2020;37(5):236–46. https://doi.org/10.4274/balkanmedj.galenos.2020.2020.4.82.
6. Schnappauf O, Aksentijevich I. Current and future advances in genetic testing in systemic autoinflammatory diseases. Rheumatology (Oxford). 2019;58:vi44–55. https://doi.org/10.1093/rheumatology/kez294.
7. Marino A, Tirelli F, Giani T, Cimaz R. Periodic fever syndromes and the autoinflammatory diseases (AIDs). J Transl Autoimmun. 2019;3:100031. https://doi.org/10.1016/j.jtauto.2019.100031.
8. Georgin-Lavialle S, Ducharme-Benard S, Sarrabay G, Savey L, Grateau G, Hentgen V. Systemic autoinflammatory diseases: clinical state of the art. Best Pract Res Clin Rheumatol. 2020;34:101529. https://doi.org/10.1016/j.berh.2020.101529.
9. Jesus AA, Goldbach-Mansky R. IL-1 blockade in autoinflammatory syndromes. Annu Rev Med. 2014;65:223–44. https://doi.org/10.1146/annurev-med-061512-150641.
10. Ter Haar NM, Oswald M, Jeyaratnam J, Anton J, Barron KS, Brogan PA, et al. Recommendations for the management of autoinflammatory diseases. Ann Rheum Dis. 2015;74:1636–44. https://doi.org/10.1136/annrheumdis-2015-207546.
11. Hosman IS, Kos I, Lamot L. Serum Amyloid A in inflammatory rheumatic diseases: a compendious review of a renowned biomarker. Front Immunol. 2021;11:631299. https://doi.org/10.3389/fimmu.2020.631299.
12. Ozen S, Demirkaya E, Erer B, Livneh A, Ben-Chetrit E, Giancane G, et al. EULAR recommendations for the management of familial Mediterranean fever. Ann Rheum Dis. 2016;75:644–51. https://doi.org/10.1136/annrheumdis-2015-208690.
13. Parlar K, Ates MB, Onal ME, Bostanci E, Azman FN, Ugurly S. Factors triggering familial Mediterranean fever attacks, do they really exist? Intern Emerg Med. 2024;19:1007–13. https://doi.org/10.1007/s11739-024-03576-w.
14. Meyer-Olson D, Witte T. Immunology: prevention of infections in patients with autoimmune diseases. Nat Rev Rheumatol. 2011;7:198–200. https://doi.org/10.10138/nrrheum.2011.14.

Pitfalls in the Management of the Rheumatic Patient as a Child

26

Abbreviations

ANA	Antinuclear antibody
AZA	Azathioprine
CS	Corticosteroids
cs/b/tsDMARDs	Conventional synthetic/biologic/targeted synthetic DMARDs
DMARDs	Disease-modifying anti-rheumatic drugs
ERA	Enthesitis-related arthritis
HCQ	Hydroxychloroquine
IL	Interleukin
JDM	Juvenile dermatomyositis
JIA	Juvenile idiopathic arthritis
MMF	Mycophenolate mofetil
MRI	Magnetic resonance imaging
MSK	Musculoskeletal
MSKUS	Musculoskeletal ultrasound
MTX	Methotrexate
NSAIDs	Non-steroidal anti-inflammatory drugs
QoL	Quality of life
RA	Rheumatoid arthritis
RF	Rheumatoid factor
RMDs	Rheumatic diseases
SLE	Systemic lupus erythematosus

E. Pelechas et al., *Pitfalls in Rheumatology*,
https://doi.org/10.1007/978-3-031-98671-0_26

26.1 Misdiagnosis and Delayed Diagnosis

Paediatric RMDs, particularly in their early stages, often present with vague, non-specific symptoms such as fever, fatigue and MSK pain. These symptoms can be easily mistaken for common viral infections, growth-related pain or even psychological stress, leading to delayed or missed diagnoses [1]. Clinicians have to be vigilant also for autoinflammatory diseases (see Chap. 25) and their symptoms. In Table 26.1, a list with the types of JIA and also juvenile SLE and Kawasaki disease, along with key diagnostic features, treatment options and long-term disabilities from delayed diagnosis, are presented.

Table 26.1 Summary of some of the diseases in childhood that may lead to devastating results in delayed diagnosis

Condition	Key features	Treatment	Disabilities in delayed diagnosis
Systemic JIA (Still's disease)	Daily spiking fevers, evanescent salmon-coloured rash (Fig. 26.1), lymphadenopathy, hepato-splenomegaly, serositis	NSAIDs, CS, IL-1 inhibitors, IL-6 inhibitors	Growth retardation, joint deformities, chronic pain, amyloidosis, severe organ damage (heart, lungs, liver)
Oligoarticular JIA	Arthritis in ≤4 joints during the first 6 months (mostly knees)	NSAIDs intra-articular CS, MTX for refractory cases	Joint contractures, limb length discrepancies, chronic pain, functional limitations, vision loss (Fig. 26.2)
Polyarticular JIA (RF-negative)	Arthritis in ≥5 joints within the first 6 months, RF-negative	NSAIDs, MTX, bDMARDs	Progressive joint damage, deformities, pain, loss of mobility, vision loss
Polyarticular JIA (RF-positive)	Arthritis in ≥5 joints within the first 6 months, RF-positive	MTX, bDMARDs	Severe joint destruction, deformities, disability, systemic complications (heart, lungs)
ERA	Arthritis and enthesitis, often affecting lower limbs associated with HLA-B27	NSAIDs, physical therapy, TNF inhibitors for sacroiliitis or refractory cases	Spinal fusion, ankylosis, severe pain, functional limitations in mobility

(continued)

Table 26.1 (continued)

Condition	Key features	Treatment	Disabilities in delayed diagnosis
Undifferentiated JIA	Arthritis that does not fit into any of the aforementioned categories or fits more than one type	Depends on symptoms but typically NSAIDs, MTX, DMARDs	Progression to severe joint damage, chronic pain and disability
Juvenile SLE	Fatigue, fever, typical rash, arthritis, renal involvement, serositis, haematologic abnormalities	CS, HCQ, immunosuppressants such as AZA, MTX, MMF, bDMARDs	Renal failure, CVD, neurological impairments, multi-organ failure
Kawasaki disease	Fever for ≥5 days, conjunctivitis, rash, cervical lymphadenopathy, lip and oral mucosa lesions	IVIG, aspirin, CS or biologics in refractory cases	Coronary artery aneurysms, myocardial infarction, cardiac arrhythmias, heart failure

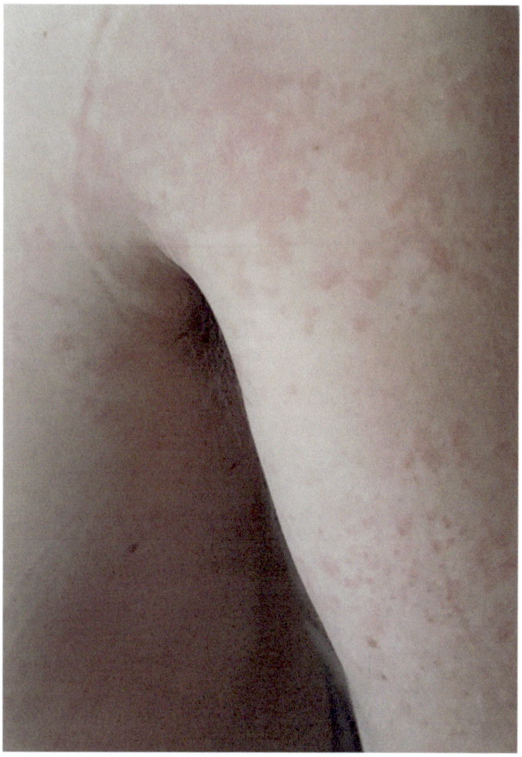

Fig. 26.1 Typical skin rash of sJIA (Still's disease). The rash is evanescent, salmon-pink, nonpruritic and maculopapular, predominantly on the extremities

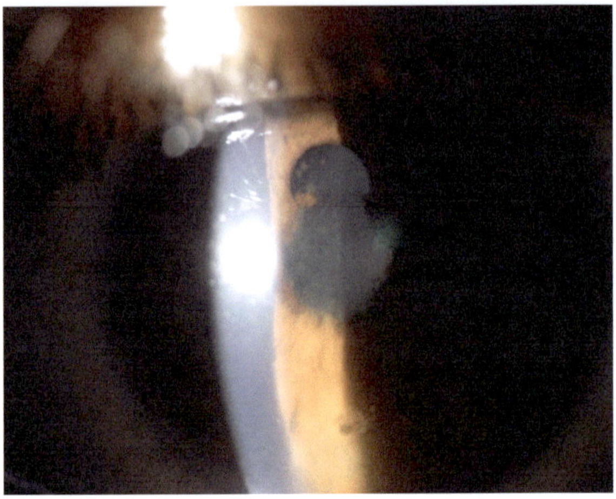

Fig. 26.2 Significant posterior synechiae in an oligoarticular JIA patient with recurrent episodes of uveitis

Consequences (a) *Delayed diagnosis*: a delay in diagnosing conditions like JIA, SLE or Kawasaki disease can result in permanent joint damage, organ involvement or severe and in some cases fatal complications like coronary artery aneurysms seen in Kawasaki disease [2]; (b) *inappropriate treatment*: misattributing symptoms to conditions such as viral infections or growing pains can lead to inappropriate treatment and progression of the underlying RMD [3].

How to Avoid This Pitfall (a) *High index of suspicion*: physicians should maintain a high index of suspicion for RMDs in children presenting with chronic or unexplained joint pain, fever or systemic symptoms lasting more than a few weeks. Special attention should be paid to patterns of pain, morning stiffness and limitations in activity; (b) *thorough evaluation*: a detailed history, including family history of autoimmune diseases, and a thorough physical examination are crucial. Persistent symptoms or symptoms not responsive to routine management should prompt further investigation, including appropriate laboratory tests (ANA and inflammatory markers) and imaging studies (MSKUS and MRI); (c) *referral to paediatric rheumatology*: early referral to a paediatric rheumatologist is essential when there is suspicion of an underlying RMD. Rheumatologists have the expertise to differentiate between various paediatric rheumatic conditions and initiate early appropriate treatment [4].

26.2 Over-Reliance on Adult Diagnostic Criteria

Paediatric RMDs do not always follow the same diagnostic criteria as their adult counterparts. Using adult criteria to diagnose or manage paediatric RMDs can lead to under-diagnosis or misclassification, especially in conditions like JIA and paediatric SLE.

Consequences (a) *Misdiagnosis*: misapplication of adult criteria can lead to under-recognition of diseases like JIA or JDM, as they often present differently in children. For example, children with JIA may not exhibit the same pattern of joint involvement as adults with RA; (b) *missed early intervention*: without early diagnosis and intervention, children with RMDs can experience long-term joint damage, growth disturbances or irreversible organ damage [5].

How to Avoid This Pitfall (a) *Paediatric-specific diagnostic criteria*: clinicians should familiarise themselves with the diagnostic criteria specific to paediatric RMDs. For example, JIA is defined by the presence of arthritis for at least 6 weeks in a child under 16 years old, and the presentation often differs from adult RA [6]; (b) *paediatric rheumatologist involvement*: collaboration with paediatric rheumatologists is critical to ensure the appropriate diagnostic approach and management of paediatric patients. Paediatric rheumatologists are trained to recognise the subtleties of disease presentation in children [7].

26.3 Failure to Recognise and Address Growth and Development Issues

Children with RMDs face unique challenges related to growth and development. Chronic inflammation, prolonged use of CS and delayed or inadequate treatment can lead to growth retardation, delayed puberty and other developmental issues.

Consequences (a) *Growth retardation*: inadequate control of chronic inflammation, particularly in diseases like JIA or SLE, can lead to impaired growth and short stature. Long-term CS use can also exacerbate growth suppression [8]; (b) *delayed puberty*: chronic illness and immunosuppressive therapy can delay the onset of puberty or may also cause infertility leading to psychological stress and impaired social development; (c) *osteoporosis*: long-term use of CS can also contribute to osteoporosis, increasing the risk of fractures in a growing child [9].

How to Avoid This Pitfall (a) *Aggressive disease control*: early and aggressive control of inflammation is critical to minimise the impact on growth and development. DMARDs of all kinds (cs, b and recently ts) should be used to control disease activity and minimise the need for long-term CS [10]; (b) *monitoring growth*: regular monitoring of growth parameters (height and weight) and puberty milestones is essential in children with RMDs. Growth should be carefully tracked, and any deviation from expected growth patterns should prompt re-evaluation of disease management; (c) *CS-sparing strategies*: minimise CS use through early initiation of DMARDs, which can control disease activity without the long-term side effects of CS. When CS are necessary, the lowest effective dose should be used for the shortest duration possible [11].

26.4 Psychosocial and Emotional Impact

Chronic RMDs can significantly impact a child's psychosocial development, self-esteem and emotional well-being. Pain, physical limitations and the stigma associated with chronic illness can lead to social isolation, anxiety and depression. These emotional aspects are often under-recognised and undertreated.

Consequences (a) *Emotional distress*: children with chronic diseases like JIA or SLE may experience emotional distress due to pain, physical limitations and social isolation. This can manifest as anxiety, depression or behavioural problems [12]; (b) *poor adherence*: emotional difficulties, particularly in adolescents, can lead to poor adherence to treatment, resulting in disease flares and worsening symptoms [13].

How to Avoid This Pitfall (a) *Holistic approach*: a holistic approach to care is needed, incorporating mental health support and addressing the child's emotional and psychological needs. Referral to a psychologist or counsellor experienced in working with chronically ill children may be necessary; (b) *support groups and social integration*: encourage participation in support groups or peer groups for children with RMDs. Social activities and integration with peers are important for a child's development and self-esteem [14]; (c) *family support*: engaging the family in the management plan and providing education on the emotional impact of chronic disease are crucial. Parents and caregivers play a key role in supporting the child's emotional and psychological well-being [15].

26.5 Challenges in Medication and Adherence

Adherence to medication regimens can be challenging in paediatric patients due to the complexity of treatment plans, the side effects of medications and the child's difficulty in understanding the importance of long-term treatment. Adolescents, in particular, may resist taking medications due to the desire for independence or fear of side effects.

Consequences (a) *Non-adherence*: poor adherence can lead to uncontrolled disease activity, increased risk of joint damage, organ involvement and overall worsening of the disease. Adolescents with SLE, for example, are at high risk of non-adherence, leading to renal flare-ups or organ damage [16]; (b) *medication side effects*: side effects of medications such as MTX, CS and in general DMARDs can cause distress and lead to non-adherence. Children may experience nausea, weight gain, mood changes or cosmetic changes that impact self-esteem and adherence.

How to Avoid This Pitfall (a) *Simplified treatment plans*: simplifying medication regimens where possible can help improve adherence. Regular communication with the child and family to discuss the importance of adherence is crucial; (b) *monitor-*

ing for side effects: regular monitoring for side effects and addressing them promptly can improve adherence. For example, providing antiemetics for nausea related to MTX or offering alternative treatments for CS side effects can help maintain compliance; (c) *age-appropriate education*: providing age-appropriate education about the disease and its treatment can empower children and adolescents to take ownership of their health. Clear, simple explanations and the use of visual aids or apps can help younger children understand their condition and treatment [7].

26.6 Impact of Chronic Disease on School and Social Activities

RMDs can interfere with a child's ability to participate in school and social activities. Chronic pain, fatigue and frequent medical appointments can lead to school absences, difficulty keeping up with academic work and limited participation in physical activities, affecting the child's academic performance and social development. They may experience social isolation as well due to physical limitations or stigma associated with their condition.

Consequences (a) *Academic difficulties*: frequent absences from school or difficulty in concentrating due to pain or fatigue can lead to academic underachievement and frustration. Children may feel left behind or isolated from their peers [17]; (b) *social isolation*: limited participation in physical activities or social events due to pain or mobility issues can lead to social isolation and difficulty forming friendships, which are critical for a child's emotional and psychological development.

How to Avoid This Pitfall (a) *Individualised education plans*: collaborating with school personnel to develop an individualised education plan or extra time for assignments, modified physical activity or tutoring support; (b) *peer support programmes*: create peer support groups that allow children to connect with others facing similar challenges [18]; (c) *school involvement*: work with schools to foster inclusive environments that accommodate the needs of children with RMDs.

26.7 Conclusion

Managing paediatric rheumatic patients involves navigating a complex landscape of diagnostics, treatment and psychosocial challenges. By recognising common pitfalls and implementing targeted strategies, healthcare providers can improve the care and outcomes for these vulnerable patients. Through education, collaboration and a commitment to holistic care, the paediatric rheumatology community can enhance the QoL for children living with chronic RMDs. Continuous improvement in practices and policies, driven by the evolving understanding of these conditions, is essential for advancing care in this field.

References

1. Woo P, Colbert RA. An overview of genetics of paediatric rheumatic diseases. Best Pract Res Clin Rheumatol. 2009;23:589–97. https://doi.org/10.1016/j.berh.2009.08.001.
2. Costello A, Rasooly I, Weiss P. Rheum fro improvement? Delayed diagnosis of juvenile idiopathic arthritis: a narrative review. Arthritis Care Res (Hoboken). 2025;77(3):283–90. https://doi.org/10.1002/acr.25438.
3. Higgins GC. Complications of treatments for pediatric rheumatic diseases. Pediatr Clin N Am. 2018;65:827–54. https://doi.org/10.1016/j.pcl.2018.04.008.
4. Martini A. Clinical approach to a child with suspected rheumatic diseases. In: Elzouki AY, Harfi HA, Nazer HM, Stapleton FB, Oh W, Whitley RJ, editors. Textbook of clinical pediatrics. Berlin, Heidelberg: Springer; 2012. https://doi.org/10.1007/978-3-642-02202-9_153.
5. Akikusa JD, Allen RC. Reducing the impact of rheumatic diseases in childhood. Best Pract Res Clin Rheumatol. 2022;16:333–45.
6. Giancane G, Consolaro A, Lanni S, Davì S, Schiappapietra B, Ravelli A. Juvenile idiopathic arthritis: diagnosis and treatment. Rheumatol Ther. 2016;3:187–207. https://doi.org/10.1007/s40744-016-0040-4.
7. McColl J, Mwizerwa O, Scott C, Tse SM, Foster HE. Pediatric rheumatology education: the virtual frontier a review. Pediatr Rheumatol Online J. 2024;22:60. https://doi.org/10.1186/s12969-024-00978-0.
8. Abdalla E, Jeyaseelan L, Ullah I, Abdwani R. Growth pattern in children with systemic lupus erythematosus. Oman Med J. 2017;32:284–90. https://doi.org/10.5001/omj.2017.56.
9. Di Marcello F, Di Donato G, d'Angelo DM, Breda L, Chiarelli F. Bone health in children with rheumatic disorders: focus on molecular mechanisms, diagnosis, and management. Int J Mol Sci. 2022;23:5725. https://doi.org/10.3390/ijms23105725.
10. Schaller JG. Aggressive treatment in childhood rheumatic diseases. Clin Exp Rheumatol. 1994;12(Suppl 10):S97–105.
11. Ravelli A, Lattanzi B, Consolaro AI, Martini A. Glucocorticoids in paediatric rheumatology. Clin Exp Rheumatol. 2011;29:S148–52.
12. Treemarcki EB, Danguecan AN, Cunningham N, Knight AM. Mental health in pediatric rheumatology: an opportunity to improve outcomes. Rheum Dis Clin N Am. 2022;48:67–90. https://doi.org/10.1016/j.rdc.2021.09.012.
13. Manatpreeprem R, Lerkvaleekul B, Vilaiyuk S. Factors associated with medication adherence among children with rheumatic diseases. Front Pharmacol. 2023;14:1149320. https://doi.org/10.3389/fphar.2023.1149320.
14. Karp N, Yazdany J, Schmajuk G. Peer support in rheumatic diseases: a narrative literature review. Patient Prefer Adherence. 2023;17:2433–49. https://doi.org/10.2147/PPA.S391396.
15. DeNardo BA, Stebulis JA, Tucker LB, Schaller JG. Parents of children with rheumatic disease as peer counsellors. Arthritis Care Res. 1995;8:120–5. https://doi.org/10.1002/art.1790080211.
16. Zigler CK, Randell RL, Reeve BB. Assessing patient-reported outcomes in pediatric rheumatic diseases: considerations and future directions. Rheum Dis Clin N Am. 2022;48:15–29. https://doi.org/10.1016/j.rdc.2021.09.008.
17. Chomistek K, Johnson N, Stevenson R, Luca N, Miettunen P, Benseler SM, et al. Patietn-reported barriers at school for children with juvenile idiopathic arthritis. ACR Open Rheumatol. 2019;1:182–7. https://doi.org/10.1002/acr2.1023.
18. Sandstrom M, Schanberg LE. Peer rejection, social behavior, and psychological adjustment in children with juvenile rheumatic disease. J Pediatr Psychol. 2004;29:29–34. https://doi.org/10.1093/jpepsy/jsh004.

Pitfalls in the Management of Elderly Rheumatic Patients

27

Abbreviations

anti-CCP	Anti-cyclic citrullinated peptide
bDMARDs	Biologic DMARDs
CPPD	Calcium pyrophosphate deposition
CRP	C-reactive protein
CS	Corticosteroids
csDMARDs	Conventional synthetic disease-modifying anti-rheumatic drugs
CVD	Cardiovascular disease
DEXA	Dual-energy X-ray absorptiometry
ESR	Erythrocyte sedimentation rate
GCA	Giant cell arteritis
GI	Gastrointestinal
HCQ	Hydroxychloroquine
HZV	Herpes zoster virus
IA	Inflammatory arthritis
IL-6i	Interleukin 6 inhibitors
LEF	Leflunomide
MRI	Magnetic resonance imaging
MSK	Musculoskeletal
MSKUS	Musculoskeletal ultrasound
MTX	Methotrexate
NSAIDs	Non-steroidal anti-inflammatory drugs
OA	Osteoarthritis
OTC	Over-the-counter
PJP	Pneumocystis jirovecii pneumonia
PMR	Polymyalgia rheumatica
PsA	Psoriatic arthritis

E. Pelechas et al., *Pitfalls in Rheumatology*,
https://doi.org/10.1007/978-3-031-98671-0_27

QoL	Quality of life
RA	Rheumatoid arthritis
RF	Rheumatoid factor
RMDs	Rheumatic diseases
SLE	Systemic lupus erythematosus
SOB	Shortness of breath
TAB	Temporal artery biopsy
TB	Tuberculosis
TNFi	Tumour necrosis factor α inhibitors

27.1 Underestimation of Disease Severity and Symptoms

Older adults often attribute their symptoms, such as joint pain, stiffness and fatigue, to aging rather than a specific disease process. Clinicians may also fall into this trap, and the incidence of many RMDs decreases with advancing age, underestimating the severity of RMD symptoms and dismissing them as "normal aging" or "arthritis" without further investigation.

Consequences (a) *Delayed diagnosis*: RMDs such as RA, PMR or GCA may be underdiagnosed or diagnosed late in elderly patients, leading to prolonged symptoms, decreased QoL and increased risk of complications [1]; (b) *progressive joint damage*: failure to identify inflammatory diseases early can lead to irreversible joint damage, particularly in diseases like RA or PsA.

How to Avoid This Pitfall (a) *Thorough evaluation*: clinicians should conduct a detailed assessment of any new MSK symptoms in older patients, rather than assuming they are age-related. Specific features like morning stiffness, joint swelling or systemic symptoms such as fever or weight loss should raise suspicion for an RMD [2]; (b) *use of diagnostic tools*: for conditions like PMR or GCA, early and appropriate diagnostic tests such as ESR, CRP and TAB or imaging (e.g. PET scan) for GCA should be ordered to confirm or rule out inflammatory conditions [3]; (c) *routine screening*: rheumatologists and primary care physicians should consider routine screening for inflammatory markers or imaging in elderly patients presenting with MSK symptoms [4].

27.2 Comorbidities Masking Rheumatic Disease

Elderly patients often have multiple comorbidities, such as CVD, diabetes or chronic lung disease, which can mask or complicate the diagnosis of RMDs. Symptoms like fatigue, malaise or SOB may be attributed to pre-existing conditions rather than to an underlying or new RMD.

Consequences (a) *Missed diagnosis*: in elderly patients, the presence of comorbidities can obscure signs of RMDs such as SLE or vasculitis, resulting in misdiagnosis or delayed treatment [5]; (b) *increased risk of complications*: comorbidities, especially CVD, may exacerbate the risks of untreated RMDs. For example, patients with RA have a higher risk of CVD events, and failure to manage inflammation adequately can increase this risk [6].

How to Avoid This Pitfall (a) *Multisystem evaluation*: physicians should maintain a broad differential diagnosis and consider the possibility that new symptoms may be related to an underlying RMD rather than attributing them solely to comorbidities; (b) *comprehensive approach*: managing elderly patients with RMDs requires a multidisciplinary approach, involving cardiologists, pulmonologists and nephrologists, especially in cases where multiple organ systems are involved; (c) *frequent monitoring*: regular follow-up and reassessment of both RMD activity and comorbid conditions can help to distinguish between disease progression and other health issues.

27.3 Over-Reliance on Corticosteroids

CS are commonly used in the management of RMDs such as PMR, RA and SLE, particularly in older patients. However, elderly patients are particularly susceptible to the side effects of long-term CS use, including osteoporosis and bone fractures (Fig. 27.1), hyperglycaemia, hypertensions, cataracts and increased infection risk.

Consequences (a) *Serious adverse effects*: prolonged use of CS in elderly patients can lead to debilitating side effects such as fractures due to osteoporosis, uncontrolled diabetes and increased susceptibility to infections; (b) *dependency on CS*: some elderly patients may become dependent on CS for symptom control, resulting in chronic use even when alternative therapies are available [7], or even after prolonged disease remission.

How to Avoid This Pitfall (a) *CS-sparing agents*: where possible, clinicians should prioritise CS-sparing agents, such as csDMARDs (MTX, LEF and HCQ) or bDMARDs (TNFi and IL-6i), to reduce or eliminate the need for long-term CS use; (b) *minimising CS use*: use the lowest effective dose of CS for the shortest duration possible. Gradual tapering should begin as soon as disease control is achieved, with close monitoring flares [8]; (c) *bone health management*: proactively manage the risk of osteoporosis in elderly patients on CS by prescribing calcium, vitamin D and bisphosphonates, and regularly assess bone density through DEXA scans [9]; (d) *patient education*: adequately inform patients about the multiple and potentially serious side effects with long-term CS use.

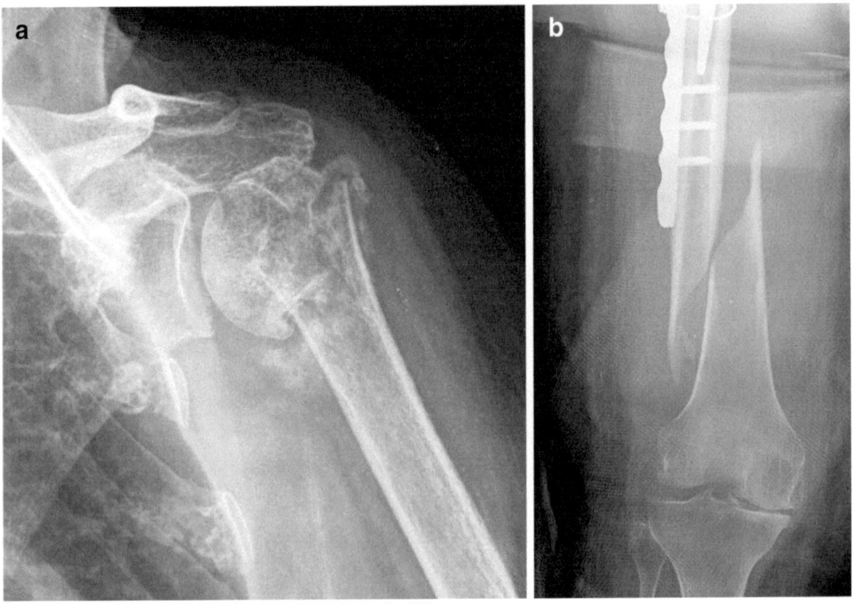

Fig. 27.1 (**a**) proximal humerus fracture in an OA patient under long-standing treatment with CS; (**b**) spiral fracture of the femoral bone in an OA patient. Note the joint space narrowing of the medial condyle and also a previous total hip arthroplasty due to hip OA

27.4 Polypharmacy and Drug Interactions

Elderly patients often take multiple medications to manage comorbidities, which increases the risk of polypharmacy and drug interactions. Common rheumatology drugs, such as NSAIDs, CS, MTX and bDMARDs, can interact with medications for hypertension, diabetes and CVD.

Consequences (a) *Adverse drug reactions*: polypharmacy increases the risk of drug toxicity, adverse effects and interactions. For example, NSAIDs can exacerbate hypertension, cause renal impairment or lead to GI bleeding, while MTX may interact with other medicines that are metabolised in the liver as well as other hepatotoxic drugs; (b) *non-adherence*: complex medication regimens can be overwhelming for elderly patients, leading to non-adherence, which may result in poorly controlled disease and adverse outcomes; (c) *polypharmacy*: due to polypharmacy and several comorbidities, there are fewer options available for disease management.

How to Avoid This Pitfall (a) *Regular medication review*: conduct regular reviews of all medications, including OTC drugs and supplements, to identify potential interactions and eliminate unnecessary drugs; (b) *simplifying treatment regimens*: simplify medication regimens where possible by reducing the number of pills or doses per day, switching to combination therapies or adjusting drug schedules to improve adherence; (c) *monitoring for interactions*: be vigilant about potential drug interactions, particularly between NSAIDs and antihypertensives, or MTX and other hepatotoxic agents. Collaborate with pharmacists and use drug interaction databases when adjusting therapy [10].

27.5 Infection Risk Due to Immunosuppressive Therapy

Elderly patients, especially those on immunosuppressive therapies such as CS, csDMARDs and bDMARDs, are at increased risk for infections. Age-related immune system decline compounds this risk, making elderly patients more vulnerable to both common and opportunistic infections. The term used for the age-related immune system decline is immunosenescence.

Consequences (a) *Serious infections*: immunosuppression can lead to severe infections, including pneumonia, sepsis and reactivation of latent infections like TB or HZV. Elderly patients are less likely to mount a robust immune response, making infections more difficult to detect and treat; (b) *hospitalisations*: infections in elderly patients on immunosuppressive therapy often require hospitalisation, leading to increased morbidity and mortality.

How to Avoid This Pitfall (a) *Infection prevention*: before initiating immunosuppressive therapy, screen for latent infection and ensure that the patient is up-to-date on vaccinations. Administer pneumococcal, influenza and HZV vaccines as appropriate, but avoid live vaccines in immunosuppressed patients; (b) *close monitoring*: monitor elderly patients on immunosuppressive therapy for early signs of infections, such as fever or respiratory symptoms. Infections in older adults may present subtly, so a high level of vigilance is required; (c) *prophylactic measures*: in certain high-risk patients, consider antimicrobial prophylaxis to prevent opportunistic infections, such as PJP [11].

27.6 Cognitive Impairment and Communication Challenges

Cognitive decline is common in elderly patients and can interfere with their ability to accurately report symptoms, follow treatment plans or adhere to complex medication regimens. In some cases, pain or discomfort may be under-reported or miscommunicated due to cognitive impairment or sensory deficits.

Consequences (a) *Inaccurate symptom reporting*: cognitive impairment can lead to under-reporting or misinterpretation of symptoms, resulting in diagnostic delays or inappropriate treatment adjustments; (b) *non-adherence to treatment*: elderly patients with cognitive decline may struggle to adhere to medication regimens or follow instructions for disease management, leading to poorly controlled disease.

How to Avoid This Pitfall (a) *Involvement of caregivers*: in patients with cognitive impairment, involving family members or caregivers in the management plan is crucial for ensuring adherence and accurate symptom reporting; (b) *simplified communication*: use clear, simple language and written instructions to improve understanding. For patients with hearing or vision loss, ensure that communication is tailored to their needs, such as providing large-print materials or using assistive hearing devices; (c) *assessing cognitive function*: regularly assess cognitive function in elderly patients, especially if there is a sudden change in disease control or adherence patterns. Cognitive screening tools can help identify patients who may need additional support [12].

27.7 Difficulty in Differentiating Between Osteoarthritis and Inflammatory Arthritis

OA is extremely common in elderly patients and can coexist with or be mistaken for IA conditions such as RA or crystal-induced arthritis (gout and CPPD). Differentiating between these conditions is often challenging, particularly in the presence of joint deformities or long-standing joint damage.

Consequences (a) *Missed diagnosis of inflammatory arthritis*: failure to distinguish IA from OA can result in untreated inflammation, joint damage and progression of diseases such as RA or PsA; (b) *overtreatment of OA*: conversely, misdiagnosing OA as an IA may lead to inappropriate use of DMARDs, exposing patients to unnecessary risks without benefits.

How to Avoid This Pitfall (a) *Careful assessment of joint symptoms*: IA typically presents with signs of inflammation such as joint swelling, warmth and morning stiffness lasting >30 min, while OA tends to cause pain that worsens with activity and improves with rest [13]; (b) *use of imaging and laboratory testing*: imaging studies, including MSKUS or MRI, can help identify synovitis or joint effusions indicative of IA. Laboratory markers such as ESR, CRP and serologic tests such as RF and anti-CCP can also aid in distinguishing inflammatory from non-inflammatory arthritis; (c) *tailored treatment*: treatment should be guided by the underlying diagnosis. For OA, focus on non-pharmacologic treatments, such as physical therapy and weight loss, and pain management, while IA requires DMARD treatments [14].

27.8 Conclusion

The management of RMDs in elderly patients is fraught with unique challenges and pitfalls, including underestimation of disease severity, comorbidities masking symptoms, over-reliance on CS and the complexities of polypharmacy and immunosuppression. A tailored approach that considers the unique needs of older adults, along with vigilant monitoring and proactive management of complications, can help to optimise outcomes and improve the QoL for elderly living with RMDs.

References

1. Raciborski F, Kłak A, Kwiatkowska B, Batko B, Sochocka-Bykowska M, Zoń-Giebel A, et al. Diagnostic delays in rheumatic diseases with associated arthritis. Rheumatologia. 2017;55:169–76. https://doi.org/10.5114/reum.2017.69777.
2. Pavlov-Dolijanovic S, Bogojevic M, Nozica-Radulovic T, Radunovic G, Mujovic N. Elderly-onset rheumatoid arthritis: characteristics and treatment options. Medicina (Kaunas). 2023;59:1878. https://doi.org/10.3390/medicina59101878.
3. Kaltsonoudis E, Pelechas E, Papoudou-Bai A, Markatseli TE, Elisaf M, Voulgari PV, et al. The impact of temporal artery biopsy for the diagnosis of giant cell arteritis in clinical practice in a tertiary university hospital. PLoS One. 2019;14:e0210845. https://doi.org/10.1371/journal.pone.0210845.
4. Singh T, Newman AB. Inflammatory markers in population studies of aging. Ageing Res Rev. 2010;10:319–29. https://doi.org/10.1016/j.arr.2010.11.002.
5. Stiebitz S, von Streng T, Strickler M. Delayed diagnosis of rheumatoid arthritis in an elderly patient presenting with weakness and desolation. BMJ Case Rep. 2021;14:e237251. https://doi.org/10.1136/bcr-2020-237251.
6. Takanashi S, Kaneko Y, Takeuchi T. Elderly patients with comorbidities in the definition of difficult-to-treat rheumatoid arthritis. Ann Rheum Dis. 2021;80:1491–3. https://doi.org/10.1136/annrheumdis-2021-220315.
7. Thomas TP. The complications of systemic corticosteroid therapy in the elderly. A retrospective study. Gerontology. 1984;30:60–5. https://doi.org/10.1159/000212608.
8. Vinicki JP, Cusa A, Domingo D, Zamora JLV, Magri S, Brigante A, et al. Effectiveness of methotrexate and leflunomide as corticoid-sparing drugs in patients with polymyalgia rheumatica. Rheumatol Adv Pract. 2024;8:rkae033.
9. Lahaye C, Tatar Z, Dubost JJ, Tournadre A, Soubrier M. Management of inflammatory rheumatic conditions in the elderly. Rheumatology (Oxford). 2018;58:748–64. https://doi.org/10.1093/rheumatology/key165.
10. Lozano-Lozano R, Vega-Morales D, Sifuentes-Martinez MR, Ornelas-Balcazar D. Prevalence of polypharmacy and drug interaction in older adults with rheumatic disease. Reumatol Clin (Engl Ed). 2024;20:249–53.
11. Kiltz U, Celik A, Tsiami S, Buehring B, Baraliakos X, Andreica I, et al. Are patients with rheumatic diseass on immunosuppressive therapies protected against preventable infections? A cross-sectional cohort study. RMD Open. 2021;7:e001499. https://doi.org/10.1136/rmdopen-2020-001499.
12. Sood A, Raji MA. Cognitive impairment in elderly patients with rheumatic disease and the effect of disease-modifying anti-rheumatic drugs. Clin Rheumatol. 2021;40:1221–31. https://doi.org/10.1007/s10067-020-05372-1.
13. Marino C, McDonald E. Osteoarthritis and rheumatoid arthritis in elderly patients. Differentiation and treatment. Postgrad Med. 1991;90:237–43. https://doi.org/10.1080/00325481.1991.11701087.
14. Pelechas E, Kaltsonoudis E, Voulgari PV, Drosos AA. Osteoarthritis. In: Illustrated handbook of rheumatic and musculo-skeletal diseases. Cham: Springer; 2023. https://doi.org/10.1007/978-3-031-47379-1_14.

Pitfalls in Raynaud's Phenomenon

28

Abbreviations

ACA	Anti-centromere antibodies
ANA	Antinuclear antibodies
CTD	Connective tissue disease
dsSScl	Diffuse cutaneous systemic sclerosis
ILD	Interstitial lung disease
lcSScl	Limited cutaneous systemic sclerosis
MCTD	Mixed connective tissue disease
MMF	Mycophenolate mofetil
MTX	Methotrexate
NVC	Nailfold videocapillaroscopy
PAH	Pulmonary arterial hypertension
PDE-5	Phosphodiesterase-5
PFTs	Pulmonary function tests
PM	Polymyositis
pRP	Primary RP
RMDs	Rheumatic diseases
RP	Raynaud's phenomenon
RTX	Rituximab
SLE	Systemic lupus erythematosus
sRP	Secondary RP
SScl	Systemic sclerosis

E. Pelechas et al., *Pitfalls in Rheumatology*,
https://doi.org/10.1007/978-3-031-98671-0_28

28.1 Understanding RP: Primary vs. Secondary

The distinction between pRP and sRP is crucial, as sRP can herald the onset of severe systemic disease. Misdiagnosis or delayed recognition of sRP can result in missed opportunities for early intervention and management of the underlying disease. RP can be classified into two major categories:

pRP Occurs in the absence of any underlying systemic disease. It is always benign, with no progression to tissue damage or systemic illness.

sRP Occurs in association with an underlying autoimmune or CTD, such as SScl, SLE or MCTD. sRP is more severe and carries a risk of complications, including digital ulcers, tissue ischaemia and gangrene that can lead to amputation of the affected anatomic structure [1]. Clinically, it is impossible to make the distinction between these two forms (Fig. 28.1).

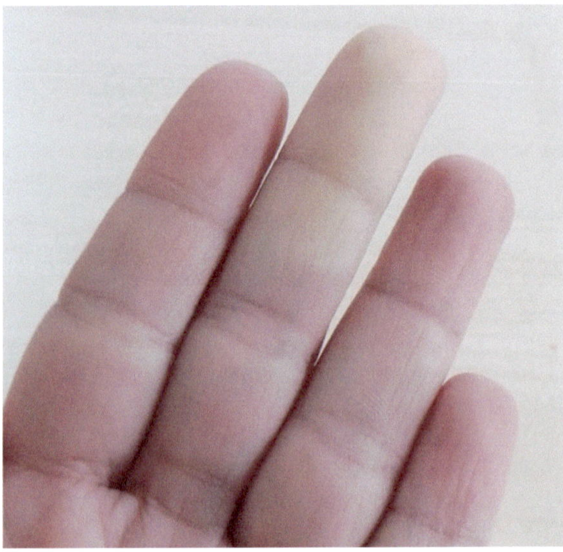

Fig. 28.1 Raynaud's phaenomenon. The third finger is mostly affected

28.2 Failure to Differentiate Between Primary and Secondary RP

The most critical pitfall in the management of RP is the failure to differentiate between primary and secondary forms. pRP is relatively benign and can be managed conservatively, while sRP requires closer monitoring and aggressive management due to its association with serious RMDs.

Overlooking Red Flags for sRP (a) *onset after 30*: pRP typically begins in adolescence or early adulthood, while sRP often starts later in life; (b) *asymmetric involvement*: pRP generally affects both hands or feet symmetrically, while sRP may present with asymmetry; (c) *severe attacks with ulcerations or gangrene*: sRP can lead to significant tissue ischaemia, resulting in digital ulcers, pitting scars, gangrene or even vasculitis in cases of MCTD or SLE. These complications are rare in pRP; (d) *associated systemic symptoms*: joint pain, muscle weakness, rashes or other signs of systemic involvement should raise concern for an underlying autoimmune disease.

When these features are present, clinicians should suspect sRP and pursue further evaluation, including laboratory testing and imaging.

Failure to Use NVC (a) *NVC*: is an essential, non-invasive tool for distinguishing pRP from sRP. Capillary changes at the nailfolds, such as enlarged or giant capillaries (Fig. 28.2), capillary dropout and haemorrhages, are commonly seen in sRP, particularly in SScl. In contrast, the capillaries appear normal in pRP [2].

Failure to perform NVC, especially in patients with new-onset RP or those with suspected CTD, can result in missed diagnoses of underlying systemic conditions.

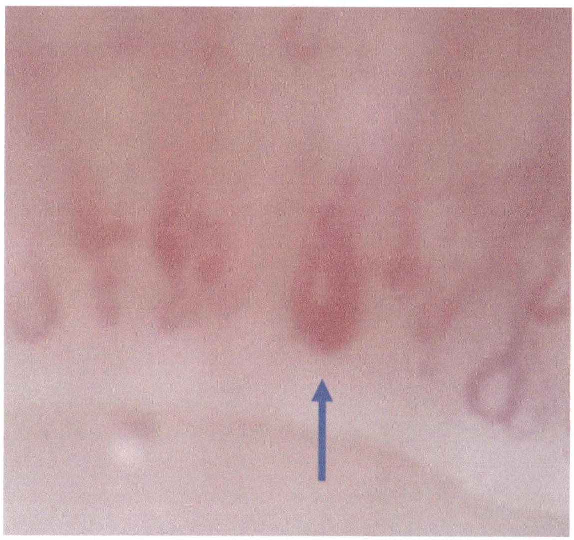

Fig. 28.2 Giant capillary in secondary Raynaud's phaenomenon >50 μm

28.3 Misdiagnosing RP in the Presence of Other RMDs

RP frequently overlaps with other autoimmune or CTDs, making it easy to misdiagnose or overlook in the context of more prominent systemic features. This pitfall is particularly relevant in diseases like SScl, SLE and MCTD.

SScl RP is often the first symptom of SScl, sometimes appearing years before other clinical manifestations. The initial subtlety of RP can lead to under-recognition, delaying the diagnosis of SScl. In dcSScl, RP is almost always present and may progress rapidly to digital ulcers, ischaemia and tissue damage if not managed appropriately. Clinicians may focus on skin thickening or internal organ involvement in SScl and overlook RP as a key early symptom, particularly in patients with more limited cutaneous involvement (such as in lcSScl) [3].

SLE RP can occur in up to 30% of patients with SLE, but it may be overshadowed by other lupus symptoms, such as arthritis, malar rash or nephritis. In such cases, RP may be mistakenly attributed to lupus vasculitis or another circulatory disorder rather than being recognised as a distinct manifestation of autoimmune disease. In SLE, the severity of RP is variable, but clinicians must be vigilant for signs of severe ischaemia or digital ulcers, which could signal a more aggressive disease course [4].

MCTD MCTD is characterised by overlapping features of SScl, SLE and PM, and RP is a near-universal feature of MCTD. However, the wide spectrum of clinical manifestations in MCTD can make RP an underappreciated aspect of the disease, leading to delayed recognition of the full clinical picture. Failure to connect RP with other autoimmune symptoms in patients with MCTD may delay diagnosis and result in suboptimal management [5].

28.4 Inadequate Evaluation of Associated Autoantibodies and Systemic Involvement

Another key pitfall is the inadequate evaluation of autoantibodies in patients presenting with RP, which can aid in distinguishing pRP from sRP and identifying the underlying RMD. A thorough assessment of systemic involvement is also essential to guide treatment and prevent complications.

Autoantibody Testing Autoantibody testing, including ANA, ACA, anti-Scl-70 (topoisomerase I) and anti-RNP antibodies, is critical in evaluating patients with RP. Positive autoantibodies, particularly at high titres, are suggestive of sRP associated with systemic autoimmune disease.

For example: (a) *ACA* are associated with lcSScl and a milder disease course but with an increased risk of PAH; (b) *anti-Scl-70 antibodies*: are linked to dcSScl and more aggressive internal organ involvement, especially ILD; (c) *anti-RNP antibodies*: are characteristic of MCTD and can help distinguish it from other CTDs.

Neglecting to asses autoantibodies in patients with RP can lead to missed diagnoses of systemic autoimmune conditions, particularly in those with subtle or early-stage disease [6].

Evaluating for Systemic Involvement sRP is often associated with systemic involvement, including pulmonary, renal and gastrointestinal complications. Failure to screen for internal organ involvement in patients with sRP is a common pitfall, especially in SScl, where lung involvement such as ILD or PAH can be life-threatening.

Routine evaluation should include PFTs and echocardiograms to assess for ILD and PAH, particularly in patients with SScl or positive autoantibodies indicative of high-risk disease [7, 8].

28.5 Inadequate Management of RP

The management of RP, particularly in the context of secondary forms, is challenging and requires a multifaceted approach. Inadequate treatment of RP can result in preventable complications, such as digital ulcers, ischaemic tissue damage and gangrene.

Suboptimal Pharmacologic Management While lifestyle modifications such as avoiding cold exposure or smoking cessation are the cornerstone of managing pRP, pharmacologic treatment is often necessary for sRP, especially in severe cases with digital ulcers or tissue ischaemia. Commonly used pharmacologic agents include [9]: (a) *calcium channel blockers*: drugs such as nifedipine and amlodipine are first-line therapy for RP, but they may be insufficient in patients with severe secondary disease. In such cases, other vasodilatory agents, such as PDE-5 inhibitors, prostaglandins or endothelin receptor antagonists, may be needed; (b) *immunosuppressive therapy*: in patients with underlying RMD, particularly SScl and SLE, immunosuppressive agents (MMF, MTX and RTX) may be required to control the underlying disease and prevent progression of RP [10].

Failure to escalate treatment in patients with severe or refractory RP, especially in those with secondary forms, can result in significant morbidity.

Under-Recognition of the Risk of Digital Ulcers Patients with sRP, particularly those with SScl, are at risk of developing digital ulcers and ischaemic complications. Digital ulcers can be painful and slow to heal, often requiring specialised wound care and aggressive pharmacologic treatment. In some cases, surgical intervention may be necessary [11].

Clinicians must remain vigilant for signs of ulceration or gangrene, particularly in patients with severe RP attacks or extensive underlying disease. A proactive approach, involving early referral to vascular specialists or rheumatologists, can prevent irreversible tissue damage.

28.6 Conclusion

RP is a common manifestation of RMDs, but its diagnosis and management are fraught with pitfalls. The failure to differentiate pRP from sRP, misdiagnosis in the presence of overlapping autoimmune diseases and inadequate evaluation of associated autoantibodies or systemic involvement can all delay appropriate treatment and worsen outcomes. Clinicians must remain vigilant for red flags suggesting sRP, utilise tools like NVC and tailor management strategies to address both vasospasm and underlying RMDs. By recognising and addressing these common pitfalls, clinicians can improve the timely diagnosis and management of RP in the context of autoimmune diseases and CTDs.

References

1. Pelechas E, Kaltsonoudis E, Voulgari PV, Drosos AA. Scleroderma. In: Illustrated handbook of rheumatic and musculo-skeletal diseases. Cham: Springer; 2023. https://doi.org/10.1007/978-3-031-47379-1_11.
2. Mannarino E, Pasqualini L, Fedeli F, Scricciolo V, Innocente S. Nailfold capillaroscopy in the screening and diagnosis of Raynaud's phenomenon. Angiology. 1994;45:37–42. https://doi.org/10.1177/000331979404500105.
3. Fernández-Codina A, Cañas-Ruano E, Pope J. Management of Raynaud's phenomenon in systemic sclerosis – a practical approach. J Scleroderma Relat Disord. 2019;4:102–10. https://doi.org/10.1177/2397198318823951.
4. Heimovski FE, Simioni J, Skare TL. Systemic lupus erythematosus and raynaud's phenomenon. An Bras Dermatol. 2015;90:837–40. https://doi.org/10.1590/abd1806-4841.20153881.
5. Grader-Beck T, Wigley FM. Raynaud's phenomenon in mixed connective tissue disease. Rheum Dis Clin N Am. 2005;31:465–81. https://doi.org/10.1016/j.rdc.2005.04.006.
6. Kallenberg CG, Pastoor GW, Wouda AA, The TH. Antinuclear antibodies in patients with Raynaud's phenomenon: clinical significance of anticetromere antibodies. Ann Rheum Dis. 1982;41:382–7. https://doi.org/10.1136/ard.41.4.382.
7. Chaisson NF, Hassoun PM. Systemic sclerosis-assciated pulmonary arterial hypertension. Chest. 2013;144:1346–56. https://doi.org/10.1378/chest.12-2396.
8. Sambataro D, Sambataro G, Pignataro F, Zanframundo G, Codullo V, Fagone E, et al. Patients with interstitial lung disease seconday to autoimmune diseases: how to recognize them? Diagnostics (Basel). 2020;10:208. https://doi.org/10.3390/diagnostics10040208.
9. Daniels J, Pauling JD, Eccleston C. Behaviour change interventions for the management of Raynaud's phenomenon: a systematic literature review. BMJ Open. 2018;8:e024528. https://doi.org/10.1136/bmjopen-2018-024528.
10. Khouri C, Lepelley M, Bailly S, Blaise S, Herrick AL, Matucci-Cerinic M, et al. Comparative efficacy and safety of treatments for secondary Raynaud's phenomenon: a systematic review and network meta-analysis of randomised trials. Lancet Rheumatol. 2019;1:e237–46. https://doi.org/10.1016/S2665-9913(19)30079-7.
11. Herrick AL. Raynaud's phenomenon and digital ulcers: advances in evaluation and management. Curr Opin Rheumatol. 2021;33:453–62. https://doi.org/10.1097/BOR.0000000000000826.

Pitfalls in Interpreting Nailfold Capillaroscopy in Rheumatic Diseases

29

Abbreviations

DM	Dermatomyositis
ILD	Interstitial lung disease
MCTD	Mixed connective tissue disease
NVC	Nailfold videocapillaroscopy
pRP	Primary Raynaud's phenomenon
RMDs	Rheumatic diseases
SLE	Systemic lupus erythematosus
sRP	Secondary RP
SScl	Systemic sclerosis

29.1 Failure to Recognise Normal Variations

Not all capillary abnormalities seen on NVC are pathologic. Normal variations in capillary morphology can occur in healthy individuals, leading to potential over-interpretation of findings.

Physiological Variability Capillary density, size and shape can vary depending on several factors, such as age, skin tone or external influences like cold exposure. Some individuals, particularly older adults, may have fewer or slightly dilated capillaries without any underlying systemic disease. (a) *dilated capillaries*: mild capillary dilation can be seen in healthy individuals, especially those exposed to frequent cold or mechanical trauma to the fingers (Fig. 29.1b); (b) *tortuosity*: slightly twisted or tortuous capillaries can be a normal finding in some people and do not necessarily indicate disease (Fig. 29.1b).

E. Pelechas et al., *Pitfalls in Rheumatology*,
https://doi.org/10.1007/978-3-031-98671-0_29

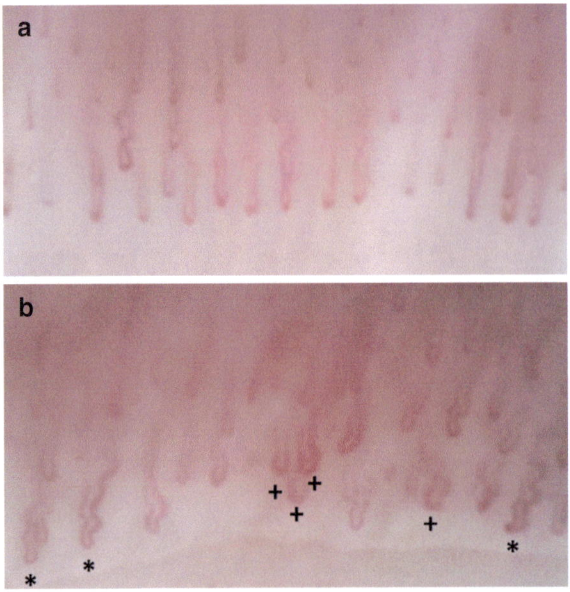

Fig. 29.1 (**a**) normal capillaroscopic pattern; (**b**) non-specific capillaroscopic findings with no underlying disease. Capillaries with an asterisk present tortuosity whereas capillaries with a cross are dilated. In such a pattern, a new capillaroscopic examination must be carried out within 1 year (magnification ×200)

How to Overcome This Pitfall Failure to recognise these normal variations may lead to an erroneous diagnosis of an RMD, causing unnecessary investigations or treatment. Clinicians should consider the full clinical context and avoid over-reliance on isolated NVC findings [1].

Inexperienced Interpretation NVC interpretation requires training and experience. Without sufficient expertise, clinicians may misinterpret subtle changes, leading to overdiagnosis or missed diagnoses. For example, distinguishing between normal dilated capillaries and pathologic giant capillaries seen in SScl can be challenging for inexperienced practitioners. Another common mistake is the erroneous distinction of traumatic haemorrhages as disease-specific haemorrhages of the capillaries.

How to Overcome This Pitfall Clinicians should undergo proper training in NVC interpretation and correlate findings with clinical and serological data [2].

29.2 Overlooking Early or Subtle Capillary Changes in Systemic Disease

One of the primary uses of NVC is to detect early capillary changes that suggest sRP and the potential development of systemic diseases, such as SScl or MCTD. However, early or subtle abnormalities may be easily overlooked.

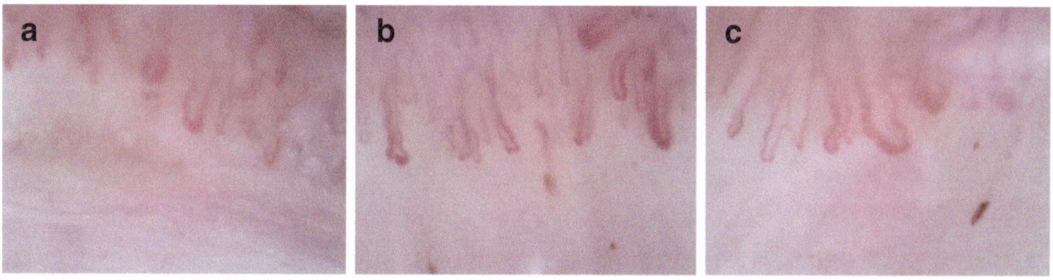

Fig. 29.2 (**a**) early scleroderma pattern with normal number of capillaries, dilatations and a giant capillary; (**b**) active scleroderma pattern with microhaemorrhages present (arrows); (**c**) late pattern with disorganization of the capillaries and diminished number of capillaries (magnification ×200)

Focusing Only on Established Patterns The classical findings in SScl, such as giant capillaries, capillary dropout and haemorrhages, may not be present in the early stages of disease. In early SScl, more subtle changes, such as mild capillary enlargement or a slight reduction in capillary density, may precede the classical SScl capillaroscopy patterns.

Failure to Recognise Evolving Changes Capillaroscopic abnormalities in systemic diseases like SScl can evolve over time. Early-stage disease may show subtle changes, while later-stage disease is marked by more significant capillary loss, disorganisation and haemorrhages. The capillaroscopic patterns in SSCs are three: early, active and late patterns (Fig. 29.2). Serial NVC is often required to capture these evolving patterns, yet clinicians may fail to re-evaluate capillaroscopy findings over time, especially in patients with progressive disease.

How to Overcome This Pitfall Regular follow-up with repeat NVC is essential in patients with suspected SScl or other autoimmune diseases to monitor for evolving capillary abnormalities. Clinicians should remain alert to subtle changes, particularly in patients with systemic symptoms but without overt capillary damage [3, 4].

29.3 Misinterpretation of Secondary Causes of Capillary Abnormalities

Capillary abnormalities can occur due to various non-RMD conditions or external factors, leading to misinterpretation if not carefully considered.

Impact of External Factors External factors such as smoking, occupational hand trauma, cold exposure and chronic hand vibrations can all lead to microvascular damage or capillary changes. These non-disease-related alterations can be mistaken for NVC findings suggestive of SScl or other autoimmune diseases. (a) *Mechanical trauma*: frequent manual labour or repetitive hand activities can lead to capillary damage, such as microhaemorrhages, that may be mistaken for NVC abnormalities seen in autoimmune diseases; (b) *cold exposure*: cold environments can cause temporary capillary dilation or spasm, mimicking features of RP on NVC.

Failing to account for these external factors can lead to an incorrect assumption that the capillary changes are due to an underlying systemic disease.

Overlap with Non-Rheumatic Conditions Certain non-autoimmune diseases or conditions can cause capillary changes that may mimic those seen in SScl or other RMDs. For example: (a) *diabetes mellitus*: can cause microvascular damage that may result in capillary abnormalities resembling those seen in autoimmune conditions; (b) *vascular diseases*: conditions like Buerger's disease in atherosclerosis can cause capillary changes, leading to potential diagnostic confusion.

How to Avoid This Pitfall Always consider the patient's history, including occupational exposures, environmental factors and comorbidities, when interpreting NVC findings. Capillaroscopic changes should be correlated with clinical and laboratory evidence of systemic disease before concluding that the findings are related to RMD [5].

29.4 Misclassification of Capillary Patterns

NVC patterns can be misclassified, particularly when atypical or mixed patterns are present. In SScl, there are three well-recognised NVC patterns: early, active and late. Misclassifying these patterns can result in inaccurate assessment of disease stage or severity.

Failure to Identify Mixed Patterns Some patients with overlapping autoimmune diseases, such as those with features of both SScl and DM, may present with mixed NCV findings. These can include a combination of giant capillaries, haemorrhages and abnormal capillary loops. Clinicians may misclassify these mixed patterns, focusing on only one disease process while missing the full spectrum of the patient's condition. For instance, anti-synthetase syndrome associated with DM can show capillary changes that are similar to SScl but with subtle differences in capillary morphology, such as more frequent haemorrhages or specific patterns of capillary dropout. On the other hand, anti-phospholipid syndrome may present with a "comb-like" pattern of haemorrhages misclassifying the findings as SScl-active pattern (Fig. 29.3).

Misclassification of Systemic Sclerosis Patterns In SScl, NVC patterns typically evolve from the early to late stage. Misclassifying the stage can impact both prognosis and treatment decisions. For example, mistaking an early scleroderma pattern (with mild capillary enlargement and a few haemorrhages) for a more advanced active pattern (with extensive haemorrhages and dropout) can result in premature escalation of treatment.

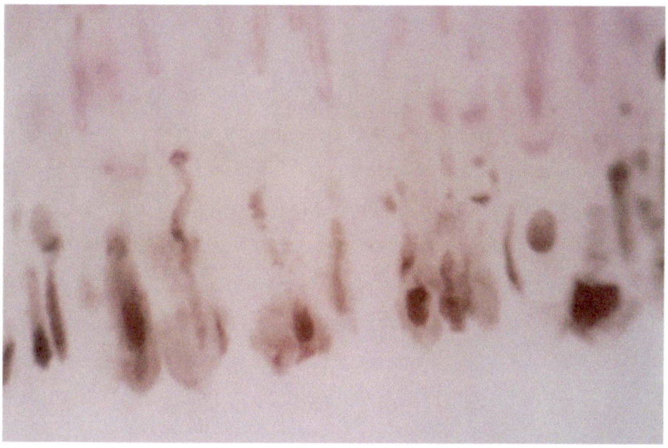

Fig. 29.3 Patient diagnosed with antiphospholipid syndrome and extensive microhaemorrhages in all capillaroscopic field

How to Avoid This Pitfall Ensure that clinicians interpreting NVC are familiar with the classification systems for capillary patterns in SScl and other RMDs. Consultation with experts may be needed in cases with atypical or mixed patterns [6, 7].

29.5 Over-Reliance on Capillaroscopy Findings in Isolation

NVC is a valuable diagnostic tool, but it should not be used in isolation. Over-reliance on capillaroscopy findings without considering the broader clinical and serological context can lead to misdiagnosis.

Neglecting Clinical Correlation NVC findings should always be interpreted in conjunction with the patient's clinical presentation, including symptoms, physical examination and laboratory data. For example, capillaroscopic abnormalities suggestive of SScl (capillary dropout and giant capillaries) should prompt evaluation for systemic features of the disease, such as skin thickening, digital ulcers or ILD. Without such correlation, NVC findings may be overinterpreted as pathologic when they are not clinically relevant.

Ignoring Autoantibody Profiles Autoantibodies play a crucial role in diagnosing and classifying RMDs. In conditions like SScl, specific autoantibodies (anti-centromere and anti-Scl-70) correlate with different clinical subtypes and disease courses. NVC findings should be integrated with autoantibody results to form a comprehensive diagnosis. Relying on NVC alone can lead to misclassification, particularly in patients with overlapping autoimmune diseases.

How to Avoid This Pitfall Capillaroscopy should be part of a multimodal approach to diagnosis, integrating clinical evaluation, autoantibody testing and imaging studies. A diagnosis of SScl or other RMDs should never be based solely on NVC findings [8, 9].

29.6 Conclusion

NVC is a powerful tool in diagnosing and managing RMDs, particularly SScl. However, its interpretation is fraught with potential pitfalls, including misclassification of normal variations, overlooking early capillary changes, misinterpreting secondary causes of capillary abnormalities and over-reliance on NVC findings in isolation. Clinicians must remain aware of these challenges and apply a comprehensive, integrated approach to diagnosis that includes clinical, serological and imaging data. With proper training and careful correlation with systemic disease features, NVC can provide valuable insights into the microvascular health of patients with RMDs, improving diagnostic accuracy and guiding appropriate management.

References

1. Komai M, Takeno D, Fujii C, Nakano J, Ohsaki Y, Shirakawa H. Nailfold capillaroscopy: a comprehensive review on its usefulness in both clinical diagnosis and improving unhealthy dietary lifestyles. Nutrients. 2024;16:1914. https://doi.org/10.3390/nu16121914.
2. Lambova SN, Muller-Ladner U. Nailfold capillaroscopy of fingers and toes – variations of normal. Curr Rheumatol Rev. 2018;14:28–35. https://doi.org/10.2174/1573397113666170726120344.
3. Cortes S, Cutolo M. Capillaroscopic patterns in rheumatic diseases. Acta Reumatol Port. 2007;32:29–36.
4. Smith V, Ickinger C, Hysa E, Snow M, Frech T, Sulli A, et al. Nailfold capillaroscopy. Best Pract Res Clin Rheumatol. 2023;37:101849. https://doi.org/10.1016/j.berh.2023.101849.
5. Cutolo M, Sulli A, Smith V. How to perform and interpret capillaroscopy. Best Pract Res Clin Rheumatol. 2013;27:237–48. https://doi.org/10.1016/j.berh.2013.03.001.
6. Pacini G, Pogna A, Pendolino M, Pizzorni C, Carmisciano L, Gotelli E, et al. Understanding the value of non-specific abnormal capillary dilations in presence of Raynaud's phenomenon: a detailed capillaroscopic analysis. RMD Open. 2022;8:e002449. https://doi.org/10.1136/rmdopen-2022-002449.
7. Smith V, Herrick AL, Ingegnoli F, Damjanov N, de Angelis R, Denton CP. Standardisation of nailfold capillaroscopy for the assessment of patients with Raynaud's phenomenon and systemic sclerosis. Autoimmun Rev. 2020;19:102458. https://doi.org/10.1016/j.autrev.2020.102458.
8. Mansueto N, Rotondo C, Corrado A, Cantatore FP. Nailfold capillaroscopy: a comprehensive review on common findings and clinical usefulness in non-rheumatic disease. J Med Investig. 2021;68:6–14. https://doi.org/10.2152/jmi.68.6.
9. Londoño-Mora JL, Leal-Vargas DD, Quintana-Lopez G. Prognostic value of capillaroscopy in organ involvement and identification of subtypes in systemic sclerosis (SS): a systematic literature review. Rev Col Reumatol (Engl Ed). 2020;27:10–25. https://doi.org/10.1016/j.rcreue.2020.06.004.

Pitfalls in Ultrasound of the Musculoskeletal System in Rheumatic Diseases

30

Abbreviations

ACR	American College of Rheumatology
CD	Colour Doppler
CT	Computed tomography
EULAR	European League Against Rheumatism
LDA	Low disease activity
MSKUS	Musculoskeletal ultrasound
OMERACT	Outcome measures in rheumatology
PD	Power Doppler
PsA	Psoriatic arthritis
RA	Rheumatoid arthritis
RMDs	Rheumatic diseases
SpA	Spondyloarthritis
T2T	Treat-to-target

30.1 Operator Dependency and Variability in Skill Level

One of the most significant limitations of MSKUS is its operator dependency. The accuracy and quality of the images are highly influenced by the experience and expertise of the clinician performing the scan [1]. Inconsistent techniques or inadequate training can lead to misinterpretation, missed diagnoses and variability in clinical decision-making [2].

How to Avoid This Pitfall (a) *Training and certification*: ensure that clinicians performing MSKUS receive formal training, ideally from accredited programmes, and maintain proficiency through regular practice. Certification programmes offered

E. Pelechas et al., *Pitfalls in Rheumatology*,
https://doi.org/10.1007/978-3-031-98671-0_30

by organisations like ACR, EULAR or national committees help standardise skills; (b) *regular practice and review*: ultrasound skills improve with experience. Regularly practicing MSKUS, reviewing images with peers and participating in quality assurance programmes can help clinicians maintain and improve their accuracy in performing and interpreting scans; (c) *use of standardised protocols*: following standardised protocols for ultrasound examination, such as those provided by EULAR or OMERACT, can reduce operator variability and ensure comprehensive evaluation [3].

30.2 Inadequate Image Acquisition

Obtaining high-quality, interpretable images requires proper technique, which can be influenced by transducer selection, image settings and patient positioning. Inadequate image acquisition can lead to poor visualisation of anatomical structures, resulting in missed pathologies or false positives.

How to Avoid This Pitfall (a) *Appropriate transducer selection*: use high-frequency linear transducers (10–18 MHz) for superficial structures like joints, tendons and ligaments. For deeper structures, such as the hip joint or deeper muscle layers, use lower-frequency transducers (5–10 MHz) to ensure adequate tissue penetration (Fig. 30.1); (b) *optimising machine settings*: adjust settings such as gain, depth and focus to obtain the best possible image. Over- or under-gained images can obscure important details, while improper depth settings may prevent accurate visualisation of deeper structures; (c) *patient positioning and probe orientation*: correct patient positioning is essential for clear imaging. For example, positioning the knee in slight flexion allows better visualisation of the joint space and synovial membrane. Ensure correct probe orientation (longitudinal and transverse) to visualise the full extent of structures like tendons and ligaments [4, 5].

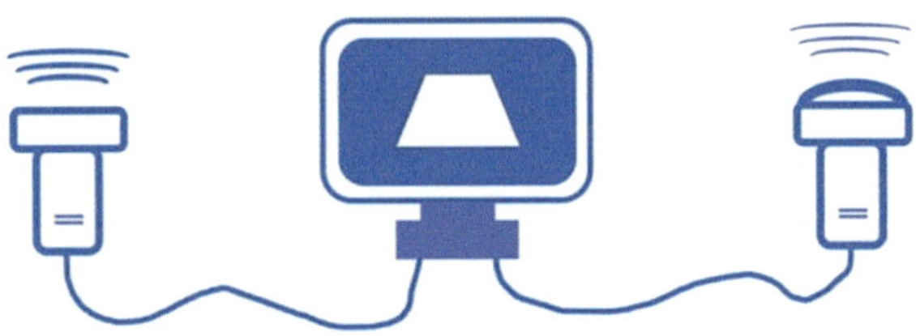

Fig. 30.1 Linear ultrasound probe on the left (high-frequency transducer for superficial structures); concave ultrasound probe on the right (lower-frequency transducer for deeper structures)

30.3 Misinterpretation of Normal Anatomic Variants

Normal anatomic structures can sometimes be mistaken for pathologies, particularly in areas prone to variability, such as the wrists, fingers and feet. This can lead to overdiagnosis of conditions such as tenosynovitis, synovitis or joint effusion in patients who may not have active disease.

Hot to Avoid This Pitfall (a) *Familiarity with normal anatomy*: develop a detailed understanding of normal MSK anatomy and variations, particularly in joints commonly involved in RMDs. Normal structures like fat pads, tendon insertions and joint recesses can sometimes mimic pathological findings like synovitis or effusion; (b) *comparison with contralateral structures*: comparing the affected side with the contralateral, unaffected side can help differentiate true pathology from normal anatomic variants. Symmetry suggests a benign or normal finding, while asymmetry is more indicative of pathology; (c) *dynamic assessment*: utilise dynamic ultrasound (moving the joint during imaging) to assess the behaviour of structures in motion. Pathological structures like synovial hypertrophy or tendon tears behave differently from normal tissues when the joint or tendons are moved [6].

30.4 Overdiagnosis of Synovitis and Enthesitis

Inflammatory conditions such as RA, PsA and SpA often manifest with synovitis or enthesitis. However, reactive changes due to mechanical stress or degenerative changes can be misinterpreted as inflammatory arthritis, leading to overdiagnosis and unnecessary treatment.

How to Avoid This Pitfall (a) *Use of Doppler imaging*: PD or CD ultrasound is essential in assessing synovitis, as it can detect increased blood flow, which is indicative of active inflammation. Reactive or mechanical synovitis often lacks significant Doppler signal, while inflammatory synovitis in conditions like RA or PsA shows increased vascularity; (b) *clinical correlation*: always correlate MSKUS findings with clinical symptoms. For example, in a patient without clinical signs of inflammatory arthritis such as prolonged morning stiffness, joint swelling or systemic symptoms, mild synovial thickening may be due to mechanical factors rather than active disease. Learn about the artifacts in the musculoskeletal ultrasound (Table 30.1); (c) *interpretation of enthesitis*: enthesophytes and cortical irregularities at entheses are often seen in degenerative conditions and should not be mistaken for inflammatory enthesitis without supporting clinical features. Doppler signal over the enthesis can help differentiate degenerative changes from active enthesitis [7, 8].

Table 30.1 Common musculoskeletal ultrasound artefacts

Acoustic shadowing (Fig. 30.2a)	Shadow behind dense structures such as calcifications
Reverberation	Repeated echoes, seen mainly with metallic objects
Acoustic enhancement (Fig. 30.2b)	Increased brightness. Fluid enhances posterior echoes
Anisotropy	Tendon appears hypoechoic because probe angle affects visualisation
Comet tail (Fig. 30.2c)	Bright lines; seen with small, strong reflectors
Mirror image	Duplicated structure; occurs near reflective interfaces

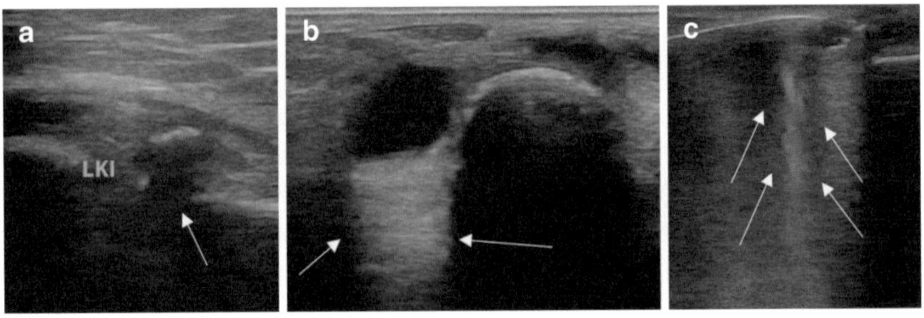

Fig. 30.2 Common artifacts: (**a**) acoustic shadowing; (**b**) acoustic enhancement; (**c**) comet tail. White arrows are showing the characteristic findings

30.5 Missed Detection of Early Inflammatory Changes

One of the key advantages of MSKUS is its ability to detect early inflammatory changes before they are visible on X-rays. However, early-stage disease can sometimes be missed, especially if the examination is too focused on advanced or obvious structural changes.

How to Avoid This Pitfall (a) *Assess for subtle findings*: in early inflammatory arthritis, look for subtle signs of synovial thickening, small joint effusions, tenosynovitis or low-grade Doppler signal in the absence of obvious structural damage. These early changes can help identify patients with active disease before radiographic damage occurs; (b) *monitor joints not just for damage but for inflammation*: particularly in diseases like early RA, structural damage may be absent, but early inflammatory changes can still be present. Prioritise inflammation over joint damage in early disease stages when making treatment decisions [9, 10].

30.6 Failure to Consider the Full Clinical Context

MSKUS provides detailed images of joints and soft tissues, but it is just one piece of the diagnostic puzzle. Relying solely on MSKUS findings without considering the full clinical context can lead to misdiagnosis or inappropriate management.

How to Avoid This Pitfall (a) *Clinical correlation is key*: always interpret MSKUS findings in the context of the patient's history, physical examination and laboratory tests. For example, tenosynovitis (Fig. 30.3) on MSKUS without clinical symptoms or elevated inflammatory markers may not necessitate aggressive treatment; (b) *multidisciplinary approach*: in cases where MSKUS findings are ambiguous or do not correlate with the clinical picture, consider consulting with radiologists or other specialists. Combining imaging findings with clinical expertise form rheumatologists, orthopaedics and radiologists leads to better diagnostic accuracy [11].

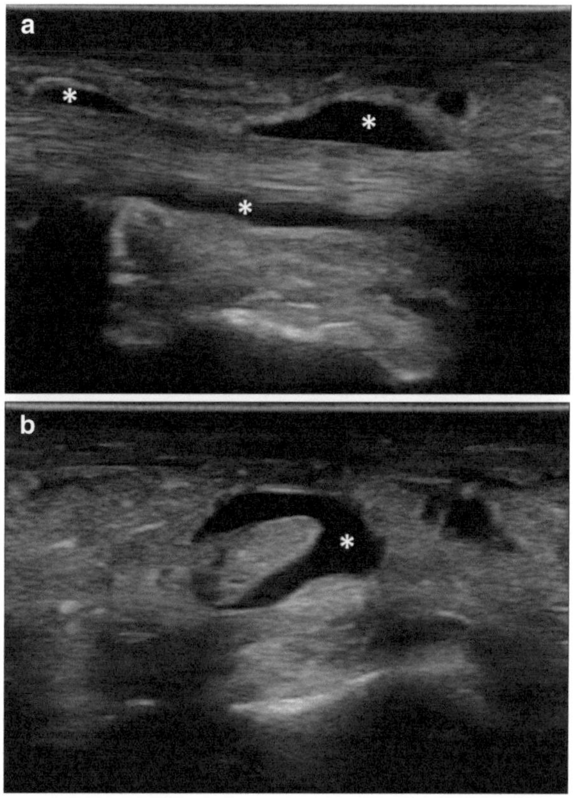

Fig. 30.3 Tenosynovitis of the tibialis posterior in longitudinal (**a**) and transverse (**b**) view. The asterisks show the increased fluid content within tendon sheath

30.7 Overuse of Ultrasound in Disease Monitoring

While MSKUS is a valuable tool for diagnosing and monitoring disease activity in RMDs, overuse or over-reliance on it can lead to unnecessary interventions or over-treatment. This is particularly relevant in conditions like RA, where clinical remission may not always correlate with complete MSKUS resolution of synovitis.

How to Avoid This Pitfall (a) *Balance imaging with clinical judgement*: MSKUS should complement, not replace, clinical assessment. In patients with well-controlled symptoms and no clinical evidence of active disease, minor residual findings on MSKUS may not warrant changes in management; (b) *define treatment goals*: clarify the therapeutic goals with patients and the healthcare team. In some cases, T2T strategies may prioritise clinical remission or LDA over complete MSKUS resolution, reducing the risk of overtreatment [12].

30.8 Inconsistent Documentation and Communication of Findings

One of the practical challenges of MSKUS is the inconsistency in how findings are documented and communicated, which can lead to confusion or misinterpretation by other healthcare providers.

How to Avoid This Pitfall (a) *Standardised reporting*: use standardised terminology and structured reporting formats to document MSKUS findings. This ensures clarity and consistency in communicating results to other clinicians. The OMERACT definitions of MSKUS pathologies such as synovitis, erosions and tenosynovitis can provide a useful framework for reporting; (b) *image archiving*: whenever possible, store key MSKUS images in the patient's medical record, especially when findings are complex or likely to change management. This allows for future comparisons and facilitates better collaboration with other clinicians [13, 14].

30.9 Conclusion

MSKUS is a powerful tool in the diagnosis and management of RMDs, but it comes with several challenges and potential pitfalls. Operator dependency, technical errors, misinterpretation of normal anatomic structures and over-reliance on imaging without clinical correlation are common issues that can lead to suboptimal outcomes. By adhering to standardised protocols, ensuring adequate training, and integrating clinical findings with imaging results, these pitfalls can be minimised.

References

1. Pelechas E, Kaltsonoudis E, Voulgari PV, Drosos AA. Musculoskeletal ultrasound in rheumatology. In: Illustrated handbook of rheumatic and musculo-skeletal diseases. Cham: Springer; 2023. https://doi.org/10.1007/978-3-031-47379-1_4.
2. Ohrndorf S, Naumann L, Grundey J, Scheel T, Scheel AK, Warner C, et al. Is musculoskeletal ultrasonography an operator-dependent method or a fast and reliably teachable diagnostic tool? Interreader agreements of three ultrasonographers with different training levels. Int J Rheumatol. 2010;2010:164518. https://doi.org/10.1155/2010/164518.
3. Terslev L, Naredo E, Aegerter P, Wakefield RJ, Backhaus M, Balint P, et al. Scoring ultrasound synovitis in rheumatoid arthritis: a EULAR-OMERACT ultrasound taskforce – Part 2: reliability and application to multiple joints of a standardised consensus-based scoring system. RMD Open. 2017;3:e000427. https://doi.org/10.1136/rmdopen-2016-000427.
4. Zander D, Hüske S, Hoffmann B, Cui XW, Dong Y, Lim A, et al. Ultrasound image optimization ("Knobology"): B-mode. Ultrasound Int Open. 2020;6:E14–24. https://doi.org/10.1055/a-1223-1134.
5. Crawford SK, Kliethermes SA, Heiderscheit BC, Bashford GR. Influence of ultrasound machine settings on quantitative measures derived from spatial frequency analysis of muscle tissue. BMC Musculoskelet Disord. 2023;24:664. https://doi.org/10.1186/s12891-023-06790-3.
6. Serafin-Król M, Maliborski A. Diagnostic errors in musculoskeletal ultrasound imaging and how to avoid them. J Ultrason. 2017;17:188–96. https://doi.org/10.15557/JoU.2017.0028.
7. Kaeley GS, Bakewell C, Deodhar A. The importance of ultrasound in identifying and differentiating patients with early inflammatory arthritis: a narrative review. Arthritis Res Ther. 2020;22:1. https://doi.org/10.1186/s13075-019-2050-4.
8. Smith E, Azzopardi C, Thaker S, Botchu R, Gupta H. Power Doppler in musculoskeletal ultrasound: used, pitfalls and principles to overcome its shortcomings. J Ultrasound. 2021;24:151–6. https://doi.org/10.1007/s40477-020-00489-0.
9. Van der Ven M, van der Veer-Meerkerk M, Cate DFT, Rasappu N, Kok MR, Csakvari D, et al. Absence of ultrasound inflammation in patients presenting with arthralgia rules out the development of arthritis. Arthritis Res Ther. 2017;19:202. https://doi.org/10.1186/s13075-017-1405-y.
10. Ciurtin C, Wyszynski K, Clarke R, Mouyis M, Manson J, Marra G. Ultrasound-detected subclinical inflammation was better reflected by the disease activity score (DAS-28) in patients with suspicion of inflammatory arthritis compared to established rheumatoid arthritis. Clin Rheumatol. 2016;35:2411–9. https://doi.org/10.1007/s10067-016-3326-6.
11. Connell MJ, Wu TS. Bedside musculoskeletal ultrasonography. Crit Care Clin. 2014;30:243–73. https://doi.org/10.1016/j.ccc.2013.10.003.
12. Patil P, Dasgupta B. Role of diagnostic ultrasound in the assessment of musculoskeletal diseases. Ther Adv Musculoskelet Dis. 2012;4:341–55. https://doi.org/10.1177/1759720X12442112.
13. Dalili D, Carne A, MacKay J, O'Connor PO, Silver D, Robinson P, et al. Musculoskeletal ultrasound imaging standards in the UK: British Society of Skeletal Radiologists (BSSR) position statement. Br J Radiol. 2021;94:20210198. https://doi.org/10.1259/bjr.20210198.
14. Azyrny Z. Standards for musculoskeletal ultrasound. J Ultrason. 2017;17:182–7. https://doi.org/10.15557/JoU.2017.0027.

MIX
Papier aus verantwortungsvollen Quellen
Paper from responsible sources
FSC® C105338
FSC
www.fsc.org

If you have any concerns about our products,
you can contact us on
ProductSafety@springernature.com

In case Publisher is established outside the EU,
the EU authorized representative is:
Springer Nature Customer Service Center GmbH
Europaplatz 3, 69115 Heidelberg, Germany

Printed by Libri Plureos GmbH
in Hamburg, Germany